Renal, Metabolic and Urologic Disorders

nova
Medicine & Health
New York

Renal, Metabolic and Urologic Disorders

The Urinary Bladder: Structure, Functions and Clinical Aspects
Nicoline J. Mikkelsen (Editor)
2020. ISBN: 978-1-53617-879-1 (Softcover)
2020. ISBN: 978-1-53617-911-8 (eBook)

Medicinal Plants for the Treatment of Metabolic Disorders. Part 1
Anaberta Cardador Martínez (Editor)
Maritza Alonzo-Macías (Editor)
Patricia Manzano, PhD (Editor)
Víctor M. Rodríguez García (Editor)
2020. ISBN: 978-1-53617-483-0 (Hardcover)
2020. ISBN: 978-1-53617-484-7 (eBook)

Medicinal Plants for the Treatment of Metabolic Disorders. Part 2
Anaberta Cardador Martínez (Editor)
Maritza Alonzo-Macías (Editor)
Patricia Manzano, PhD (Editor)
Víctor M. Rodríguez García (Editor)
2020. ISBN: 978-1-53618-061-9 (Hardcover)
2020. ISBN: 978-1-53618-062-6 (eBook)

Medicinal Plants for the Treatment of Metabolic Disorders. Part 2
Anaberta Cardador Martínez (Editor)
Maritza Alonzo-Macías (Editor)
Patricia Manzano, PhD (Editor)
Víctor M. Rodríguez García (Editor)
2020. ISBN: 978-1-53618-064-0 (Hardcover)
2020. ISBN: 978-1-53618-065-7978 (eBook)

More information about this series can be found at
https://novapublishers.com/product-category/series/renal-metabolic-and-urologic-disorders/

Warren Y. Salinas
Editor

Hyperuricemia

Symptoms, Diagnosis and Treatment

nova
Medicine & Health
New York

Library of Congress Cataloging-in-Publication Data

ISBN: 979-8-89113-239-9

Published by Nova Science Publishers, Inc. † New York

Contents

Preface

This book contains five chapters that detail hyperuricemia. Chapter One proposes a preventive method for hyperuricemia through the evaluation of recent dietary habits in the Japanese adult population (aged $\geq$ 20 years). Chapter Two describes the importance of diet and proper choice of foods to control serum uric acid concentration for the prevention and management of hyperuricemia. Chapter Three details the importance of nutrient intake for the prevention and management of hyperuricemia in the general population (especially adults), referencing the results of clinical research reported. Chapter Four presents the current knowledge on the interactions between hyperuricemia and the kidney and the role of the immune response in this relationship. Lastly, Chapter Five explains the main surgical techniques for the treatment of uric acid stones.

Chapter 1

Dietary Modification for the Prevention of Hyperuricemia in the Japanese Adult Population in 2019

Takashi Koguchi*, **PhD**
Department of Human Education, Kokugakuin Tochigi Junior College, Tochigi-shi, Tochigi, Japan

Abstract

Hyperuricemia is recognized as a lifestyle-related disease. A high serum uric acid (SUA) concentration (hyperuricemia) is frequently associated with gout. In Japan, the prevalence of gout has increased markedly since the 1960s. This phenomenon is thought to be attributed to the Westernization in the Japanese diet since 1955. The objective of this article is to propose a preventive method for hyperuricemia through the evaluation of recent dietary habits in the Japanese adult population (aged ≥ 20 years). The author used the data of the National Health and Nutrition Survey in Japan for serum uric acid (SUA) concentrations and the rate of hyperuricemia in Japanese adult population (2010-2019) and the intake of nutrients and food (2001-2019). The increase in the rate of hyperuricemia in Japanese adult women (aged ≥ 20 years) between 2010 and 2019 was higher than in Japanese adult men (aged ≥ 20 years). The correlation between the rate of hyperuricemia and the daily intake of nutrient (i.e., animal protein, total fat, animal fat, vegetable fat, saturated fatty acids, n-6 polyunsaturated fatty acids, cholesterol, pantothenic acid, sodium, salt, potassium, phosphorus) or food (i.e., total meat, total

* Corresponding author's email: echo130@nifty.com.

In: Hyperuricemia
Editor: Warren Y. Salinas
ISBN: 979-8-89113-239-9

seafood, eggs, milk and dairy products, oils and fats, total grains, seaweed, total legumes, seeds and nuts) or the mean ratio of energy intake from carbohydrate in total energy intake (carbohydrates/energy) or the mean ratio of energy intake from fat in total energy intake (fat/energy) was stronger in Japanese adult women than in Japanese adult men. The modification of food intake for the prevention of hyperuricemia in the Japanese adult population (aged $\geq$ 20 years) in 2019 was suggested as follows:

- limiting or decreasing alcohol beverage consumption:
- limiting or decreasing intake of purine-rich food (e.g., meat, seafood and organ meats), animal fats, saturated fatty acids, cholesterol, high-fructose food, sugar-sweetened beverages, confectioneries (sugary foods including desserts and sweets), salt, oils and fats;
- avoiding overdose of total sugars, foods rich in vitamin A, vitamin B_5 (pantothenic acid), folate, vitamin B_{12}, sodium, phosphorus, and copper;
- replacement of saturated fatty acids (e.g., dairy fats, meat fat) with mono- and polyunsaturated fatty acids (particularly n-3 polyunsaturated fatty acids) (e.g., macadamia nuts, almonds, peanuts and peanut butter, olive oil, canola oil, avocados);
- increasing the intake of fiber-rich foods (e.g., cereals, whole grains, high-fiber bread), milk and dairy products (particularly low-fat dairy products), mushrooms, seaweed, legumes, seeds and nuts, fruit, vegetables, which contain rich in carbohydrate (particularly dietary fiber), vitamin A, vitamin E, vitamin B_1, vitamin B_2, vitamin B_6, folate, vitamin B_{12}, vitamin C, calcium, potassium, magnesium, zinc, and polyphenol;
- recognizing the intake of eggs, milk and dairy products (particularly low-fat dairy products), coffee, cocoa, tea, and probiotics;
- and the maintenance of good hydration.

The above dietary modifications may play a helpful role in the prevention of hyperuricemia in the Japanese adult population.

Keywords: adequate intake, dietary reference intakes, food, gout, hyperuricemia, Japanese diet, nutrient, recommended dietary allowance, uric acid

Introduction

Hyperuricemia is recognized as a lifestyle-related disease. The prevalence of hyperuricemia has increased in various regions over the last 30 years and was different among populations or regions (Roman 2019). In Japan, the prevalence of hyperuricemia has increased for six decades; that is to say, the Japanese Society of Gout and Nucleic Acid Metabolism (2002) has stated that the incidence rate of hyperuricemia has increased from about 5% in adult men in the 1960s to about 15% in the 1970s to the early 1980s and about 20% in the late 1980s to 1990s. Two large-scale surveys reported that the prevalence of hyperuricemia affected about32.5% or 26.2% of adult men in the early 2000s (Tomita and Mizuno 2006; Fujimori et al. 2006). Recently, Hisatome et al. (2018) have stated that the prevalence of hyperuricemia affected about 30% of adult men. The number of asymptomatic hyperuricemia was estimated to be over ten million in 2016 (Japan Preventive Association of Lifestyle Related Disease 2023).

A high serum uric acid (SUA) concentration (hyperuricemia) is frequently associated with gout (Khanna et al. 2012) and is a risk factor for gout (as uratosis) (Saag and Choi 2006; Hisatome et al. 2018; Cabău et al. 2020; Li, Zhang and Zeng 2020). Hyperuricemia is considered the precursor of gout (Choi, Mount and Reginato 2005; Saag and Choi 2006). The global burden of gout is substantial and seems to have been increasing in many parts of the world, including Japan over the past 50 years (Kuo et al.2015; Mikanagi 1963; Nishioka, Mikanagi and Hirose 1974). In Japan, a remarkable increase in gout patients has been observed since the 1960s (Mikanagi 1963; Nishioka, Mikanagi and Hirose 1974). In particular, the increase in gout patients was remarkable after 1965 (Nishioka, Mikanagi and Hirose 1974). The 1960s was a time when the post-war chaos calmed down, and eating habits became stable (The Ministry of Agriculture, Forestry and Fisheries 2020). The Japanese food menu has shown a rapid increase in the variety of dishes due to the Westernization of meals from 1955 to 1965 (The Ministry of Agriculture, Forestry and Fisheries 2020; Yanagimoto 2004). In the last five or six decades, it is thought that the Japanese diet has become more westernized and dietary habits have changed. The number of gout patients among Japanese people in

2022 was higher compared to that in 2019 and increased 5.12-fold compared to that in 1986 (1986: 0.255 million; 2016: 1.105 million; 2019: 1.254 million; 2022: 1.305 million) (The Ministry of Health, Labour and Welfare. Household Statistics Office 2023).

Asymptomatic hyperuricemia is a biomarker of both increased risk for and presence of vascular disease (e.g., hypertension, coronary artery disease, kidney disease), and it may also have certain causal effects on vascular disease, hypertension, and progression of chronic kidney disease (CKD) (Feig, Kang and Johnson 2008). Asymptomatic hyperuricemia also induced by urate can contribute to the development of obesity, CKD, diabetes mellitus, and hypertension by stimulating inflammation (Joosten et al. 2020). The Japanese Society of Gout and Uric & Nucleic Acids Guidelines for Management of Hyperuricemia and Gout established by Hisatome et al. (2018) has stated that hyperuricemia and/or gout is associated with CKD, urolithiasis, hypertension, and cardiovascular disease (CVD). In Japan, the number of patients with gout, hypertension, diabetes mellitus, dyslipidemia, and kidney disease increased between 1998 and 2022, respectively and the number of patients with myocardial infarction tended to increase between 1998 and 2022 (The Ministry of Health, Labour and Welfare. Household Statistics Office. 2023).

Epidemiological studies have shown that dietary factors affect SUA levels parallel to the direction of the risk of hyperuricemia (Choi 2010). Recognizing dietary patterns, adopting choice and moderate intakes of serum uric acid (SUA) lowering foods is important for the prevention and management of hyperuricemia. In the previous chapters (Koguchi 2023), the author described the association between dietary nutrients, foods or dietary patterns and hyperuricemia based on the results of clinical research (clinical trials and epidemiological studies). As based on the premise of the results of a clinical research reported about the association between dietary nutrients, foods or dietary patterns and hyperuricemia and daily food intake, the aim of this article is to suggest dietary modification for the prevention of hyperuricemia in the Japanese adult population (aged ≥ 20 years) in 2019 through the evaluation of the intake of nutrients in the Japanese adult population (aged ≥ 20 years) by comparing with Dietary Reference Intakes set by the Institute of Medicine of the National Academy of Sciences in the US (2011; 2019; 2021). Furthermore, this article proposes a common preventive method for hyperuricemia and some of its comorbidities, such as CVD, obesity, and hypertension, which explains the possible role of dietary habits through the improvement in the Japanese adult population's nutrient intake.

Methods

Serum uric acid concentration and rate of hyperuricemia

The serum uric acid (SUA) concentrations and the rate of hyperuricemia in the Japanese adult population was reviewed by the National Health and Nutrition Survey Japan (2010-2019), performed by the Ministry of Health, Labour and Welfare in Japan (The Ministry of Health, Labour and Welfare, Health Service Bureau 2020; The Ministry of Health, Labour and Welfare, Japan 2023; National Institute of Health and Nutrition 2023). We defined hyperuricemia as SUA concentrations > 7.0 mg/ dL (416.4 μmol/L) for men and ≥ 6.0 mg/dL (356.9 μmol/L) for women.

Trends in nutrient or food intake in the Japanese adult population

The intake of nutrients or foods was searched in the National Health and Nutrition Survey, Japan (2001-2019) performed by the Ministry of Health, Labour and Welfare in Japan (The Ministry of Health, Labour and Welfare, Health Service Bureau 2020; The Ministry of Health, Labour and Welfare, Japan 2023; National Institute of Health and Nutrition 2023). Data was extracted from a series of Japanese national nutrition surveys that have been carried out every year throughout Japan since 1946 (National Institute of Health and Nutrition 2023). In these surveys, food consumption by families enrolled in the study was assessed by weighing food items consumed on three consecutive weekdays (until 1994) or one weekday (from 1995). The daily nutrient or food intakes of Japanese people are presented as the mean values reported by the National Health and Nutrition Survey Japan (2001-2019) (The Ministry of Health, Labour and Welfare, Health Service Bureau 2020).

The Ministry of Health, Labour and Welfare in Japan not conducted investigations into the daily intake of sugars, glucose, fructose, sucrose, purines, polyphenols, total water, alcohol, sugar-sweetened beverages and probiotics among Japanese people.

Dietary Reference Intakes for the Japanese adult population

Dietary reference intakes definitions set by the Institute of Medicine of the National Academy of Sciences in the US (Institute of Medicine of the National Academy of Sciences 2021) are as follows: (1) the Estimated Average Requirement (EAR) indicates the average daily nutrient intake level that is estimated to meet the requirements of half of the healthy individuals in a particular life stage and gender group; (2) the Recommended Dietary Allowance (RDA) indicates the average daily nutrient intake level that is sufficient to meet the nutrient requirements of nearly all (97-98%) healthy individuals in a particular life stage and gender group; (3) the Adequate Intake (AI) indicates that the recommended average daily intake level based on observed or experimentally determined approximations or estimates of nutrient intake by a group (or groups) of apparently healthy people that are assumed to have an adequate intake, used when an RDA cannot be determined; and (4) the Tolerable Upper Intake Level (UL) indicates the highest average daily nutrient intake level that is likely to pose no risk of adverse health effects to almost all individuals in the general population. As intake increases above the UL, the potential risk of adverse effects may increase.

Food Composition

The food composition was extracted from a standard table of food composition in Japan -2020- (Eighth Revised Edition) from the Council for Science and Technology, Ministry of Education, Culture, Sports, Science and Technology in Japan. The Ministry of Education, Culture, Sports, Science and Technology in Japan (2023) and the US Department of Health & Human Services. National Institutes of Health. The Office of Dietary Supplements (2023). Foods rich in dietary nutrients using the data of food composition announced by the Council for Science and Technology, Ministry of Education, Culture, Sports, Science and Technology in Japan (2023) and US Department of Health & Human Services. National Institutes of Health. The Office of Dietary Supplements (2023) are shown in the previous reports (Koguchi 2021; Koguchi 2022; Koguchi 2023).

Statistical Analysis

The correlation is efficient and the significance of the rate of hyperuricemia and nutrients or food intake from 2010 to 2019 was analyzed by Pearson Product-Moment Correlation. A SigmaPlot 12.0 software program (version 12.0, Systat Software Inc, San Jose, CA) was used for statistical analysis. Differences were considered significant at $p < 0.05$.

Results

Serum uric acid concentration in Japanese adult population

Mean SUA concentrations in Japanese adult men and Japanese adult women in 1989-2019 were shown in Table 1. Mean SUA concentrations in Japanese adult men (aged ≥ 30 years) was 5.5 mg/dL (327.2 µmol/L) in 1989 and was 5.6 mg/dL (333.1 µmol/L) in 1990. Mean SUA concentrations in Japanese adult men (aged ≥ 20 years) was 5.8 mg/dL (345.0 µmol/L) in 2010, 2011, 2013, 2014, 2017, 2018, and 2019 and was 5.9 mg/dL (351.0 µmol/L) in 2015 (The Ministry of Health, Labour and Welfare 2023). Mean SUA concentration in Japanese adult women (aged ≥ 30 years) was 4.0 mg/dL (237.9 µmol/L) in 1989 and 1990. Mean SUA concentrations in Japanese adult women (aged ≥ 20 years) was 4.4 mg/dL (261.7 µmol/L) in 2010, 2013 and 4.5 mg/dL (267.7 µmol/L) in 2011, 2014, 2015, 2017 and was 4.6 mg/dL (273.6 µmol/L) in 2018 and 2019 (The Ministry of Health, Labour and Welfare 2023). Mean SUA concentrations in Japanese adult men in 1989-2019 were higher than those in Japanese adult women, respectively (The Ministry of Health, Labour and Welfare 2023).

Table 1. Serum uric acid concentrations in the Japanese adult population

	Year									
Gender	1989*	1990*	2010**	2011**	2013**	2014**	2015**	2017**	2018**	2019**
	Mean serum uric acid concentration (mg/dL)									
Men	5.5	5.6	5.8	5.8	5.8	5.8	5.9	5.8	5.8	5.8
Women	4.0	4.0	4.4	4.5	4.4	4.5	4.5	4.5	4.6	4.6

* Japanese adult men and women (aged ≥ 30 years).

** Japanese adult men and women (aged ≥ 20 years).

Rate of hyperuricemia in the Japanese adult population

The rate of hyperuricemia in the Japanese adult population in 1989-2019 was shown in Table 2. The rate of hyperuricemia, defined as serum uric acid (SUA) level > 7.0 mg/dL (416.4 μmol/L) in men and ≥ 6.0 mg/dL (356.9 μmol/L) in women, in the National Health and Nutrition Survey Japan (1946-2019) performed by the Ministry of Health, Labour and Welfare in Japan (The Ministry of Health, Labour and Welfare, Health Service Bureau 2020; The Ministry of Health, Labour and Welfare, Japan 2023; National Institute of Health and Nutrition. 2023). The rate of hyperuricemia was higher in Japanese adult men than in Japanese adult women (Table 2). The rate of hyperuricemia in the Japanese adult population (men or women) (aged ≥ 30 years) in 1990 was higher than in 1989.

The rate of hyperuricemia in Japanese adult men (aged ≥ 20 years) and Japanese adult women (aged ≥ 20 years) in 2010s were 15.8-18.6% and 7.0-10.4%, respectively (The Ministry of Health, Labour and Welfare 2023) (Table 2). The rate of hyperuricemia in Japanese adult men remained substantial in 2013-2019 (The Ministry of Health, Labour and Welfare, Health Service Bureau 2020; The Ministry of Health, Labour and Welfare, Japan 2023; National Institute of Health and Nutrition 2023). The rate of hyperuricemia in Japanese adult women (aged ≥ 20 years) in 2019 was higher compared to that in 2010 (2010: 7.0%; 2019: 9.9%).

The increase in the rate of hyperuricemia in Japanese adult women between 2010 and 2019 was higher than in Japanese adult men.

Table 2. Rate of hyperuricemia in the Japanese adult population

	Year									
Gender	1989*	1990*	2010**	2011**	2013**	2014**	2015**	2017**	2018**	2019**
	Rate of hyperuricemia (%)									
Men	12.2	14.1	18.0	18.3	15.8	16.9	18.6	16.9	16.8	16.8
Women	4.7	5.3	7.0	8.2	7.8	9.4	9.5	10.4	10.4	9.9

* Japanese adult men and women (aged ≥ 30 years).

** Japanese adult men and women (aged ≥ 30 years).

Dietary nutrient intake among the Japanese adult population (aged ≥ 20 years)

The Institute of Medicine of the National Academy of Sciences in the US (2021) has set Dietary Reference Intakes values: the Estimated Average Requirement (EAR), the Recommended Dietary Allowance (RDA), the Adequate Intake (AI), the Tolerable Upper Intake Level (UL), the Acceptable Macronutrient Distribution Ranges (AMDRs) apply to vitamins, minerals, macronutrients, and energy across different life stage and gender groups. Nutrient intake in the Japanese adult population (aged ≥ 20 years) in 2019 was assessed using the Dietary Reference Intakes definitions established by the Institute of Medicine of the National Academy of Sciences in the US (Institute of Medicine of the National Academy of Sciences 2021).

Energy

The balance of the caloric ratio of protein, fat, and carbohydrates in the Japanese adult population (aged ≥ 20 years) in 2019 was carbohydrates: 56.4%, protein: 15.2%, and fat: 28.4%. In comparison to the caloric ratio of protein, fat, and carbohydrates in the Japanese adult population (aged ≥ 20 years) in 2002, in the Japanese diet of the adult population (aged ≥ 20 years) in 2019, the mean ratio of energy intake from fat in total energy intake (fat/energy) increased by 4.1% and the mean ratio of energy intake from carbohydrates in total energy intake (carbohydrates/energy) decreased by 4.1%. These results suggests that the balance of the caloric ratio of protein, fat, and carbohydrates in the Japanese adult population (aged ≥ 20 years) in 2019 was weighted toward fat in the Japanese adult population (aged ≥ 20 years). The Japanese adult population (aged ≥ 20 years) need to decrease fat (especially saturated fatty acids and cholesterol) intake.

With regards to Japanese adult men (aged ≥ 20 years), the mean ratio of energy intake from carbohydrates, protein, and fat in total energy intake was 57.8%, 14.8%, 27.4%, respectively. Compared to the caloric ratio of protein, fat, and carbohydrates in the Japanese adult population (aged ≥ 20 years) in 2002, in the Japanese diet of Japanese adult population (aged ≥ 20 years) in 2019, the mean ratio of energy intake from fat in total energy intake (fat/energy) increased by 4.0% and the mean ratio of energy intake from protein in total energy intake (protein/energy) and the mean ratio of energy intake from carbohydrates in total energy intake (carbohydrates/energy) decreased by 0.1% and 3.9%, respectively.

Regarding Japanese adult women (aged ≥ 20 years), the mean ratio of energy intake from carbohydrates, protein, and fat in total energy intake was 55.3%, 15.5%, and 29.2%, respectively. Compared to the caloric ratio of protein, fat, and carbohydrates in the Japanese adult population (aged ≥ 20 years) in 2002, in the Japanese diet of Japanese adult population (aged ≥ 20 years) in 2019, the mean ratio of energy intake from fat in total energy intake (fat/energy) increased by 4.2% and the mean ratio of energy intake from carbohydrates in total energy intake (carbohydrates/energy) decreased by 4.2%.

The energy-providing nutrient balance (percentages of carbohydrates, protein, and fat in the total energy intake) in the Japanese adult population, Japanese adult men, and Japanese adult women were within the Acceptable Macronutrient Distribution Ranges (AMDRs) established by the Institute of Medicine of the National Academy of Sciences in the US (carbohydrates: 45-65%; protein: 10-35%; fat: 20-35%) (Institute of Medicine of the National Academy of Sciences 2021).

Carbohydrates

Total Carbohydrates

The daily carbohydrate intake of the Japanese adult population (aged ≥ 20 years) in 2019 was lower compared to that in 2002 and 2010 (2002: 274.5 g/day; 2010: 259.8 g/day; 2019: 248.7 g/day).

The daily carbohydrate intake among the Japanese adult men (aged ≥ 20 years) in 2019 was lower compared to that in 2002 and 2010 (2002: 302.2 g/day; 2010: 288.2 g/day; 2019: 275.3 g/day). The daily carbohydrate intake did not exhibit a significant correlation with the rate of hyperuricemia in Japanese adult men (aged ≥ 20 years) from 2010 to 2019 ($r = 0.088$, $p=0.836$). The daily carbohydrate intake of adult women (aged ≥ 20 years) in 2019 was lower compared to that in 2002 and 2010 (2002: 250.9 g/day; 2010: 235.5 g/day; 2019: 225.5 g/day). The daily carbohydrate intake did not exhibit a significant correlation with the rate of hyperuricemia in Japanese adult women (aged ≥ 20 years) from 2010 to 2019 ($r = -0.593$, $p=0.121$).

The mean ratio of energy intake from carbohydrates in total energy intake (carbohydrates/energy)

The mean ratio of energy intake from carbohydrates in total the energy intake (carbohydrate/energy) of the Japanese adult population (aged ≥ 20 years) in 2019 was lower compared to that in 2002 and 2010 (2002: 60.5%; 2010: 60.0%; 2019: 56.4%).

The carbohydrates/energy of Japanese adult men (aged ≥ 20 years) in 2019 was lower compared to that in 2002 and 2010 (2002: 61.7%; 2010: 61.3%; 2019: 57.8%). The carbohydrates/energy did not show a significant correlation with the rate of hyperuricemia in Japanese adult men (aged ≥ 20 years) from 2010 to 2019 (r= 0.387, p=0.343).

The carbohydrates/energy of Japanese adult women (aged ≥ 20 years) in 2019 was lower compared to that in 2002 and 2010 (2002: 59.5%; 2010: 58.8%; 2019: 55.3%). The carbohydrates/energy were negatively correlated with the rate of hyperuricemia in Japanese adult women (aged ≥ 20 years) from 2010 to 2019 (r= -0.818, p=0.013). These results suggest that the correlation of the carbohydrates/energy with the rate of hyperuricemia varies with gender and is stronger in Japanese adult women than in Japanese adult men.

A cross-sectional study from China showed that every 10 g increase in energy-adjusted carbohydrate intakes and dietary fiber intakes decreased hyperuricemia risk by 5% and 13%, respectively (Zhang et al. 2023). Increased intake of fiber-rich foods (e.g., whole grains, legumes, seeds and nuts, fruit, vegetables) appears to be important for the prevention of hyperuricemia.

The Institute of Medicine of the National Academy of Sciences in the US (2021) has determined that the Acceptable Macronutrient Distribution Ranges (AMDRs), which is defined as a range of intakes for a particular energy source that is associated with the reduced risk of chronic disease, while providing adequate intakes of essential nutrients. For carbohydrates, both adults (aged ≥ 19 years) and children (aged 1-18 years) is 45-65% of total calories. It appears better to increase the mean ratio of energy intake from carbohydrates in total energy intake (carbohydrates/energy) to around 60-65%. The carbohydrates/energy appears to be appropriate or it appears better to increase it slightly.

Sugars

The Ministry of Health, Labour and Welfare in Japan has not investigated the daily sugars, glucose, fructose, and sucrose intake among the Japanese people.

Increased intake of sugars was associated with an increased hyperuricemia risk (Tappy et al. 2018). Tappy et al. (2018) have proposed to set a maximum limit to the intake of total sugars containing fructose (sucrose, glucose fructose syrups, honey or other syrups, and natural concentrates, etc.) of 100 g/day.

The recommendation for added sugars, as established by the Institute of Medicine of the National Academy of Sciences in the US suggests limiting their intake to a maximal intake of no more than 25 percent total energy (Institute of Medicine of the National Academy of Sciences 2021). The World Health Organization (WHO) recommends reducing the intake of free sugars to less than 10% of total energy intake in both adults and children and suggests a further reduction of the intake of free sugars to below 5% of total energy intake (World Health Organization 2015; World Health Organization 2023). It should pay attention to excessive intake of total sugars.

As stated in the reviews (Choi 2010; Sun and Empie 2012; Dornas et al. 2015; Ekpenyong and Daniel 2015; Kakutani-Hatayama et al. 2015; Caliceti et al. 2017; Koguchi 2018), excessive intake of fructose and fructose-rich foods (e.g., high-fructose corn syrup and sugar-sweetened beverages, soft drinks) may lead to hyperuricemia. It seems that limiting or decreasing intake of fructose in the Japanese adult population may play an important role in the prevention of hyperuricemia.

Foods high in fructose are as follows: raisins, date palms, dried figs, dried mangos, dried tomatoes, dried kanpyo, dried apricots, dried prunes, ginger powders, grapes, apples, dried bananas, lychees, cherimoyas, pears, cherries, kiwifruit, quinces, gooseberries, persimmons, figs, mangos, blueberries (The Council for Science and Technology, Ministry of Education, Culture, Sports, Science and Technology in Japan 2023).

Fiber

The daily intake of dietary fiber among the Japanese adult population (aged $\geq$ 20 years) in 2019 was higher compared to that in 2002 and 2010 (2002: 14.8 g/day; 2010: 14.6 g/day; 2019: 18.8 g/day).

The daily intake of dietary fiber among the Japanese adult men (aged $\geq$ 20 years) in 2019 was higher compared to that in 2002 and 2010 (2002: 14.9 g/day; 2010: 14.9 g/day; 2019: 19.9 g/day). The daily intake of dietary fiber did not exhibit a significant correlation with the rate of hyperuricemia in Japanese adult men (aged $\geq$ 20 years) from 2010 to 2019 ($r= -0.259$, $p=0.536$).

The daily intake of dietary fiber among the Japanese adult women (aged $\geq$ 20 years) in 2019 was higher compared to that in 2002 and 2010 (2002: 14.7

g/day; 2010: 14.3 g/day; 2019: 18.0 g/day). The daily intake of dietary fiber did not show a significant correlation with the rate of hyperuricemia in Japanese adult women (aged ≥ 20 years) from 2010 to 2019 ($r = 0.420$, $p = 0.300$).

The daily intake of dietary fiber in the Japanese adult population (aged ≥ 20 years), Japanese adult men (aged ≥ 20 years), and Japanese adult women (aged ≥ 20 years) in 2019 were 18.8 g/day, 19.9 g/day, and 18.0 g/day, respectively. The US Department of Agriculture (USDA) has recommended that dietary fiber intake is 14 g/1000kcal, for an average-aged adult, this means a daily intake of 25 g (female) or 38 g (male) in the US (US Department of Agriculture 2023). The Adequate Intakes (AIs) for total fiber in the US population (aged ≥ 1 year) established by the Institute of Medicine of the National Academy of Sciences in the US is 14 g/1,000 kcal [men (aged 14-50 years): 38 g/day; men (aged ≥ 51 years): 30 g/day; women (aged 9-18 years): 26 g/day; women (aged 19-50 years): 25 g/day; women (aged ≥ 51 years): 21 g/day] (Institute of Medicine of the National Academy of Sciences 2021). The daily dietary fiber intake for Japanese adult men and women (aged ≥ 20 years) was below the recommendation by the US Department of Agriculture (USDA) and the Institute of Medicine of the National Academy of Sciences in the US (US Department of Agriculture 2023).

As stated in the reviews (Ekpenyong and Daniel 2015; Kakutani-Hatayama et al. 2015; Koguchi 2018; Bouike, Nakata and Moriwaki 2021) and the previous reports (Koguchi 2023), an increased intake of dietary fiber appears to be important for the prevention of hyperuricemia through reduced serum uric acid (SUA) concentrations.

Judging from the data of food composition (The Council for Science and Technology, Ministry of Education, Culture, Sports, Science and Technology in Japan 2023; US Department of Health & Human Services; National Institutes of Health; Office of Dietary Supplements 2023), it is important for the Japanese adult population (aged ≥ 20 years) to eat seeds and nuts (pumpkin seeds, chia seeds, almonds, pistachio nuts, hazelnuts, peanuts), whole grains (high-fiber bran ready-to-eat cereals, shredded wheat ready-to-eat cereals, whole grain bread, oats, barley, rye), legumes (navy beans, small white beans, yellow beans, cranberry beans, adzuki beans, French beans, split peas, chickpeas, lentils, pinto beans), seaweed, mushrooms (wood ear, shiitake mushrooms, maitake mushrooms), potatoes (konjac, potato with skin), fruit (avocados, apples, raspberries, blackberries, prunes, oranges, bananas, guavas), and vegetables (artichokes, pumpkins, tomatoes, broccoli, carrots, sweet corn, pears)

To consume more dietary fiber in order to meet the Tentative Dietary Goal for Preventing Lifestyle-related Diseases (DG) established by the Adequate Intakes (AIs), established by the Institute of Medicine of the National Academy of Sciences in the US (2021).

Protein

Total protein

The daily total protein intake of the Japanese adult population (aged ≥ 20 years) in 2019 was lower compared to that in 2002 and was higher compared to that in 2010 (2002: 73.3 g/day; 2010: 68.1 g/day; 2019: 72.2 g/day).

The daily total protein intake among the Japanese adult men (aged ≥ 20 years) in 2019 was lower compared to that in 2002 and was higher compared to that in 2010 (2002: 80.3 g/day; 2010: 74.5 g/day; 2019: 78.8 g/day). The daily intake of total protein did not demonstrate a significant correlation with the rate of hyperuricemia in Japanese adult men (aged ≥ 20 years) from 2010 to 2019 ($r= -0.596$, $p=0.119$).

The daily total protein intake among the Japanese adult women (aged ≥ 20 years) in 2019 was lower compared to that in 2002 and was higher compared to that in 2010 (2002: 67.3 g/day; 2010: 62.6 g/day; 2019: 66.4 g/day). The daily intake of total protein tended to be positively correlated with the rate of hyperuricemia in Japanese adult women (aged ≥ 20 years) from 2010 to 2019 ($r= 0.687$, $p=0.060$). These results suggest that the correlation between the daily total protein intake with rate of hyperuricemia tends to vary with gender.

The Recommended Dietary Allowances (RDAs) for protein in US adults (aged ≥ 19 years) established by the Institutes of Medicine is 0.8 g/kg body weight for the reference of body weight (Institute of Medicine of the National Academy of Sciences 2021; Institute of Medicine, Food and Nutrition Board 2011). In healthy adult men and women, protein intake should not exceed the World Health Organization (WHO) recommendation (0.83 g/ kg body weight/day for adults) (World Health Organization, Food and Agriculture Organization, and United Nations University 2007).

The mean ratio of energy intake from protein in total energy intake (protein/energy)

The mean ratio of energy intake from protein in the total energy intake (protein/energy) among the Japanese adult population (aged ≥ 20 years) in 2019 was higher compared to that in 2010 and was about the same as that in 2002 (2002: 15.2%; 2010: 14.8%; 2013: 14.8%; 2019: 15.2%).

The ratio of protein to energy (protein/energy) among Japanese adult men (aged ≥ 20 years) in 2019 was lower compared to that in 2002 and was higher compared to that in 2010 (2002: 14.9%; 2010: 14.4%; 2019: 14.8%). The protein/energy did not exhibit a significant correlation with the rate of hyperuricemia in Japanese adult men (aged ≥ 20 years) from 2010 to 2019 (r= -0.667, p=0.072).

The protein/energy of Japanese adult women (aged ≥ 20 years) in 2019 was higher compared to that in 2010 and was about the same as that in 2002 (2002: 15.5%; 2010: 15.1%; 2019: 15.5%). The protein/energy did not show a significant correlation with the rate of hyperuricemia in Japanese adult women (aged ≥ 20 years) from 2010 to 2019 (r= 0.480, p=0.228).

A cross-sectional study from China demonstrated that for every 10 g increase in energy-adjusted protein intake, there was a 17% increase in the risk of hyperuricemia (Zhang et al., 2023). This highlights the need to be cautious about excessive protein intake. .

The ratio of protein to energy (protein/energy) among Japanese adult men and women (aged ≥ 20 years) fell within the range defined by the Acceptable Macronutrient Distribution Ranges (AMDRs) established by the Institute of Medicine of the National Academy of Sciences in the US [adults (aged ≥ 19 years): 10-35 percent of total calories] (Institute of Medicine of the National Academy of Sciences 2021). The protein/energy of Japanese adult men and women (aged ≥ 20 years) appears to be appropriate or it appears better to increase it slightly.

Animal Protein

The daily intake of animal protein by the Japanese adult population (aged ≥ 20 years) in 2019 was higher compared to that in 2002 and 2010 (2002: 39.1 g/day; 2010: 35.8 g/day; 2019: 40.1 g/day).

The daily intake of animal protein by Japanese adult men (aged ≥ 20 years) in 2019 was higher compared to that in 2002 and 2010 (2002: 43.6 g/day; 2010: 39.7 g/day; 2019: 44.3 g/day). The daily intake of animal protein did not show a significant correlation with the rate of hyperuricemia in Japanese adult men (aged ≥ 20 years) from 2010 to 2019 (r= -0.520, p=0.187).

The daily intake of animal protein by Japanese adult women (aged ≥ 20 years) in 2019 was higher compared to that in 2002 and 2010 (2002: 35.2 g/day; 2010: 32.5 g/day; 2019: 36.4 g/day).

The daily intake of animal protein showed a positive correlation with the rate of hyperuricemia in Japanese adult women (aged ≥ 20 years) from 2010 to 2019 (r= 0.712, p=0.048). These results suggest that the correlation between daily animal protein intake with the rate of hyperuricemia tends to vary with gender and is stronger in Japanese adult women than in Japanese adult men.

As stated in the reviews (Choi 2010; Ekpenyong and Daniel 2015; Kakutani-Hatayama et al. 2015; Koguchi 2018; Bouike, Nakata and Moriwaki 2021) and the previous reports (Koguchi 2023), intake of protein from milk proteins (casein and lactalbumin) may have a protective effect for hyperuricemia.

A cross-sectional study from China revealed that every 10 g increase in energy-adjusted animal protein intakes led to an 18% increase in the risk of hyperuricemia (Zhang et al. 2023). It should pay attention to excessive intake of animal protein.

Vegetable Protein

The daily intake of vegetable protein by the Japanese adult population (aged ≥ 20 years) in 2019 was lower compared to that in 2002 and 2010 (2002: 34.2 g/day; 2010: 32.3 g/day; 2019: 32.1 g/day).

The daily vegetable protein among the Japanese adult men (aged ≥ 20 years) in 2019 was lower compared to that in 2002 and 2010 (2002: 36.7 g/day; 2010: 34.8 g/day; 2019: 34.5 g/day). The daily intake of vegetable protein did not exhibit a significant correlation with the rate of hyperuricemia in Japanese adult men (aged ≥ 20 years) from 2010 to 2019 (r= -0.330, p=0.425).

The daily vegetable protein intake among Japanese adult women (aged ≥ 20 years) in 2019 was lower compared to that in 2002 and 2010 (2002: 32.0 g/day; 2010: 30.1 g/day; 2019: 30.0 g/day). The daily intake of vegetable protein did not demonstrate a significant correlation with the rate of hyperuricemia in Japanese adult women (aged ≥ 20 years) from 2010 to 2019 (r= 0.414, p=0.308).

Vegetable sources of protein [e.g., wheat gluten (Jenkins et al. 2001), rice endosperm protein (Hosojima et al. 2016)] decreased serum uric acid (SUA) concentrations. A conscious intake of wheat, gluten and rice endosperm protein seems to be important for the prevention of hyperuricemia.

Fat

Total fat

The daily intake of total fat among the Japanese adult population (aged ≥ 20 years) in 2019 was higher compared to that in 2002 and 2010 (2002: 53.0 g/day; 2010: 52.7 g/day; 2019: 61.2 g/day).

The daily intake of total fat by Japanese adult men (aged ≥ 20 years) in 2019 was higher compared to that in 2002 and 2010 (2002: 57.1 g/day; 2010: 56.9 g/day; 2019: 66.3 g/day). The daily intake of total fat did not exhibit a significant correlation with the rate of hyperuricemia in Japanese adult men (aged ≥ 20 years) from 2010 to 2019 ($r = -0.393$, $p=0.336$).

The daily intake of total fat by Japanese adult women (aged ≥ 20 years) in 2019 was higher compared to that in 2002 and 2010 (2002: 49.5 g/day; 2010: 49.1 g/day; 2019: 56.7 g/day). The daily intake of total fat showed a positive correlation with the rate of hyperuricemia in Japanese adult women (aged ≥ 20 years) from 2010 to 2019 ($r = 0.837$, $p=0.009$). These results suggest that the correlation between daily intake of total fat with the rate of hyperuricemia tends to vary with gender and is stronger in Japanese adult women than in Japanese adult men.

The Estimated Average Requirements (EARs), the Recommended Dietary Allowances (RDAs), the Adequate Intakes (AIs), and the Tolerable Upper Intake Levels (ULs) for total fat for individuals aged 1 year and older in the U.S. established by the Institutes of Medicine has not been set (Institute of Medicine of the National Academy of Sciences 2021; Institute of Medicine, Food and Nutrition Board 2011).

The mean ratio of energy intake from fat in total energy intake (fat/energy)

The mean ratio of energy intake from fat in total energy intake (fat/energy) of Japanese adult population (aged ≥ 20 years) in 2019 was higher compared to that in 2002 and 2010 (2002: 24.3%; 2010: 25.2%; 2019: 28.4%).

The fat/energy of Japanese adult men (aged ≥ 20 years) in 2019 was higher compared to that in 2002 and 2010 (2002: 23.4%; 2010: 24.3%; 2019: 27.4%). The ratio of fat to energy (fat/energy) did not exhibit a significant correlation with the rate of hyperuricemia in Japanese adult men (aged ≥ 20 years) from 2010 to 2019 ($r = -0.358$, $p=0.384$).

The ratio of fat to energy (fat/energy) among Japanese adult women (aged ≥ 20 years) in 2019 was higher compared to that in 2002 and 2010 (2002:

25.0%; 2010: 26.1%; 2019: 29.2%). The ratio of fat/energy was positively correlated with the rate of hyperuricemia in Japanese adult women (aged ≥ 20 years) from 2010 to 2019 (r= 0.846, p=0.0081). These results suggest that the correlation between the ratio of fat to energy (fat/energy) and the rate of hyperuricemia tends to vary with gender and is stronger in Japanese adult women than in Japanese adult men.

The ratio of fat to energy (fat/energy) in the Japanese adult population (aged ≥ 20 years), Japanese adult men (aged ≥ 20 years), and Japanese adult women (aged ≥ 20 years) in 2019 was 28.4% of energy, 27.4% of energy, and 29.2% of energy, respectively. Although the fat/energy of Japanese adult men and women (aged ≥ 20 years) were within the range of the Acceptable Macronutrient Distribution Ranges (AMDRs) established by the Institute of Medicine of the National Academy of Sciences in the US [adults (aged ≥ 19 years): 20-35 percent of total calories] (Institute of Medicine of the National Academy of Sciences 2021), it seems better to decrease the mean ratio of energy intake from fat in total energy intake (fat/energy). In an epidemiological study, the increased intake of fat was associated with increased SUA concentrations (Zykova et al. 2015). Zhu et al. (2016) reported that the excessive intake of fat was a risk factor of hyperuricemia in middle-aged and elderly people in China. A cross-sectional study from China showed that every 10 g increase in energy-adjusted fat intakes caused a 10% increase in hyperuricemia risk (Zhang et al. 2023).

Animal fat

The daily animal fat intake among the Japanese adult population (aged ≥ 20 years) in 2019 was higher compared to that in 2002 and 2010 (2002: 26.1 g/day; 2010: 26.1 g/day; 2019: 31.9 g/day).

The daily animal fat intake among Japanese adult men (aged ≥ 20 years) in 2019 was higher compared to that in 2002 and 2010 (2002: 28.8 g/day; 2010: 28.9 g/day; 2019: 35.2 g/day). The daily animal fat intake did not exhibit a significant correlation with the rate of hyperuricemia in Japanese adult men (aged ≥ 20 years) from 2010 to 2019 (r= -0.413, p=0.310).

The daily animal fat intake among the Japanese adult women (aged ≥ 20 years) in 2019 was higher compared to that in 2002 and 2010 (2002: 23.8 g/day; 2010: 23.7 g/day; 2019: 28.9 g/day). The daily animal fat intake was positively correlated with the rate of hyperuricemia in Japanese adult women (aged ≥ 20 years) from 2010 to 2019 (r= 0.797, p=0.018). These results suggest that the correlation between the daily animal fat intake with the rate of hyperuricemia tends to vary with gender and is stronger in Japanese adult women than in Japanese adult men.

As stated in the previous reports (Koguchi 2023), limiting, or decreasing the intake of animal fat may play an important role in the prevention of hyperuricemia.

Vegetable fat

The daily vegetable fat intake among the Japanese adult population (aged ≥ 20 years) in 2019 was higher compared to that in 2002 and 2010 (2002: 26.9 g/day; 2010: 26.5 g/day; 2019: 29.3 g/day).

The daily vegetable fat intake among the Japanese adult men (aged ≥ 20 years) in 2019 was higher compared to that in 2002 and 2010 (2002: 28.3 g/day; 2010: 28.0 g/day; 2019: 31.1 g/day). The daily intake of vegetable fat did not show a significant correlation with the rate of hyperuricemia in Japanese adult men (aged ≥ 20 years) from 2010 to 2019 ($r = -0.316$, $p=0.386$).

The daily vegetable fat intake among the Japanese adult women (aged ≥ 20 years) in 2019 was higher compared to that in 2002 and 2010 (2002: 25.7 g/day; 2010: 25.3 g/day; 2019: 27.7 g/day). The daily intake of vegetable fat was positively correlated with the rate of hyperuricemia in Japanese adult women (aged ≥ 20 years) from 2010 to 2019 ($r= 0.886$, $p=0.003$). These results suggest that the correlation between the daily vegetable fat intake with the rate of hyperuricemia tends to vary with gender and is stronger in Japanese adult women than in Japanese adult men.

Saturated fatty acids

The daily saturated fatty acid intake among the Japanese adult population (aged ≥ 20 years) in 2019 was higher compared to that in 2002 and 2010 (2002: 13.4 g/day; 2010: 13.9 g/day; 2019: 17.9 g/day).

The daily saturated fatty acid intake among Japanese adult men (aged ≥ 20 years) in 2019 was higher compared to that in 2002 and 2010 (2002: 14.1 g/day; 2010: 14.8 g/day; 2019: 19.1 g/day). The daily saturated fatty acids intake did not exhibit a significant correlation with the rate of hyperuricemia in Japanese adult men (aged ≥ 20 years) from 2010 to 2019 ($r= -0.381$, $p=0.352$).

The daily saturated fatty acid intake among the Japanese adult women (aged ≥ 20 years) in 2019 was higher compared to that in 2002 and 2010 (2002: 12.7 g/day; 2010: 13.2 g/day; 2019: 16.7 g/day). The daily intake saturated fatty acids was positively correlated with the rate of hyperuricemia in Japanese adult women (aged ≥ 20 years) from 2010 to 2019 ($r= 0.758$, $p=0.029$). These results suggest that the correlation between the daily intake of saturated fatty acids and the rate of hyperuricemia tends to vary with gender and is stronger in Japanese adult women than in Japanese adult men.

As stated in the previous reports (Koguchi 2023), limiting or decreasing the intake of saturated fatty acids may play an important role in the prevention of hyperuricemia.

The Estimated Average Requirements (EARs), the Recommended Dietary Allowances (RDAs), the Adequate Intakes (AIs), and the Tolerable Upper Intake Levels (ULs) for saturated fatty acids in the US population established by the Institutes of Medicine has not been set (Institute of Medicine of the National Academy of Sciences 2021; Institute of Medicine, Food and Nutrition Board 2011). The Institute of Medicine of the National Academy in the US has stated that the recommendation for saturated fatty acids is to keep it as low possible while maintaining a nutritionally adequate diet (Institute of Medicine of the National Academy of Sciences 2021).

n-3 Polyunsaturated Fatty Acids

The daily n-3 polyunsaturated fatty acid intake among the Japanese adult population (aged ≥ 20 years) in 2019 was higher than in 2010 (2010: 2.33 g/day; 2019: 2.46 g/day).

The daily n-3 polyunsaturated fatty acid intake by Japanese adult men (aged ≥ 20 years) in 2019 was higher than in 2010 (2010: 2.57 g/day; 2019: 2.68 g/day). The daily n-3 polyunsaturated fatty acids intake did not exhibit a significant correlation with the rate of hyperuricemia in Japanese adult men (aged ≥ 20 years) from 2010 to 2019 ($r= -0.109$, $p=0.798$).

The daily n-3 polyunsaturated fatty acid intake by Japanese adult women (aged ≥ 20 years) in 2019 was higher than in 2010 (2010: 2.13 g/day; 2019: 2.27 g/day). The daily intake of n-3 polyunsaturated fatty acids did not exhibit a significant correlation with the rate of hyperuricemia in Japanese adult women (aged ≥ 20 years) from 2010 to 2019 ($r= 0.395$, $p=0.333$).

The mean ratio of energy intake from n-3 polyunsaturated fatty acids in total energy intake (n-3 polyunsaturated fatty acid/energy) of Japanese adult men (aged ≥ 20 years) and Japanese adult women (aged ≥ 20 years) in 2019 was 1.13% and 1.19%, respectively. The Institute of Medicine of the National Academy of Sciences in the US (2021) has determined that the Acceptable Macronutrient Distribution Ranges (AMDRs) for n-3 polyunsaturated fatty acids (α-linolenic acid) for both adults (aged ≥ 19 years) and children (aged 4-18 years) is 0.6-1.2% of total calories. The daily intake of n-3 polyunsaturated fatty acid seems to be appropriate for Japanese adult men and women (aged ≥ 20 years).

n-6 Polyunsaturated Fatty Acids

The daily intake of n-6 polyunsaturated fatty acid among the Japanese adult population (aged ≥ 20 years) in 2019 was higher compared to that in 2010 (2010: 9.29 g/day; 2019: 10.66 g/day).

The daily intake of n-6 polyunsaturated fatty acids among the Japanese adult men (aged ≥ 20 years) in 2019 was higher compared to that in 2010 (2010: 10.11 g/day; 2019: 11.61 g/day). The daily intake of n-6 polyunsaturated fatty acids intake did not exhibit a significant correlation with the rate of hyperuricemia in Japanese adult men (aged ≥ 20 years) from 2010 to 2019 (r= -0.404, p=0.321).

The daily intake of n-6 polyunsaturated fatty acids by Japanese adult women (aged ≥ 20 years) in 2019 was higher compared to that in 2010 (2010: 8.58 g/day; 2019: 9.84 g/day). The daily intake of n-6 polyunsaturated fatty acids was positively correlated with the rate of hyperuricemia in Japanese adult women (aged ≥ 20 years) from 2010 to 2019 (r= 0.768, p=0.026). These results suggest that the correlation of the daily intake of n-6 polyunsaturated fatty acids with the rate of hyperuricemia tends to vary with gender and is stronger in Japanese adult women than in Japanese adult men.

The mean ratio of energy intake from n-6 polyunsaturated fatty acids in the total energy intake (n-6 polyunsaturated fatty acid/energy) of Japanese adult men (aged ≥ 20 years) and Japanese adult women (aged ≥ 20 years) in 2019 were 4.88% and 5.16%, respectively. The Institute of Medicine of the National Academy of Sciences in the US (2021) has determined that the Acceptable Macronutrient Distribution Ranges (AMDRs) for n-6 polyunsaturated fatty acids (linoleic acid) both adults (aged ≥ 19 years) and children (aged 4-18 years) is 5-10% of total calories. The daily intake of n-6 polyunsaturated fatty acid appears to be appropriate for Japanese adult women and it appears better to increase it slightly for Japanese adult men.

Cholesterol

The daily intake of cholesterol by the Japanese adult population (aged ≥ 20 years) in 2019 was higher compared to that in 2002 and 2010 (2002: 335 mg/day; 2010: 307 mg/day; 2019: 340 mg/day).

The daily intake of cholesterol among the Japanese adult men (aged ≥ 20 years) in 2019 was higher compared to that in 2002 and 2010 (2002: 364 mg/day; 2010: 331 mg/day; 2019: 366 mg/day). The daily cholesterol intake did not exhibit a significant correlation with the rate of hyperuricemia in Japanese adult men (aged ≥ 20 years) from 2010 to 2019 (r= -0.359, p=0.383).

The daily intake of cholesterol among the Japanese adult women (aged ≥ 20 years) in 2019 was higher compared to that in 2002 and 2010 (2002: 309 mg/day; 2010: 285 mg/day; 2019: 317 mg/day). The daily cholesterol intake was positively correlated with the rate of hyperuricemia in Japanese adult women (aged ≥ 20 years) from 2010 to 2019 (r= 0.710, p=0.048). These results suggest that the correlation between the daily cholesterol intake with the rate of hyperuricemia tends to vary with gender and is stronger in Japanese adult women than in Japanese adult men.

As stated in the previous reports (Koguchi 2023), limiting or decreasing intake of cholesterol may play an important role in the prevention of hyperuricemia.

The Estimated Average Requirement (EAR), the Recommended Dietary Allowances (RDAs), the Adequate Intakes (AIs), and the Tolerable Upper Intake Levels (ULs) for cholesterol in the US population established by the Institutes of Medicine has not been set (Institute of Medicine of The National Academy 2021). The Institute of Medicine of the National Academy of Sciences in the US (2021) has stated that recommendation for dietary cholesterol is as low possible while consuming a nutritionally adequate diet.

Foods high in cholesterol are as follows: liver, egg yolk, dried herring roe, dried squid, anchovy, sardines, shrimp, abalone, salmon, mackerel, sea urchin, carp, sweet fish, lobster, full-fat dairy products (Institute of Medicine of the National Academy of Sciences 2021; The Council for Science and Technology, Ministry of Education, Culture, Sports, Science and Technology in Japan 2023).

Alcohol

As stated in the reviews (Choi 2010; Ekpenyong and Daniel 2015; Kakutani-Hatayama et al. 2015; Koguchi 2018; Bouike, Nakata and Moriwaki 2021) and the previous reports (Koguchi 2023), limiting or decreasing intake of alcohol in Japanese adult population may play an important role in the prevention of hyperuricemia.

Water Intake

The Ministry of Health, Labour and Welfare in Japan has not investigated the daily water intake among the Japanese people.

The mean total water intake of Japanese adults (aged 30-76 years), Japanese men (aged 30-76 years), and Japanese women (aged 30-69 years) was 2230 g/day, 2423 g/day, and 2037 g/day, respectively (Tani et al. 2015). Since the density of the drinking water is unknown, it is not possible to compare the total water intake of the Japanese adult population with the Adequate Intakes (AIs) established by the Institute of Medicine of the National Academy of Sciences in the U.S. [Total water intake: males (aged 14-18 years): 3.3 L g/day (approximately 2.6 L as total beverages, including drinking water); males (aged $\geq$ 19 years): 3.7 L/day (approximately 3.0 L as total beverages, including drinking water); females (aged 14-18 years): 2.3 L/day (approximately 1.8 L as total beverages, including drinking water); females (aged $\geq$ 19 years): 2.7 L/day (approximately 2.2 L as total beverages, including drinking water)] (Institute of Medicine of the National Academy of Sciences 2021).

Purine

The Ministry of Health, Labour and Welfare in Japan has not investigated the daily purine intake among the Japanese people.

As stated in the reviews (Choi 2010; Ekpenyong and Daniel 2015; Kakutani-Hatayama et al. 2015; Koguchi 2018; Bouike, Nakata and Moriwaki 2021) and the previous reports (Koguchi 2023), limiting or decreasing intake of purines in the Japanese adult population may play an important role in the prevention of hyperuricemia.

Polyphenol

The Ministry of Health, Labour and Welfare in Japan has not investigated the daily polyphenol intake among the Japanese people.

As stated in the previous reports (Koguchi 2023), conscious intake of polyphenols seems to be important for the prevention of hyperuricemia through reduced serum uric acid (SUA) concentrations. However, dietary polyphenol intake in the US was ~1 g/day (Kuhnau 1976). Since it has reported that excessive intake of some polyphenols resulted in growth of depression in animals (Yoon and Baek 2005), it must take care of excessive intake of polyphenols.

Vitamins

Vitamin A and β-carotene

The daily intake of vitamin A (retinol equivalent) among the Japanese adult population (aged ≥ 20 years) in 2019 was lower than in 2002 and was higher than in 2010 (2002: 953 μgRAE; 2010: 534 μgRAE; 2019: 547 μgRAE).

The daily vitamin A (retinol equivalent) intake among the Japanese adult men (aged ≥ 20 years) in 2019 was lower than in 2002 and was higher than in 2010 (2002: 965 μgRAE; 2010: 550 μgRAE; 2019: 564 μgRAE). The intake of vitamin A did not show a significant correlation with the rate of hyperuricemia in Japanese adult men (aged ≥ 20 years) from 2010 to 2019 ($r= 0.481$, $p=0.227$).

The daily intake of vitamin A (retinol equivalent) among the Japanese adult women (aged ≥ 20 years) in 2019 was lower than in 2002 and was higher than in 2010 (2002: 942 μgRAE; 2010: 520 μgRAE; 2019: 532 μgRAE). The intake of vitamin A did not show a significant correlation with the rate of hyperuricemia in Japanese adult women (aged ≥ 20 years) from 2010 to 2019 ($r= 0.177$, $p=0.676$).

The daily intake of vitamin A (retinol equivalent) among the Japanese men (aged 15-69 years) and women (aged 15-49 years) were 451-596 μgRAE/day and 409-458 μgRAE/day, respectively, and were below the Estimated Average Requirements (EARs) established by the Institute of Medicine of the National Academy of Sciences in the US [men (aged 15-69 years): 625-630 μgRAE/day; women (aged 15-49 years): 485-500 μgRAE/day] (Institute of Medicine of the National Academy of Sciences 2021). Thus the daily intake of vitamin A (retinol equivalent) among Japanese men (aged 15-69 years) and women (aged 15-49 years) were below the Recommended Dietary Allowances (RDAs) for vitamin A established by the Institute of Medicine of the National Academy of Sciences in the US [men (aged ≥ 14 years): 900 μgRAE/day; women (aged ≥ 14 years): 700 μgRAE/day] (Institute of Medicine of the National Academy of Sciences 2021; US Department of Health & Human Services; National Institutes of

Health; Office of Dietary Supplements 2023). The daily intake of vitamin A (retinol equivalent) among Japanese men (aged ≥ 14 years) and women (aged ≥ 14 years) were below the Recommended Dietary Allowances (RDAs) established by the Institute of Medicine of the National Academy of Sciences in the US (2021).

Judging from the data of food composition (The Council for Science and Technology, Ministry of Education, Culture, Sports, Science and Technology in Japan 2023; US Department of Health & Human Services; National Institutes of Health; Office of Dietary Supplements 2023), it is important for Japanese people (aged ≥ 14 years) to eat organ meats (liver, breast), seafood (salmon, tuna, herring, firefly squid, eel, conger eel, sablefish), potatoes, whole grains (fortified ready-to-eat cereals), nuts (pistachio nuts), legumes (black-eyed peas, baked beans), seaweed, fruit (apricots, mangos, cantaloupes), vegetables (spinach, carrots, peppers, broccoli, Jew's mallows, perillas), dairy products (milk, cheese, yogurt), eggs, green tea to take in more vitamin A to reach the Recommended Dietary Allowances (RDAs) established by the Institute of Medicine of the National Academy of Sciences in the US (2021). Serum vitamin A (retinol) levels were positively associated with SUA concentrations (Ford and Choi 2013; Kim et al. 2020; Liu et al. 2021) and hyperuricemia risk (Kim et al. 2020). To avoid high serum vitamin A levels in the general population and not exceed the Tolerable Upper Intake Levels (ULs) for vitamin A, one must pay attention to vitamin A intake. .

Vitamin D

The daily intake of vitamin D in the Japanese adult population (aged ≥ 20 years) in 2019 was lower compared to that in 2002 and 2010 (2002: 8.8 μg/day; 2010: 7.7 μg/day; 2019: 7.2 μg/day).

The daily intake of vitamin D for Japanese adult men (aged ≥ 20 years) in 2019 was lower compared to that in 2002 and 2010 (2002: 9.6 μg/day; 2010: 8.4 μg/day; 2019: 7.9 μg/day). The intake of vitamin D did not show a significant correlation with the rate of hyperuricemia in Japanese adult men (aged ≥ 20 years) from 2010 to 2019 ($r= 0.206$, $p=0.625$).

The daily intake of vitamin D for Japanese adult women (aged ≥ 20 years) in 2019 was lower compared to that in 2002 and 2010 (2002: 8.1 μg/day; 2010: 7.2 μg/day; 2019: 6.6 μg/day). The intake of vitamin D did not show a significant correlation with the rate of hyperuricemia in Japanese adult women (aged ≥ 20 years) from 2010 to 2019 ($r= -0.460$, $p=0.252$).

The daily intake of vitamin D among the Japanese adult population (aged ≥ 20 years), Japanese adult men (aged ≥ 20 years), and Japanese adult women (aged ≥ 20 years) in 2019 were 7.2 µg/day, 7.9 µg/day, and 6.6 µg/day, respectively. The Recommended Dietary Allowances (RDAs) for vitamin D in men and women (aged 19-70 years), men and women (aged ≥ 71 years) established by the Food and Nutrition Board at Institute of Medicine in the US are 15 µg/day and 20 µg/day, respectively (Institute of Medicine, Food and Nutrition Board 2011). The Adequate Intakes (AIs) for vitamin D in the U.S. for men and women aged 0-50 years, men and women (aged 51-70) years, and men and women (aged ≥ 71 years) and older were established by the Institute of Medicine of the National Academy of Sciences are 5 µg/day, 10 µg/day and 15 µg/day, respectively (Institute of Medicine of the National Academy of Sciences 2021). The daily intake for vitamin D among the Japanese men (aged 7-49 years) and Japanese women (aged 7-19 years, aged 40-49 years) were 5.5-6.4 µg/day, 5.3-5.8 µg/day and 5.3 µg/day, respectively, and were above the Adequate Intakes (AIs) established by the Institute of Medicine of the National Academy of Sciences in the US [men (aged 0-50 years): 5 µg/day; women (aged 0-50 years): 5 µg/day] (Institute of Medicine of the National Academy of Sciences 2021). Whereas the daily intake of vitamin D among the Japanese men (aged 50-69 years, aged ≥ 75 years) and Japanese women (aged 20-39 years, aged 50-69 years, aged ≥ 70 years) were 8.0-9.0 µg/day, 13.4 µg/day, 4.6-4.9 µg/day, 5.4-7.1 µg/day, and 8.4 µg/day, respectively, and were below the Adequate Intakes (AIs) established by the Institute of Medicine of the National Academy of Sciences in the US [men (aged 50-69 years): 10.0 µg/day; men (aged ≥ 75 years): 15.0 µg/day; women (aged 20-39 years): 5.0 µg/day; women (aged 50-69 years): 10.0 µg/day; women (aged ≥ 70 years): 10.0-15.0 µg/day] (Institute of Medicine of the National Academy of Sciences 2021).

Judging from the data of food composition (The Council for Science and Technology, Ministry of Education, Culture, Sports, Science and Technology in Japan 2023; US Department of Health & Human Services; National Institutes of Health; Office of Dietary Supplements 2023) and the roles of vitamin D in the body (promotion of calcium absorption, reduction of inflammation, modulation of such processes as cell growth, neuromuscular and immune function, and glucose metabolism) (US Department of Health & Human Services; National Institutes of Health; Office of Dietary Supplements 2023), it is important for Japanese adult men (aged 50-69 years, aged ≥ 75 years) and Japanese adult women (aged 20-39 years, aged 50-69 years, aged ≥ 70 years) to eat fish (salmon, trout, swordfish, sturgeon, cisco, whitefish, mackerel, tuna, sardines, rockfish, tilapia, flatfish), fish oil (cod liver), mushrooms, milks (whole milk, whole chocolate milk, soy milk, almond milk), dairy products (yogurt), cereals (fortified ready-to-eat cereals), eggs to take in more vitamin D to reach the Adequate Intakes (AIs) set by the Institute of Medicine of the National Academy of Sciences in the US [men (aged 50-69 years): 10.0 μg/day; men (aged ≥ 75 years): 15.0 μg/day; women (aged 20-39 years): 5.0 μg/day; women (aged 50-69 years): 10.0 μg/day; women (aged ≥ 70 years): 10.0-15.0 μg/day] (Institute of Medicine of the National Academy of Sciences 2021). However, it must be careful not to exceed the Tolerable Upper Intake levels (ULs) of the daily vitamin D intake. An overdose of vitamin D-rich foods and/or supplementation should be avoided to prevent exceeding the Tolerable Upper Intake Levels (ULs). The Tolerable Upper Intake levels (ULs) for vitamin D in men (aged ≥ 1 year), women (aged ≥ 1 year), pregnancy (aged ≤ 18 years and aged 19-50 years), and lactation (aged ≤ 18 years and aged 19-50 years) are 50 μg/day, respectively (Institute of Medicine of the National Academy of Sciences 2021).

Vitamin E

The daily intake of vitamin E among the Japanese adult population (aged ≥ 20 years) in 2019 was lower compared to that in 2002 and 2010 (2002: 8.4 mg/day; 2010: 8.3 mg/day; 2019: 6.9 mg/day).

The daily intake of vitamin E among Japanese adult men (aged ≥ 20 years) in 2019 was lower compared to that in 2002 and 2010 (2002: 8.8 mg/day; 2010: 8.3 mg/day; 2019: 7.2 mg/day). The daily intake of vitamin E did not exhibit a significant correlation with the rate of hyperuricemia in Japanese adult men (aged ≥ 20 years) from 2010 to 2019 ($r= 0.552$, $p=0.156$).

The daily intake of vitamin E among Japanese adult women (aged ≥ 20 years) in 2019 was lower compared to that in 2002 and 2010 (2002: 8.0 mg/day; 2010: 8.3 mg/day; 2019: 6.6 mg/day). The daily intake of vitamin E did not exhibit a significant correlation with the rate of hyperuricemia in Japanese adult women (aged ≥ 20 years) from 2010 to 2019 ($r= -0.590$, $p=0.124$).

The average daily vitamin E intake among the Japanese men (aged ≥ 20 years) and women (aged ≥ 20 years) in 2019 were 7.2 mg/day and 6.6 mg/day, respectively. The Estimated Average Requirements (EARs) and the Recommended Dietary Allowances (RDAs) for vitamin E in men (aged ≥ 14 years) and women (aged ≥ 14 years) established by the Institute of Medicine of the National Academy of Sciences in the US are 12 mg/day and 15 mg/day, respectively (Institute of Medicine of the National Academy of Sciences 2021). Judging from the Dietary Reference Intakes established by the Institute of Medicine of the National Academy of Sciences in the US (2021), Japanese men (aged ≥ 15 years) and women (aged ≥ 15 years) need to take in more vitamin E to reach the Recommended Dietary Allowances (RDAs).

As stated in the previous reports (Koguchi 2023), an increased intake of vitamin E appears to be important for the prevention of hyperuricemia through reduced serum uric acid (SUA) concentrations.

Judging from the data of food composition (The Council for Science and Technology, Ministry of Education, Culture, Sports, Science and Technology in Japan 2023; U.S. Department of Health & Human Services; National Institutes of Health; Office of Dietary Supplements 2023), it is important for Japanese men (aged ≥ 15 years) and women (aged ≥ 15 years) to eat wheat germ, seeds and nuts (sunflower seeds, almonds, hazelnuts, peanuts), vegetables (spinach, broccoli, tomatoes), and fruit (kiwi fruits, mangos) to take in more vitamin E to reach the Recommended Dietary Allowances (RDAs) established by the Institute of Medicine of the National Academy of Sciences in the US (2021). An overdose of vitamin E-rich foods and/or supplementation should be avoided to prevent exceeding the Tolerable Upper Intake Levels (ULs). The Tolerable Upper Intake levels (ULs) for vitamin E intake in men and women (aged 14-18 years), men and women (aged ≥ 19 years), pregnancy and lactation (aged ≤ 18 years), and pregnancy and lactation (aged 19-50 years) are 800 mg/day, 1,000 mg/day, 800 mg/day, and 1,000 mg/day, respectively (Institute of Medicine of the National Academy of Sciences 2021).

Vitamin K

The daily intake of vitamin K among the Japanese adult population (aged ≥ 20 years) in 2019 was lower compared to that in 2002 and was higher compared to that in 2010 (2002: 277 μg/day; 2010: 240 μg/day; 2019: 250 μg/day).

The daily intake of vitamin K among Japanese adult men (aged ≥ 20 years) in 2019 was lower compared to that in 2002 and was higher compared to that in 2010 (2002: 280 μg/day; 2010: 246 μg/day; 2019: 258 μg/day). The daily intake of vitamin K did not exhibit a significant correlation with the rate of hyperuricemia in Japanese adult men (aged ≥ 20 years) from 2010 to 2019 ($r= 0.026$, $p=0.952$).

The daily intake of vitamin K among Japanese adult women (aged ≥ 20 years) in 2019 was lower compared to that in 2002 and was higher compared to that in 2010 (2002: 274 μg/day; 2010: 235 μg/day; 2019: 243 μg/day). The daily intake of vitamin K did not exhibit a significant correlation with the rate of hyperuricemia in Japanese adult women (aged ≥ 20 years) from 2010 to 2019 ($r= 0.653$, $p=0.079$).

The daily intake of vitamin K among the Japanese adult population (aged ≥ 20 years), Japanese adult men (aged ≥ 20 years), and Japanese adult women (aged ≥ 20 years) in 2019 were 250 μg/day, 258 μg/day, and 243 μg/day, respectively. The Adequate Intakes (AIs) for vitamin K in the US men (aged ≥ 19 years) and women (aged ≥ 19 years) established by the Institute of Medicine of the National Academy of Sciences in the US are 120 μg/day and 90 μg/day, respectively (Institute of Medicine of the National Academy of Sciences 2021). This suggests that the daily intake of vitamin K in Japanese men (aged ≥ 14 year) and women (aged ≥ 14 year) appears to be very unlikely to cause a deficiency.

Conscious intake of vitamin K-rich foods (e.g., natto, collards, turnip greens, spinach, kales, broccoli, soybeans, edamame, pumpkins, okra, pine nuts, blueberries, iceberg lettuces, chicken breast, grapes, cashews, carrots, chicken liver, ground beef) (The Council for Science and Technology, Ministry of Education, Culture, Sports, Science and Technology in Japan 2023; US Department of Health & Human Services; National Institutes of Health; Office of Dietary Supplements 2023) appears to be important.

Thiamin (Vitamin B_1)

The daily intake of vitamin B_1 among the Japanese adult population (aged ≥ 20 years) in 2019 was higher compared to that in 2002 and was lower compared to that in 2010 (2002: 0.87 mg/day; 2010: 1.60 mg/day; 2019: 0.95 mg/day).

The daily intake of vitamin B_1 among Japanese adult men (aged ≥ 20 years) in 2019 was higher compared to that in 2002 and was lower compared to that in 2010 (2002: 0.93 mg/day; 2010: 1.54 mg/day; 2019: 1.03 mg/day). The daily intake of vitamin B_1 did not exhibit a significant correlation with the rate of hyperuricemia in Japanese adult men (aged ≥ 20 years) from 2010 to 2019 (r= 0.559, p=0.149).

The daily intake vitamin B_1 among Japanese adult men (aged ≥ 20 years) in 2019 was higher compared to that in 2002 and was lower compared to that in 2010 (2002: 0.81 mg/day; 2010: 1.65 mg/day; 2019: 0.88 mg/day). The daily intake of vitamin B_1 tended to be negatively correlated with the rate of hyperuricemia in Japanese adult women (aged ≥ 20 years) from 2010 to 2019 (r= -0.688, p=0.059). These results suggest that the correlation between the daily vitamin B_1 intake with the rate of hyperuricemia tends to vary with gender.

The daily intake of vitamin B_1 among Japanese adult men (aged ≥ 20 years) and Japanese adult women (aged ≥ 20 years) in 2019 were 1.03 mg/day and 0.88 mg/day, respectively. The Recommended Dietary Allowances (RDAs) for vitamin B_1 in US men (aged ≥ 14 years), women (aged 14-18 years) and women (aged ≥ 19 years) established by the Institute of Medicine of the National Academy of Sciences in the US are 1.2 mg/day, 1.0 mg/day, and 1.1 mg/day, respectively (Institute of Medicine of the National Academy of Sciences 2021). Therefore, the daily intake of vitamin B_1 for Japanese men (aged ≥ 15 years) and women (aged ≥ 15 years) were below the Recommended Dietary Allowances (RDAs).

As stated in the previous reports (Koguchi 2023), the increased intake of vitamin B_1 appears to be important for the prevention of hyperuricemia through reduced serum uric acid (SUA) concentrations.

Judging from the data of food composition (The Council for Science and Technology, Ministry of Education, Culture, Sports, Science and Technology in Japan 2023; US Department of Health & Human Services; National Institutes of Health; Office of Dietary Supplements 2023), it is important for Japanese people (aged ≥ 15 years) to eat meats (pork), seafood (mussels, trout, tuna, walleye pollock, eel), mushrooms (maitake mushrooms), grains (white rice, egg noodle, bread), whole grains (whole wheat, brown rice, oatmeal, fortified ready-to-eat cereals), seeds (sunflower seeds, sesame seeds, chia seeds), legumes (black beans, soybeans), fruit (avocados), vegetables (broccoli), dairy products (milk), eggs to take in more vitamin B_1 to reach the Recommended Dietary Allowances (RDAs) established by the Institute of Medicine of the National Academy of Sciences in the US (Institute of Medicine of the National Academy of Sciences 2021).

Riboflavin (Vitamin B_2)

The daily intake of vitamin B_2 among the Japanese adult population (aged ≥ 20 years) in 2019 was lower compared to that in 2002 and 2010 (2002: 1.21 mg/day; 2010: 1.52 mg/day; 2019: 1.19 mg/day).

The daily intake of vitamin B_2 among Japanese adult men (aged ≥ 20 years) in 2019 was lower compared to that in 2002 and 2010 (2002: 1.26 mg/day; 2010: 1.45 mg/day; 2019: 1.25 mg/day). The daily intake of vitamin B_2 did not exhibit a significant correlation with the rate of hyperuricemia in Japanese adult men (aged ≥ 20 years) from 2010 to 2019 ($r= 0.605, p=0.112$).

The daily intake of vitamin B_2 among Japanese adult women (aged ≥ 20 years) in 2019 was lower compared to that in 2002 and 2010 (2002: 1.17 mg/day; 2010: 1.59 mg/day; 2019: 1.13 mg/day). The daily intake of vitamin B_2 tended to be negatively correlated with the rate of hyperuricemia in Japanese adult women (aged ≥ 20 years) from 2010 to 2019 ($r= -0.673$, p=0.067). These results suggest that the correlation between the daily vitamin B_2 intake with the rate of hyperuricemia tends to vary with gender.

The daily intake of vitamin B_2 among Japanese men (aged 20-59 years) and women (aged 20-59 years) in 2019 were 1.10-1.20 mg/day and 0.97-1.09 mg/day, respectively, and were below the Recommended Dietary Allowances (RDAs) established by the Institute of Medicine of the National Academy of Sciences in the US [men (aged $\geq$ 19 years): 1.30 mg/day; women (aged $\geq$ 19 years): 1.10 mg/day] (Institute of Medicine of the National Academy of Sciences 2021). The daily vitamin B_2 intake among the Japanese adult men (aged $\geq$ 75 years) and adult women (aged $\geq$ 75 years) were 1.31 mg/day and 1.18 mg/day, respectively, and were above the Recommended Dietary Allowances (RDAs) established by the Institute of Medicine of the National Academy of Sciences in the US [men (aged $\geq$ 19 years): 1.30 mg/day; women (aged $\geq$ 19 years): 1.10 mg/day] (Institute of Medicine of the National Academy of Sciences 2021).

The Institute of Medicine of the National Academy of Sciences in the US (2021) has not set the Tolerable Upper Intake Levels (ULs) for riboflavin (vitamin B_2).

As stated in the previous reports (Koguchi 2023), conscious intake of vitamin B_2 seems to be important for the prevention of hyperuricemia through reduced serum uric acid (SUA) concentrations.

Judging from the data of food composition (The Council for Science and Technology, Ministry of Education, Culture, Sports, Science and Technology in Japan 2023; US Department of Health & Human Services; National Institutes of Health; Office of Dietary Supplements 2023), it is important for Japanese men (aged 20-59 years) and women (aged 20-59 years) to eat organ meats (kidneys, liver), seafood (clams, salmon, cod), mushrooms (maitake mushrooms, shiitake mushrooms), grains (white rice, egg noodle, bread), whole grains (whole wheat, brown rice, oats, fortified ready-to-eat cereals), seeds (sunflower seeds, almonds), legumes (kidney beans), seaweed, vegetables (asparaguses, tomatoes, cauliflowers), dairy products (milk, cheese, yogurt), eggs to take in more vitamin B_2 to reach the Recommended Dietary Allowances (RDAs) established by the Institute of Medicine of the National Academy of Sciences in the US (Institute of Medicine of the National Academy of Sciences 2021).

Niacin

The daily intake of niacin equivalent (niacin) among the Japanese adult population (aged $\geq$ 20 years) in 2019 was higher compared to that in 2002 and

2010 (2002: 27.9 mg NE /day; 2010: 26.2 mg NE /day; 2019: 31.3 mg NE /day).

The daily intake of niacin equivalent (niacin) among Japanese adult men (aged ≥ 20 years) in 2019 was higher compared to that in 2002 and 2010 (2002: 30.9 mg NE /day; 2010: 29.0 mg NE /day; 2019: 34.5 mg NE /day). The daily niacin intake did not exhibit a significant correlation with the rate of hyperuricemia in Japanese adult men (aged ≥ 20 years) from 2010 to 2019 ($r=-0.314$, $p=0.449$).

The daily intake of niacin equivalent (niacin) among Japanese adult women (aged ≥ 20 years) in 2019 was higher compared to that in 2002 and 2010 (2002: 25.2 mg NE /day; 2010: 23.8 mg NE /day; 2019: 28.5 mg NE /day). The daily intake of niacin did not exhibit a significant correlation with the rate of hyperuricemia in Japanese adult women (aged ≥ 20 years) from 2010 to 2019 ($r= 0.571$, $p=0.139$).

The daily intake of niacin in men (aged ≥ 1 years) and women (aged ≥ 1 years) established by the Institute of Medicine of the National Academy of Sciences in the US were above the Recommended Dietary Allowances (RDAs), respectively [men (aged ≥ 1 year): 6.0-16.0 mg NE /day; women (aged ≥ 1 year): 6.0-14.0 mg NE /day; men (aged ≥ 14 years): 16.0 mg NE /day; women (aged ≥ 14 years): 14.0 mg NE /day] (Institute of Medicine of the National Academy of Sciences 2021). The Tolerable Upper Intake levels (ULs) for niacin in men (aged ≥ 19 years) and women (aged ≥ 19 years) established by the Institute of Medicine of the National Academy of Sciences in the US are 35.0 mg NE /day, respectively (Institute of Medicine of the National Academy of Sciences 2021). The daily niacin intake among Japanese adult men (aged 40 to 49 years) and Japanese adult men (aged 60-69 years) were 35.4 mg NE /day and 35.6 mg NE /day, respectively. It seems that the daily niacin intake among the Japanese people except for adult men (aged 40-49 years and aged 60-69 years) in 2019 are appropriate.

Pantothenic Acid (Vitamin B_5)

The daily pantothenic acid intake among the Japanese adult population (aged ≥ 20 years) in 2019 was lower compared to that in 2002 and was higher compared to that in 2010 (2002: 5.66 mg/day; 2010: 5.23 mg/day; 2019: 5.65 mg/day).

The daily pantothenic acid intake among the Japanese adult men (aged ≥ 20 years) in 2019 was higher compared to that in 2002 and 2010 (2002: 6.03 mg/day; 2010: 5.61 mg/day; 2019: 6.05 mg/day). The daily pantothenic acid intake did not exhibit a significant correlation with the rate of hyperuricemia in Japanese adult men (aged ≥ 20 years) from 2010 to 2019 (r= -0.508, p=0.199).

The daily pantothenic acid intake among the Japanese adult women (aged ≥ 20 years) in 2019 was lower compared to that in 2002 and was higher compared to that in 2010 (2002: 5.34 mg/day; 2010: 4.90 mg/day; 2019: 5.30 mg/day). The daily pantothenic acid intake was positively correlated with the rate of hyperuricemia in Japanese adult women (aged ≥ 20 years) from 2010 to 2019 (r= 0.815, p=0.014). These results suggest that the correlation between the daily pantothenic acid intake with the rate of hyperuricemia tends to vary with gender and is stronger in Japanese adult women than in Japanese adult men.

The daily intake of pantothenic acid among Japanese men (aged ≥ 20 years) and women (aged ≥ 20 years) were above the Adequate Intakes (AIs) established by the Institute of Medicine of the National Academy of Sciences in the US [men (aged ≥ 14 years): 5.0 mg/day; women (aged ≥ 14 years): 5.0 mg/day] (Institute of Medicine of the National Academy of Sciences 2021). The daily intake of pantothenic acid among Japanese adult men (aged ≥ 20 years) and Japanese adult women (aged ≥ 20 years) appears to be very unlikely to cause a deficiency.

The Institute of Medicine of the National Academy of Sciences in the US (2021) has not set the Tolerable Upper Intake Levels (ULs) for pantothenic acid.

Serum vitamin B_5 (pantothenic acid) was positively associated with SUA concentrations (Liu et al. 2021). It must pay attention to vitamin B_5 (pantothenic acid) intake to avoid high serum vitamin B_5 (pantothenic acid) levels in general population.

Foods high in pantothenic acid are as follows: organ meats (beef liver, pork liver, chicken liver, chicken breast, beef kidney, pork kidney), seafood (tuna, anchovy), mushrooms (shitake mushrooms, mushrooms), potatoes, whole grains (breakfast cereals), seeds (sunflower seeds), soy products (natto), fruit (avocados), dairy products (milk, Greek yogurt), eggs, beverages (green tea), seasonings and condiments (baker's yeast) (The Council for Science and Technology, Ministry of Education, Culture, Sports, Science and Technology in Japan 2023; US Department of Health & Human Services; National Institutes of Health; Office of Dietary Supplements 2023).

Vitamin B$_6$

The daily intake of vitamin B$_6$ among the Japanese adult population (aged $\geq$ 20 years) in 2019 was lower compared to that in 2002 and 2010 (2002: 1.21 mg/day; 2010: 1.87 mg/day; 2019: 1.20 mg/day).

The daily intake of vitamin B$_6$ among the Japanese adult men (aged $\geq$ 20 years) in 2019 was lower compared to that in 2002 and 2010 (2002: 1.31 mg/day; 2010: 1.75 mg/day; 2019: 1.30 mg/day). The daily intake of vitamin B$_6$ did not exhibit a significant correlation with the rate of hyperuricemia in Japanese adult men (aged $\geq$ 20 years) from 2010 to 2019 (r= 0.583, p=0.129).

The daily intake of vitamin B$_6$ among Japanese adult women (aged $\geq$ 20 years) in 2019 was the same as that in 2002 and was lower compared to that in 2010 (2002: 1.12 mg/day; 2010: 1.85 mg/day; 2019: 1.12 mg/day). The daily intake of vitamin B$_6$ tended to be negatively correlated with the rate of hyperuricemia in Japanese adult women (aged $\geq$ 20 years) from 2010 to 2019 (r= -0.698, p=0.054). These results suggest that the correlation between the daily vitamin B$_6$ intake with the rate of hyperuricemia tends to vary with gender.

The daily intake of vitamin B$_6$ among Japanese men (aged 20-49 years), men (aged $\geq$ 50 years), women (aged 19-49 years), and women (aged $\geq$ 50 years) in Japan were 1.12-1.25 mg/day, 1.23-1.42 mg/day, 0.91-1.01 mg/day, and 1.05-1.23 mg/day, respectively. The daily intake of vitamin B$_6$ among Japanese adult men (aged $\geq$ 20 years) and adult women (aged $\geq$ 20 years) were below the Recommended Dietary Allowances (RDAs) established by the Institute of Medicine of the National Academy of Sciences in the US [men (aged 14-50 years): 1.3 mg/day; men (aged $\geq$ 51 years): 1.7 mg/day; women (aged 19-50 years): 1.3 mg/day; women (aged $\geq$ 51 years): 1.5 mg/day] (Institute of Medicine of the National Academy of Sciences 2021).

Judging from the data of food composition (The Council for Science and Technology, Ministry of Education, Culture, Sports, Science and Technology in Japan 2023; US Department of Health & Human Services; National Institutes of Health; Office of Dietary Supplements 2023), it is important for Japanese men (aged $\geq$ 20 years) and women (aged $\geq$ 20 years) to eat meats (turkey, chicken, pork fin), organ meats (chicken breast, beef liver, pork liver), seafood (tuna, salmon, skipjack, sardines, mackerel, Nile tilapia), grains (white rice, buckwheat), whole grains (fortified ready-to-eat cereals), potatoes, seeds and nuts (sunflower seeds, squid, pistachio nuts, sesame seeds), legumes (chickpeas), seaweed, vegetables (onions, garlic, tomatoes, peppers), fruit (bananas, raisins, watermelons), dairy products (cheese), soy products (tofu) to take in more vitamin B$_6$ to reach the Recommended Dietary Allowances

(RDAs) set by the Institute of Medicine of the National Academy of Sciences in the US However, it is important to be cautious not to exceed the Tolerable Upper Intake levels (ULs) of the daily vitamin B_6 intake. An overdose of vitamin B_6-rich foods and/or supplementation should be avoided so as not to exceed the Tolerable Upper Intake Levels (ULs). The Tolerable Upper Intake levels (ULs) for vitamin B_6 in men and women (aged 14-18 years), men and women (aged ≥ 19 years), pregnancy and lactation (aged ≤ 18 years), and pregnancy and lactation (aged 19-50 years) are 80 mg/day, 100 mg/day, 80 mg/day, and 100 mg/day, respectively (Institute of Medicine of the National Academy of Sciences 2021).

Folate (Vitamin B_9)

The daily intake of folate among the Japanese adult population (aged ≥ 20 years) in 2019 was lower compared to that in 2002 and was higher compared to that in 2010 (2002: 325 µg/day; 2010: 297 µg/day; 2019: 302 µg/day).

The daily intake of folate among Japanese adult men (aged ≥ 20 years) in 2019 was lower compared to that in 2002 and was higher compared to that in 2010 (2002: 333 µg/day; 2010: 305 µg/day; 2019: 310 µg/day). The daily intake of folate did not exhibit a significant correlation with the rate of hyperuricemia in Japanese adult men (aged ≥ 20 years) from 2010 to 2019 (r= 0.166, p=0.694).

The daily intake of folate among Japanese adult women (aged ≥ 20 years) in 2019 was lower compared to that in 2002 and was higher compared to that in 2010 (2002: 318 µg/day; 2010: 289 µg/day; 2019: 295 µg/day). The daily intake of folate did not exhibit a significant correlation with the rate of hyperuricemia in Japanese adult women (aged ≥ 20 years) from 2010 to 2019 (r= 0.606, p=0.112).

The daily intake of folate among the Japanese adult men (aged ≥ 20 years) and Japanese adult women (aged ≥ 20 years) in 2019 were below the Recommended Dietary Allowances (RDAs) established by the Institute of Medicine of the National Academy of Sciences in the US [males and females (aged ≥ 14 years): 400 µg DFE (dietary folate equivalents: 1 DFE = 1µg food folate = 0.6 µg of folic acid from fortified food or as a supplement consumed with food = 0.5 µg of folic acid from a supplement taken on an empty stomach); pregnancy (aged ≤ 18 years and aged 19-50 years): 600µg DFE; lactation (aged ≤ 18 years and aged 19-50 years): 500µg DFE] (Institute of Medicine of the National Academy of Sciences 2021).

As stated in the previous reports (Koguchi 2018; Koguchi 2023), the increased intake of folate seems to be important for the prevention of hyperuricemia through reduced serum uric acid (SUA) concentrations.

Judging from the data of food composition (The Council for Science and Technology, Ministry of Education, Culture, Sports, Science and Technology in Japan 2023; US Department of Health & Human Services; National Institutes of Health; Office of Dietary Supplements 2023), it is important for Japanese adult men (aged ≥ 20 years) and Japanese adult women (aged ≥ 20 years) to eat meats (beef), organ meats (liver, breast), seafood (crab, halibut, sardines, sea urchin), mushrooms (maitake mushrooms, shiitake mushrooms), grains (white rice, spaghetti, bread, wheat), whole grains (fortified ready-to-eat cereals), seeds (sunflower seeds, peanuts), legumes (black-eyed peas, kidney beans, green peas, soybeans, chickpeas), seaweed, fruit (avocados, oranges, papayas, bananas, mangos), vegetables (asparaguses, spinach, brussels sprouts, lettuces, broccoli, mustard greens, Jew's mallows), dairy products (milk), eggs, green tea to take in more folate to reach the Recommended Dietary Allowances (RDAs) established by the Institute of Medicine of the National Academy of Sciences in the US (2021).

Since serum vitamin B_9 was positively associated with SUA concentrations (Liu et al. 2021), one must pay attention to folate intake to avoid high serum folate levels in the general population and to ensure it does not exceed the Tolerable Upper Intake Levels (ULs) for folate in the general population. . The Tolerable Upper Intake levels (ULs) of folate in males and females (aged 14-18 years), males and females (aged ≥ 19 years), pregnancy and lactation (aged ≤ 18 years), and pregnancy and lactation (aged 19-50 years) are 800 μg DFE, 1.000 μg DFE, 800 μg DFE, and 1.000 μg DFE, respectively (Institute of Medicine of the National Academy of Sciences 2021).

Vitamin B_{12}

The daily intake of vitamin B_{12} among the Japanese adult population (aged ≥ 20 years) in 2019 was lower compared to that in 2002 and was higher compared to that in 2010 (2002: 7.7 μg/day; 2010: 6.3 μg/day; 2019: 6.5 μg/day).

The daily intake of vitamin B_{12} among the Japanese adult men (aged ≥ 20 years) in 2019 was lower compared to that in 2002 and was higher compared to that in 2010 (2002: 8.7 μg/day; 2010: 7.1 μg/day; 2019: 7.3 μg/day). The daily intake of vitamin B_{12} did not exhibit a significant correlation with the rate of hyperuricemia in Japanese adult men (aged ≥ 20 years) from 2010 to 2019 (r= -0.049, p=0.909).

The daily intake of vitamin B_{12} among Japanese adult women (aged ≥ 20 years) in 2019 was lower compared to that in 2002 and was higher compared to that in 2010 (2002: 7.0 µg/day; 2010: 5.6 µg/day; 2019: 5.9 µg/day). The daily vitamin B_{12} intake did not exhibit a significant correlation with the rate of hyperuricemia in Japanese adult women (aged ≥ 20 years) from 2010 to 2019 (r= -0.240, p=0.566).

The daily intake of vitamin B_{12} among the Japanese adult men (aged ≥ 20 years) and Japanese adult women (aged ≥ 20 years) in 2019 were above the Recommended Dietary Allowances (RDAs) established by the Institute of Medicine of the National Academy of Sciences in the US [men and women (aged ≥ 14 years): 2.4 µg/day; pregnancy (aged ≤ 18 years and aged 19-50 years): 2.6 µg/day; lactation (aged ≤ 18 years and aged 19-50 years): 2.8 µg/day] (Institute of Medicine of the National Academy of Sciences 2021). The daily intake of vitamin B_{12} appears to be appropriate or it appears better to increase it slightly.

The Institute of Medicine of the National Academy of Sciences in the U.S. (2021) has not set the Tolerable Upper Intake Levels (ULs) for vitamin B_{12}.

Foods high in vitamin B_{12} are as follows: meats (beef, turkey), organ meats (beef liver, chicken liver), seafood (clams, tuna, salmon, anchovy, sweetfish, lamprey), whole grains (breakfast cereals), legumes and soybean processed foods (tempeh), seaweed, dairy products (milk, yogurt, cheese), eggs, seasonings and condiments (nutritional yeast) (The Council for Science and Technology, Ministry of Education, Culture, Sports, Science and Technology in Japan 2023; U.S. Department of Health & Human Services; National Institutes of Health; Office of Dietary Supplements 2023).

Vitamin C

The daily intake of vitamin C among the Japanese adult population (aged ≥ 20 years) in 2019 was lower compared to that in 2002 and 2010 (2002: 107 mg/day; 2010: 115 mg/day; 2019: 99 mg/day).

The daily vitamin C intake among the Japanese adult men (aged ≥ 20 years) in 2019 was lower compared to that in 2002 and 2010 (2002: 101 mg/day; 2010: 109 mg/day; 2019: 96 mg/day). The daily intake of vitamin C tended to be positively correlated with the rate of hyperuricemia in Japanese adult men (aged ≥ 20 years) from 2010 to 2019 (r= 0.698, p=0.054).

The daily intake of vitamin C among Japanese adult women (aged ≥ 20 years) in 2019 was lower compared to that in 2002 and 2010 (2002: 112 mg/day; 2010: 121 mg/day; 2019: 101 mg/day). The daily vitamin C intake did not exhibit a significant correlation with the rate of hyperuricemia in Japanese adult women (aged ≥ 20 years) from 2010 to 2019 (r= -0.628, p=0.095). These results suggest that the correlation between daily vitamin C intake and the rate of hyperuricemia tends to vary with gender.

The Recommended dietary allowances (RDAs) for vitamin C in men (aged ≥ 19 years), women (aged ≥ 19 years), pregnancy (aged 19-50 years), and lactation (aged 19-50 years) established by the Institute of Medicine of the National Academy of Sciences in the US (2021) are 90.0 mg/day, 75.0 mg/day, 85.0 mg/day, and 120 mg/day, respectively. The daily vitamin C intake among the Japanese men (aged 20-59 years) and women (aged 20-49 years) were 62.0-82.0 mg/day and 62.0-74.0 mg/day, respectively, and were below the Recommended Dietary Allowances (RDAs) established by the Institute of Medicine of the National Academy of Sciences in the US (2021). Whereas the daily intake of vitamin C among Japanese men (aged ≥ 60 years) and women (aged ≥ 50 years) were 102.0-126.0 mg/day and 88.0-129.0 mg/day, respectively, and exceeded the Recommended Dietary Allowances (RDAs) established by the Institute of Medicine of the National Academy of Sciences in the US (2021). Smokers require 35 mg/day more vitamin C than nonsmokers (Institute of Medicine of the National Academy of Sciences 2021).

As stated in the reviews (Choi 2010; Ekpenyong and Daniel 2015; Kakutani-Hatayama et al. 2015; Koguchi 2018; Bouike, Nakata and Moriwaki 2021) and the previous reports (Koguchi 2023), conscious intake of vitamin C seems to be important for the prevention of hyperuricemia through reduced serum uric acid (SUA) concentrations.

Judging from the data of food composition (The Council for Science and Technology, Ministry of Education, Culture, Sports, Science and Technology in Japan 2023; US Department of Health & Human Services; National Institutes of Health; Office of Dietary Supplements 2023), it is important for Japanese men (aged 20-59 years), Japanese women (aged 20-49 years), and lactation (aged 19-50 years) to eat seaweed, fruit (acerolas, guavas, kiwi fruits, lemons, strawberries, papayas, blackcurrants), vegetables (kales, peppers, parsley, broccoli, tomatoes, cauliflowers, peas, eggplants, brussels sprouts, Chinese cabbages, mustard spinach) to take in more vitamin C to reach the Recommended Dietary Allowances (RDAs) established by the Institute of Medicine of the National Academy of Sciences in the US (2021). From the results of the articles (Huang et al. 2005; Gao et al. 2008), though the Recommended Dietary Allowances (RDAs) for vitamin C established by the Institute of Medicine of the National Academy of Sciences in the US (2021) were below 500.0 mg/day, it appears that the Japanese adult population (aged ≥ 20 years) with higher SUA levels need to take in more vitamin C.

Terkeltaub and Edwards (2013, 148-149) have stated that it is not known if combined effects on urine pH, oxalate generation, and uricosuria of high vitamin C intake can promote urolithiasis. The Institute of Medicine of the National Academy of Sciences in the US (2021) has shown the Tolerable Upper Intake Levels (ULs) for healthy individuals [men and women (aged 14-18 years): 1800 mg/day; men and women (aged ≥ 19 years): 2000 mg/day; pregnancy and lactation (aged ≤ 18 years): 1800 mg/day; and pregnancy and lactation (aged 19-50 years): 2000 mg/day]. An overdose of vitamin C-rich foods and/or supplementation should be avoided so as not to exceed the Tolerable Upper Intake Levels (ULs).

Minerals

Sodium and salt

The daily intake of sodium among the Japanese adult population (aged ≥ 20 years) in 2019 was lower compared to that in 2002 and 2010 (2002: 4.71 g/day; 2010: 4.16 g/day; 2019: 3.96 g/day).

The daily intake of sodium among Japanese adult men (aged ≥ 20 years) in 2019 was lower compared to that in 2002 and 2010 (2002: 5.05 g/day; 2010: 4.51 g/day; 2019: 4.31 g/day). The daily intake of sodium did not exhibit a significant correlation with the rate of hyperuricemia in Japanese adult men (aged ≥ 20 years) from 2010 to 2019 ($r= 0.414$, $p=0.308$).

The daily intake of sodium among Japanese adult men (aged ≥ 20 years) in 2019 was lower compared to that in 2002 and 2010 (2002: 4.41 g/day; 2010: 3.87 g/day; 2019: 3.65 g/day). The daily intake of sodium was negatively correlated with the rate of hyperuricemia in Japanese adult women (aged ≥ 20 years) from 2010 to 2019 ($r= -0.818$, $p=0.013$). These results suggest that the correlation between the daily sodium intake with the rate of hyperuricemia tends to vary with gender and is stronger in Japanese adult women than in Japanese adult men.

The Institute of Medicine of the National Academy of Sciences in the U.S. (2021) and the Institute of Medicine of the National Academies of Sciences, Engineering, and Medicine in the U.S. (2019) have not set the

Estimated Average Requirements (EARs) and the Recommended Dietary Allowances (RDAs).

The daily sodium intake among the Japanese adult men (aged ≥ 20 years) and Japanese adult women (aged ≥ 20 years) in 2019 were above the Adequate Intakes (AIs) [men and women (aged 9-50 years): 1500 mg/day; men and women (aged 51-70 years): 1.3 g/day; men and women (aged ≥ 71 years): 1.2 g/day; pregnancy and lactation (aged ≤ 18 years and 19-50 years): 1.5 g/day] and the Tolerable Upper Intake Levels (ULs) [men and women (aged ≥ 14 years): 2.3 mg/day; pregnancy and lactation (aged ≤ 18 years and 19-50 years): 2.3 mg/day] (Institute of Medicine of the National Academy of Sciences 2021; Institute of Medicine of the National Academies of Sciences, Engineering, and Medicine 2019). It seems that the daily sodium intake among the Japanese adult men and women in 2002, 2010, and 2019 are excessive.

Salt

The daily intake of salt among the Japanese adult population (aged ≥ 20 years) in 2019 was lower compared to that in 2002 and 2010 (2002: 12.0 g/day; 2010: 10.8 g/day; 2019: 10.1 g/day).

The daily intake of salt among Japanese adult men (aged ≥ 20 years) in 2019 was lower compared to that in 2002 and 2010 (2002: 12.8 g/day; 2010: 11.4 g/day; 2019: 10.9 g/day). The daily intake of salt did not exhibit a significant correlation with the rate of hyperuricemia in Japanese adult men (aged ≥ 20 years) from 2010 to 2019 ($r= 0.480$, $p=0.228$).

The daily intake of salt among Japanese adult women (aged ≥ 20 years) in 2019 was lower compared to that in 2002 and 2010 (2002: 11.2 g/day; 2010: 9.8 g/day; 2019: 9.3 g/day). The daily intake of salt was negatively correlated with the rate of hyperuricemia in Japanese adult women (aged ≥ 20 years) from 2010 to 2019 ($r= -0.859$, $p=0.006$). These results suggest that the correlation between daily salt intake with the rate of hyperuricemia tends to vary with gender and is stronger in Japanese adult women than in Japanese adult men.

The World Health Organization recommendations for a healthy diet (World Health Organization 2023) state that salt intake should be kept to less than 5 g/day. . It seems that the daily intake of salt among the Japanese adult men and women in 2019 are excessive.

Calcium

The daily intake of calcium among the Japanese adult population (aged ≥ 20 years) in 2019 was lower compared to that in 2002 and 2010 (2002: 532 mg/day; 2010: 502 mg/day; 2019: 498 mg/day).

The daily calcium intake among the Japanese adult men (aged ≥ 20 years) in 2019 was lower compared to that in 2002 and was the same as that in 2010 (2002: 535 mg/day; 2010: 503 mg/day; 2019: 503 mg/day). The daily intake of calcium did not exhibit a significant correlation with the rate of hyperuricemia in Japanese adult men (aged ≥ 20 years) from 2010 to 2019 (r= -0.244, p=0.560).

The daily calcium intake among the Japanese adult women (aged ≥ 20 years) in 2019 was lower compared to that in 2002 and 2010 (2002: 529 mg/day; 2010: 501 mg/day; 2019: 494 mg/day). The daily intake of calcium did not exhibit a significant correlation with the rate of hyperuricemia in Japanese adult women (aged ≥ 20 years) from 2010 to 2019 (r= 0.259, p=0.536).

The daily intake of calcium among Japanese men (aged ≥ 1 year) and women (aged ≥ 1 year) were 395-676 mg/day and 391-594 mg/day, respectively, and were below the Adequate Intakes (AIs) established by the Institute of Medicine of the National Academy of Sciences in the US [men and women (aged 19-50 years): 1,000 mg/day; men and women (aged ≥ 51 years): 1,200 mg/day; pregnancy and lactation (aged 19-50 years): 1,000 mg/day] (Institute of Medicine of the National Academy of Sciences 2021). It seems that Japanese population (aged ≥ 1 year) need to take in more calcium.

As stated in the previous reports (Koguchi 2023), increased intake of calcium seems to be important for the prevention of hyperuricemia through reduced serum uric acid (SUA) concentrations.

Judging from the data of food composition (The Council for Science and Technology, Ministry of Education, Culture, Sports, Science and Technology in Japan 2023; US Department of Health & Human Services; National Institutes of Health; Office of Dietary Supplements 2023), it is important for Japanese people (aged ≥ 15 years) to eat seafood (sardines), cereals (fortified ready-to-eat cereals), milks (almond milk, low-fat milk, skim milk, whole butter milk, whole chocolate milk), vegetables (spinach, okra, curly kale), dairy products (milk, cheese, yogurt), soy products (soy milk, tofu) to take in more calcium to reach the Adequate Intakes (AIs) established by the Institute of Medicine of the National Academy of Sciences in the U.S. (Institute of Medicine of the National Academy of Sciences 2021).

Potassium

The daily intake of potassium among the Japanese adult population (aged ≥ 20 years) in 2019 was lower compared to that in 2002 and was higher compared to that in 2010 (2002: 2452 mg/day; 2010: 2260 mg/day; 2019: 2350 mg/day).

The daily intake of potassium among Japanese adult men (aged ≥ 20 years) in 2019 was lower compared to that in 2002 and was higher compared to that in 2010 (2002: 2529 mg/day; 2010: 2350 mg/day; 2019: 2439 mg/day). The daily intake of potassium did not exhibit a significant correlation with the rate of hyperuricemia in Japanese adult men (aged ≥ 20 years) from 2010 to 2019 ($r= -0.344$, $p=0.419$).

The daily intake of potassium among the Japanese adult women (aged ≥ 20 years) in 2019 was lower compared to that in 2002 and was higher compared to that in 2010 (2002: 2386 mg/day; 2010: 2182 mg/day; 2019: 2273 mg/day). The daily intake of potassium was positively correlated with the rate of hyperuricemia in Japanese adult women (aged ≥ 20 years) from 2010 to 2019 ($r= 0.733$, $p=0.039$). These results suggest that the correlation between daily potassium intake and the rate of hyperuricemia tends to vary with gender and is stronger in Japanese adult women than in Japanese adult men.

The daily intake of potassium among Japanese adult men (aged ≥ 20 years) and Japanese adult women (aged ≥ 20 years) in 2019 were below the Adequate Intakes (AIs) established by the Institute of Medicine of the National Academies of Sciences, Engineering, and Medicine in the US [men (aged ≥ 19 years): 3400 mg/day; women (aged ≥ 19 years): 2600 mg/day] (Institute of Medicine of the National Academies of Sciences, Engineering, and Medicine 2019).

Judging from the data of food composition (The Council for Science and Technology, Ministry of Education, Culture, Sports, Science and Technology in Japan 2023; US Department of Health & Human Services; National Institutes of Health; Office of Dietary Supplements 2023), it is important for Japanese men (aged ≥ 20 years) and women (aged ≥ 20 years) to eat meats (poultry), seafood (tuna, halibut, cod, trout, rockfish), nuts, whole grains (brown and wild rice, brown cereal, whole-wheat bread and pasta), potatoes, legumes (peas, lima beans, pinto beans, kidney beans, soybeans, lentils), mushrooms, fruit (bananas, oranges, apricots, grapefruits, cantaloupes), vegetables (spinach, broccoli, cucumbers, zucchinis, pumpkins, leafy greens), coffee to take in more potassium to reach the Adequate Intakes (AIs) established by the Institute of Medicine of the National Academies of Sciences, Engineering, and Medicine in the US (Institute of Medicine of the

National Academies of Sciences, Engineering, and Medicine 2019). It is encouraged to replace meat with fish and legumes.

Magnesium

The daily intake of magnesium among the Japanese adult population (aged ≥ 20 years) in 2019 was lower compared to that in 2002 and was higher compared to that in 2010 (2002: 268 mg/day; 2010: 245 mg/day; 2019: 255 mg/day).

The daily intake of magnesium among Japanese adult men (aged ≥ 20 years) in 2019 was lower compared to that in 2002 and was higher compared to that in 2010 (2002: 284 mg/day; 2010: 260 mg/day; 2019: 270 mg/day). The daily intake of magnesium did not exhibit a significant correlation with the rate of hyperuricemia in Japanese adult men (aged ≥ 20 years) from 2010 to 2019 ($r = -0.293$, $p = 0.480$).

The daily intake of magnesium among Japanese adult women (aged ≥ 20 years) in 2019 was lower compared to that in 2002 and was higher compared to that in 2010 (2002: 254 mg/day; 2010: 232 mg/day; 2019: 242 mg/day). The intake of daily magnesium did not exhibit a significant correlation with the rate of hyperuricemia in Japanese adult women (aged ≥ 20 years) from 2010 to 2019 ($r = 0.597$, $p = 0.118$).

The daily intake of magnesium among Japanese adult men (aged ≥ 20 years) and Japanese adult women (aged ≥ 20 years) in 2019 were below the Recommended Dietary Allowances (RDAs) established by the Institute of Medicine of the National Academy of Sciences in the US [men (aged ≥ 14 years): 400-420 mg/day; women (aged ≥ 14 years): 310-360 mg/day] (Institute of Medicine of the National Academy of Sciences 2021).

As stated in the previous reports (Koguchi 2023), an increased intake of magnesium appears to be important for the prevention of hyperuricemia through reduced serum uric acid (SUA) concentrations.

Judging from the data of food composition (The Council for Science and Technology, Ministry of Education, Culture, Sports, Science and Technology in Japan 2023; US Department of Health & Human Services; National Institutes of Health; Office of Dietary Supplements 2023), it is important for Japanese adult men (aged ≥ 20 years) and Japanese adult women (aged ≥ 20 years) to eat meats (beef), organ meats (chicken breast), seafood (salmon, sardines), seeds and nuts (pumpkin seeds, chia seeds, sunflower seeds, almonds, peanuts, cashew nuts, sesame seeds, flaxseeds), grains (white rice, bread), whole grains (brown rice, cereals, fortified ready-to-eat cereals, whole-wheat bread, oatmeal), potatoes, legumes (black beans, kidney beans, edamame), seaweeds, fruit (bananas, raisins, avocados, apples), vegetables (spinach, broccoli, carrots, parsley), dairy products (milk, yogurt), soy products (soy milk), tea, green tea to take in more magnesium to reach the Recommended Dietary Allowances (RDAs) established by the Institute of Medicine of the National Academy of Sciences in the US (Institute of Medicine of the National Academy of Sciences 2021).

Phosphorus

The daily intake of phosphorus among the Japanese adult population (aged ≥ 20 years) in 2019 was lower compared to that in 2002 and was higher compared to that in 2010 (2002: 1046 mg/day; 2010: 963 mg/day; 2019: 1012 mg/day).

The daily intake of phosphorus among the Japanese adult men (aged ≥ 20 years) in 2019 was lower compared to that in 2002 and was higher compared to that in 2010 (2002: 1128 mg/day; 2010: 1037 mg/day; 2019: 1084 mg/day). The daily intake of phosphorus did not exhibit a significant correlation with the rate of hyperuricemia in Japanese adult men (aged ≥ 20 years) from 2010 to 2019 (r= -0.583, p=0.129).

The daily intake of phosphorus among Japanese adult women (aged ≥ 20 years) in 2019 was lower compared to that in 2002 and was higher compared to that in 2010 (2002: 976 mg/day; 2010: 900 mg/day; 2019: 948 mg/day). The daily intake of phosphorus was positively correlated with the rate of hyperuricemia in Japanese adult women (aged ≥ 20 years) from 2010 to 2019 (r= 0.717, p=0.045). These results suggest that the correlation between daily phosphorus intake and the rate of hyperuricemia tends to vary with gender and is stronger in Japanese adult women than in Japanese adult men.

The daily intake of phosphorus among Japanese adult men (aged ≥ 20 years) and Japanese adult women (aged ≥ 20 years) in 2019 were above the Recommended Dietary Allowances (RDAs) for phosphorus established by the Institute of Medicine of the National Academy of Sciences in the US [men (aged ≥ 19 years): 700 mg/day; women (aged ≥ 19 years): 700 mg/day] and was below the Tolerable Upper Intake Levels (ULs) established by the Institute of Medicine of the National Academy of Sciences in the US [men and women (aged 9-70 years): 4000 mg/day; men and women (aged ≥ 71 years): 3000 mg/day: pregnancy (aged 9-70 years): 3500 mg/day; lactation: 4000 mg/day] (Institute of Medicine of the National Academy of Sciences 2021). It appears that the Japanese adult population (aged ≥ 20 years) need to decrease the intake of phosphorus to reach the Recommended Dietary Allowances (RDAs) established by the Institute of Medicine of the National Academy of Sciences in the US (Institute of Medicine of the National Academy of Sciences 2021).

It appears important to reduce the intake of one serving of high-phosphorus food (e.g., yogurt, milk, cheese, salmon, scallops, sardines, flying fish, dried squid, chicken, lentils, cashew nuts, potatoes) (The Council for Science and Technology, Ministry of Education, Culture, Sports, Science and Technology in Japan 2023; US Department of Health & Human Services; National Institutes of Health. Office of Dietary Supplements 2023).

Iron

The daily intake of iron among the Japanese adult population (aged ≥ 20 years) in 2019 was lower compared to that in 2002 and was the same as that in 2010 (2002: 8.4 mg/day; 2010: 7.9 mg/day; 2019: 7.9 mg/day).

The daily intake of iron among Japanese adult men (aged ≥ 20 years) in 2019 was lower compared to that in 2002 and was the same as that in 2010 (2002: 8.8 mg/day; 2010: 8.3 mg/day; 2019: 8.3 mg/day). The daily intake of iron did not exhibit a significant correlation with the rate of hyperuricemia in Japanese adult men (aged ≥ 20 years) from 2010 to 2019 ($r= 0.023$, $p=0.957$).

The daily intake of iron among Japanese adult women (aged ≥ 20 years) in 2019 was lower compared to that in 2002 and 2010 (2002: 8.1 mg/day; 2010: 7.6 mg/day; 2019: 7.5 mg/day). The daily intake of iron did not exhibit a significant correlation with the rate of hyperuricemia in Japanese adult women (aged ≥ 20 years) from 2010 to 2019 ($r= 0.058$, $p=0.891$).

The daily intake of iron among the Japanese men (aged 15-49 years) and women (aged 15-59 years) in 2019 were 7.2-7.9 mg/day and 6.2-7.2 mg/day, respectively, and were below the Recommended Dietary Allowances (RDAs) established by the Institute of Medicine of the National Academy of Sciences in the US [men (aged 14-18 years): 11 mg/day; men (aged ≥ 15 years): 8 mg/day; women (aged 14-18 years): 15 mg/day; women (aged 19-50 years): 18 mg/day; women (aged ≥ 51 years): 8 mg/day] (Institute of Medicine of the National Academy of Sciences 2021). Whereas the daily iron intake for Japanese adult men (aged ≥ 50 years) and Japanese adult women (aged ≥ 60 years) ranged from 8.1-9.0 mg/day and 8.2-8.4 mg/day, respectively, it exceeded the Recommended Dietary Allowances (RDAs) and remained below the Tolerable Upper Intake Levels (ULs) established by the Institute of Medicine of the National Academy of Sciences in the US [men (aged ≥ 14 years): 45.0 mg/day; women (aged ≥ 14 years): 45.0 mg/day] (Institute of Medicine of the National Academy of Sciences 2021).

Judging from the data of food composition (The Council for Science and Technology, Ministry of Education, Culture, Sports, Science and Technology in Japan 2023; US Department of Health & Human Services; National Institutes of Health; Office of Dietary Supplements 2023), it is important for Japanese men (aged 15-49 years) and women (aged 15-59 years) including women with menstruation (aged ≥ 40 years) to eat lean meat and meats (poultry), organ meats (liver), seafood (oysters, sardines, tuna, sweetfish, abalone, clams, firefly squid), potatoes (konjac), nuts (cashew nuts, pistachio nuts, sesame seeds, flaxseeds), grains (white rice, bread, spaghetti), whole grains (brown rice, iron-fortified ready-to-eat cereals and breads), mushrooms (wood ear), legumes (kidney beans, white beans, lentils, peas, green peas), seaweed, fruit (raisins, cantaloupes), vegetables (spinach, broccoli, parsley), dairy products (milk, cheese), soy products (tofu), eggs, and tea to take in more iron to reach the Recommended Dietary Allowances (RDAs) established by the Institute of Medicine of the National Academy of Sciences in the US (Institute of Medicine of the National Academy of Sciences 2021). One must be careful not to exceed the Tolerable Upper Intake Levels (ULs) of the daily iron intake in Japanese adult men (aged ≥ 50 years) and Japanese adult women (aged ≥ 60 years).

Copper

The daily intake of copper among the Japanese adult population (aged ≥ 20 years) in 2019 was lower compared to that in 2002 and 2010 (2002: 1.27 mg/day; 2010: 1.15 mg/day; 2019: 1.14 mg/day).

The daily intake of copper among Japanese adult men (aged ≥ 20 years) in 2019 was lower compared to that in 2002 and 2010 (2002: 1.38 mg/day; 2010: 1.25 mg/day; 2019: 1.23 mg/day). The daily intake of copper did not exhibit a significant correlation with the rate of hyperuricemia in Japanese adult men (aged ≥ 20 years) from 2010 to 2019 ($r= -0.333$, $p=0.420$).

The daily intake of copper among Japanese adult women (aged ≥ 20 years) in 2019 was lower compared to that in 2002 and was higher compared to that in 2010 (2002: 1.18 mg/day; 2010: 1.06 mg/day; 2019: 1.07 mg/day). The daily intake of copper did not exhibit a significant correlation with the rate of hyperuricemia in Japanese adult women (aged ≥ 20 years) from 2010 to 2019 ($r= 0.640$, $p=0.087$).

The daily intake of copper among the Japanese adult men (aged ≥ 20 years) and Japanese adult women (aged ≥ 20 years) in 2019 was 1.23 mg/day and 1.07 mg/day, respectively. The daily intake of copper among Japanese adult men (aged ≥ 20 years) and Japanese adult women (aged ≥ 20 years) in

2019 exceeded the Recommended Dietary Allowances (RDAs) established by the Institute of Medicine of the National Academy of Sciences in the US [men (aged ≥ 19 years): 0.90 mg/day; women (aged ≥ 19 years): 0.90 mg/day; pregnancy (aged 19-50 years): 1.0 mg/day] (Institute of Medicine of the National Academy of Sciences 2021) and were below the Tolerable Upper Intake Levels (ULs) established by the Institute of Medicine of the National Academy of Sciences in the US [men (aged ≥ 19 years): 10.0 mg/day; women (aged ≥ 19 years): 10.0 mg/day] (Institute of Medicine of the National Academy of Sciences 2021). It appears that an overdose of copper can occur due to improper use of supplementation. In healthy men and women, taking of copper supplementation should be approached with caution to avoid exceeding the Tolerable Upper Intake Levels (ULs).

Zinc

The daily intake of zinc among the Japanese adult population (aged ≥ 20 years) in 2019 was lower compared to that in 2002 and was higher compared to that in 2010 (2002: 8.5 mg/day; 2010: 7.9 mg/day; 2019: 8.4 mg/day).

The daily intake of zinc among the Japanese adult men (aged ≥ 20 years) in 2019 was lower compared to that in 2002 and was higher compared to that in 2010 (2002: 9.4 mg/day; 2010: 8.8 mg/day; 2019: 9.2 mg/day). The daily intake of zinc did not exhibit a significant correlation with the rate of hyperuricemia in Japanese adult men (aged ≥ 20 years) from 2010 to 2019 ($r=-0.458$, $p=0.254$).

The daily intake of zinc among Japanese adult women (aged ≥ 20 years) in 2019 was lower compared to that in 2002 and was higher compared to that in 2010 (2002: 7.8 mg/day; 2010: 7.2 mg/day; 2019: 7.7 mg/day). The daily intake of zinc did not exhibit a significant correlation with the rate of hyperuricemia in Japanese adult women (aged ≥ 20 years) from 2010 to 2019 ($r= 0.652$, $p=0.080$).

The daily intake of zinc among Japanese adult men (aged ≥ 20 years) in 2019 was below the Estimated Average Requirements (EARs) established by the Institute of Medicine of the National Academy of Sciences in the US [men (aged ≥ 20 years): 9.4 mg/day] (Institute of Medicine of the National Academy of Sciences 2021).

The daily intake of zinc among Japanese adult men (aged ≥ 20 years), Japanese adult women (aged 20-59 years), and Japanese adult women (aged ≥ 70 years) in 2019 were 8.9-9.8 mg/day, 7.3-7.8 mg/day, and 7.7 mg/day, respectively and were below the Recommended Dietary Allowances (RDAs) established by the Institute of Medicine of the National Academy of Sciences in the US [men (aged ≥ 14 years): 11.0 mg/day; women (aged 14-18 years): 9.0 mg/day; women (aged ≥ 19 years): 8.0 mg/day] (Institute of Medicine of the National Academy of Sciences 2021). The daily intake of zinc among the Japanese adult women (aged 60-69 years) in 2019 was 8.0 mg/day and reach the Recommended Dietary Allowances (RDAs) established by the Institute of Medicine of the National Academy of Sciences in the US (Institute of Medicine of the National Academy of Sciences 2021).

As stated in the previous reports (Koguchi 2018; Koguchi 2023), an increased intake of zinc seems to be important for the prevention of hyperuricemia.

Judging from the data of food composition (The Council for Science and Technology, Ministry of Education, Culture, Sports, Science and Technology in Japan 2023; US Department of Health & Human Services; National Institutes of Health; Office of Dietary Supplements 2023), it is important for Japanese men (aged ≥ 20 years) and women (aged 20-59 years, aged ≥ 70 years) to eat meats (beef, chicken), processed meats (beef chuck, beef patty, beef jerky, pork chop), organ meats (liver, breast), seafood (oysters, crab, lobster, blue mackerel, anchovy, sardines, snail, scallop, lamprey), seeds and nuts (pumpkin seeds, cashew nuts, almonds, sesame seeds, flaxseeds, chia seeds), whole grains (fortified ready-to-eat cereals, oatmeal), mushrooms (maitake mushrooms), legumes (kidney beans, baked beans, chickpeas, green peas), seaweed, dairy products (low-fat milk, cheese, yogurt) to take in more zinc to reach the Recommended Dietary Allowances (RDAs) established by the Institute of Medicine of the National Academy of Sciences in the US (2021). An overdose of zinc-rich foods and/or supplementation should be avoided so as not to exceed the Tolerable Upper Intake Levels (ULs).
The Tolerable Upper Intake Levels (ULs) established by the Institute of Medicine of the National Academy in men (aged 14-18 years), men (aged ≥ 19 years), women (aged 14-18 years), women (aged ≥ 19 years), and pregnancy and lactation (aged 19-50 years) are 34.0 mg/day, 40.0 mg/day, 34.0 mg/day, 40.0 mg/day, and 40.0 mg/day, respectively (Institute of Medicine of the National Academy of Sciences 2021).

Food

Meat

The daily intake of total meat among the Japanese adult population (aged ≥ 20 years) in 2019 was higher compared to that in 2001 and 2010 (2001: 74.0 g/day; 2010: 79.6 g/day; 2019: 101.0 g/day).

The daily intake of total meat among Japanese adult men (aged ≥ 20 years) in 2019 was higher compared to that in 2001 and 2010 (2001: 87.6 g/day; 2010: 93.4 g/day; 2019: 117.4 g/day). The daily intake of total meat did not show a significant correlation with the rate of hyperuricemia in Japanese adult men (aged ≥ 20 years) from 2010 to 2019 (r= -0.479, p=0.229).

The daily intake of total meat among Japanese adult women (aged ≥ 20 years) in 2019 was higher compared to that in 2001 and 2010 (2001: 62.4 g/day; 2010: 67.8 g/day; 2019: 86.7 g/day). The daily intake of total meat was positively correlated with the rate of hyperuricemia in Japanese adult women (aged ≥ 20 years) from 2010 to 2019 (r= 0.857, p=0.007). These results suggest that the correlation between daily intake of total meat and the rate of hyperuricemia tends to vary with gender and is stronger in Japanese adult women than in Japanese adult men.

As stated in the reviews (Choi 2010; Ekpenyong and Daniel 2015; Kakutani-Hatayama et al. 2015; Koguchi 2018; Bouike, Nakata and Moriwaki 2021) and the previous reports (Koguchi 2023), limiting or decreasing the intake of meat in the Japanese adult population (especially women) may play an important role in the prevention of hyperuricemia.

Seafood

The daily intake of total seafood (fish and shellfish) among the Japanese adult population (aged ≥ 20 years) in 2019 was lower compared to that in 2001 and 2010 (2001: 102.9 g/day; 2010: 78.2 g/day; 2019: 68.5 g/day).

The daily intake of total seafood (fish and shellfish) of Japanese adult men (aged ≥ 20 years) in 2019 was lower compared to that in 2001 and 2010 (2001: 116.3 g/day; 2010: 87.4 g/day; 2019: 76.3 g/day). The daily intake of total seafood (fish and shellfish) did not show a significant correlation with the rate of hyperuricemia in Japanese adult men (aged ≥ 20 years) from 2010 to 2019 (r= 0.258, p=0.538).

The daily intake of total seafood (fish and shellfish) of Japanese adult women (aged ≥ 20 years) in 2019 was lower compared to that in 2001 and 2010 (2001: 91.6 g/day; 2010: 70.4 g/day; 2019: 61.7 g/day). The daily intake of total seafood (fish and shellfish) was negatively correlated with the rate of hyperuricemia in Japanese adult women (aged ≥ 20 years) from 2010 to 2019 (r= -0.882, p=0.004). These results suggest that the correlation between the daily intake of total seafood (fish and shellfish) with the rate of hyperuricemia tends to vary with gender and is stronger in Japanese adult women than in Japanese adult men.

As stated in the reviews (Choi 2010; Ekpenyong and Daniel 2015; Kakutani-Hatayama et al. 2015; Koguchi 2018; Bouike, Nakata and Moriwaki 2021) and the previous reports (Koguchi 2023), limiting or decreasing the intake of seafood may play an important role in the prevention of hyperuricemia.

The daily intake of seafood of Japanese adult men (aged ≥ 20 years) seems to be appropriate and it seems better for Japanese adult women to increase it slightly.

Eggs

The daily intake of eggs among the Japanese adult population (aged ≥ 20 years) in 2019 was higher compared to that in 2001 and 2010 (2001: 36.6 g/day; 2010: 35.0 g/day; 2019: 41.4 g/day).

The daily intake of eggs among Japanese adult men (aged ≥ 20 years) in 2019 was higher compared to that in 2001 and 2010 (2001: 38.8 g/day; 2010: 37.6 g/day; 2019: 43.5 g/day). The daily intake of eggs did not exhibit a significant correlation with the rate of hyperuricemia in Japanese adult men (aged ≥ 20 years) from 2010 to 2019 ($r= -0.273$, $p=0.512$).

The daily intake of eggs among Japanese adult women (aged ≥ 20 years) in 2019 was higher compared to that in 2001 and 2010 (2001: 34.7 g/day; 2010: 32.8 g/day; 2019: 39.4 g/day). The daily intake of eggs was positively correlated with the rate of hyperuricemia in Japanese adult women (aged ≥ 20 years) from 2010 to 2019 ($r= 0.731$, $p=0.039$). These results suggest that the correlation between the daily egg intake with the rate of hyperuricemia tends to vary with gender and is stronger in Japanese adult women than in Japanese adult men.

In epidemiological studies, increased egg intake was associated with decreased serum uric acid (SUA) concentrations (Chuang et al. 2011; Major et al. 2018) and hyperuricemia risk (Chang 2011). Conscious intake of milk and dairy products seems to be important for the prevention of hyperuricemia through reduced serum uric acid (SUA) concentrations.

Considering the mean ratio of energy intake from protein in total energy intake (protein/energy) and the daily vitamin A, vitamin D, vitamin B_1, pantothenic acid, folate, phosphorus, iron intake, the daily egg intake appears to be appropriate or it appears better to increase it slightly.

Milk and Dairy products

The daily intake of milk and dairy products of Japanese adult population (aged ≥ 20 years) in 2019 was lower compared to that in 2001 and was higher compared to that in 2010 (2001: 143.1 g/day; 2010: 91.9 g/day; 2019: 110.7 g/day).

The daily intake of milk and dairy products among Japanese adult men (aged ≥ 20 years) in 2019 was lower compared to that in 2001 and was higher compared to that in 2010 (2001: 126.3 g/day; 2010: 81.2 g/day; 2019: 103.1 g/day). The daily intake of milk and dairy products did not show a significant correlation with the rate of hyperuricemia in Japanese adult men (aged ≥ 20 years) from 2010 to 2019 ($r = -0.427$, $p = 0.292$).

The daily intake of milk and dairy products of Japanese adult women (aged ≥ 20 years) in 2019 was lower compared to that in 2001 and was higher compared to that in 2010 (2001: 157.2 g/day; 2010: 100.9 g/day; 2019: 117.4 g/day). The daily intake of milk and dairy products was positively correlated with the rate of hyperuricemia in Japanese adult women (aged ≥ 20 years) from 2010 to 2019 ($r = 0.826$, $p = 0.012$). These results suggest that the correlation between daily intake of milk and dairy products and the rate of hyperuricemia tends to vary with gender and is stronger in Japanese adult women than in Japanese adult men.

As stated in the reviews (Choi 2010; Ekpenyong and Daniel 2015; Kakutani-Hatayama et al. 2015; Koguchi 2018; Bouike, Nakata and Moriwaki 2021) and the previous reports (Koguchi 2023), conscious intake of milk and dairy products seems to be important for the prevention of hyperuricemia through reduced serum uric acid (SUA) concentrations.

Considering the results from the balance of the caloric ratio of protein, fat and carbohydrates in the Japanese adult population (aged ≥ 20 years) in 2019 (protein: 15.2%, fat: 28.4%, and carbohydrates: 56.4%) and the daily vitamin A, vitamin D, vitamin B_1, vitamin B_2, vitamin B_6, pantothenic acid, folic acid, calcium, magnesium, phosphorus, iron, zinc, purine intake, it is important for Japanese adult population to consume low-fat dairy products. The daily intake of milk and dairy products (especially low-fat dairy products) appears to be appropriate or it appears better to increase it slightly.

Seasonings, Condiments, and Spices

The daily intake of seasonings, condiments, and spices among the Japanese adult population (aged ≥ 20 years) in 2019 was lower compared to that in 2001 and 2010 (2001: 91.3 g/day; 2010: 91.6 g/day; 2019: 64.9 g/day).

The daily intake of seasonings, condiments, and spices among Japanese adult men (aged ≥ 20 years) in 2019 was lower compared to that in 2001 and 2010 (2001: 101.4 g/day; 2010: 102.5 g/day; 2019: 70.3 g/day). The daily intake of seasonings, condiments, and spices did not show a significant correlation with the rate of hyperuricemia in Japanese adult men (aged ≥ 20 years) from 2010 to 2019 (r= 0.349, p=0.396).

The daily intake of seasonings, condiments, and spices among Japanese adult women (aged ≥ 20 years) in 2019 was lower compared to that in 2001 and 2010 (2001: 82.7 g/day; 2010: 82.3 g/day; 2019: 60.3 g/day). The daily intake of seasonings, condiments, and spices did not show a significant correlation with the rate of hyperuricemia in Japanese adult women (aged ≥ 20 years) from 2010 to 2019 (r= -0.621, p=0.101).

Spices (such as capers, caraways, cloves, and cumin) contain polyphenols that suppress uric acid (UA) production by inhibiting xanthine oxidase activity (INRA 2023). It appears important to use these spices when cooking dishes in order to maintain serum uric acid (SUA) concentrations at normal levels in healthy individuals. .

Oils and Fats

The daily intake of oils and fats among the Japanese adult population (aged ≥ 20 years) in 2019 was lower compared to that in 2001 and was higher compared to that in 2010 (2001: 11.2 g/day; 2010: 10.0 g/day; 2019: 11.1 g/day).

The daily intake of oils and fats of Japanese adult men (aged ≥ 20 years) in 2019 was the same as that in 2001 and was higher compared to that in 2010 (2001: 12.6 g/day; 2010: 11.0 g/day; 2019: 12.6 g/day). The daily intake of oils and fats did not show a significant correlation with the rate of hyperuricemia in Japanese adult men (aged ≥ 20 years) from 2010 to 2019 (r= -0.461, p=0.251).

The daily intake of oils and fats of Japanese adult women (aged ≥ 20 years) in 2019 was higher compared to that in 2001 and 2010 (2001: 10.0 g/day; 2010: 9.0 g/day; 2019: 10.3 g/day). The daily intake of oils and fats was positively correlated with the rate of hyperuricemia in Japanese adult women (aged ≥ 20 years) from 2010 to 2019 (r= 0.925, p=0.001). These results suggest that the correlation between the daily intake of oils and fats with the rate of hyperuricemia tends to vary with gender and is stronger in Japanese adult women than in Japanese adult men.

Compared to the ideal balance of the caloric ratio of protein, fat, and carbohydrates for Japanese people (protein: 15%, fat: 25%, and carbohydrates: 60%) (The Ministry of Agriculture, Forestry and Fisheries 2020), the balance in the Japanese adult population (aged ≥ 20 years) in 2019 was weighted toward fat (protein: 15.2%, fat: 28.4%, and carbohydrates: 56.4%). It seems advisable to reduce the daily intake of oils and fats until the mean ratio of energy intake from fat in total energy intake (fat/energy) becomes 25%.

Confectioneries (Japanese sweets, cakes, pastries, biscuits, candies, etc.)

The daily intake of confectioneries among the Japanese adult population (aged ≥ 20 years) in 2019 was higher compared to that in 2001 and 2010 (2001: 23.4 g/day; 2010: 23.2 g/day; 2019: 24.4 g/day).

The daily intake of confectioneries among Japanese adult men (aged ≥ 20 years) in 2019 was higher compared to that in 2001 and 2010 (2001: 18.3 g/day; 2010: 19.0 g/day; 2019: 21.7 g/day). The daily intake of confectioneries was negatively correlated with the rate of hyperuricemia in Japanese adult men (aged ≥ 20 years) from 2010 to 2019 (r= -0.770, p=0.025).

The daily intake of confectioneries among Japanese adult women (aged ≥ 20 years) in 2019 was lower compared to that in 2001 and was higher compared to that in 2010 (2001: 27.8 g/day; 2010: 26.7 g/day; 2019: 26.8 g/day). The daily intake of confectioneries did not show a significant correlation with the rate of hyperuricemia in Japanese adult women (aged ≥ 20 years) from 2010 to 2019 (r= 0.591, p=0.123). These results suggest that the correlation between the daily intake of confectioneries and the rate of hyperuricemia tends to vary with gender and is stronger in Japanese adult men than in Japanese adult women.

As stated in the reviews (Choi 2010; Ekpenyong and Daniel 2015; Kakutani-Hatayama et al. 2015; Koguchi 2018; Bouike, Nakata and Moriwaki 2021) and the previous reports (Koguchi 2023), limiting or decreasing the intake of confectioneries in Japanese adult population (especially women) may play an important role in the prevention of hyperuricemia.

Beverages

The daily beverage consumption of Japanese adult population (aged ≥ 20 years) in 2019 was higher compared to that in 2001 and 2010 (2001: 586.8 g/day; 2010: 663.5 g/day; 2019: 673.5 g/day).

The daily beverage consumption among Japanese adult men (aged ≥ 20 years) in 2019 was higher compared to that in 2001 and 2010 (2001: 685.2 g/day; 2010: 741.6 g/day; 2019: 771.0 g/day). The daily beverage consumption did not exhibit a significant correlation with the rate of hyperuricemia in Japanese adult men (aged ≥ 20 years) from 2010 to 2019 (r= 0.584, p=0.128).

The daily beverage consumption among Japanese adult women (aged ≥ 20 years) in 2019 was higher compared to that in 2001 and lower compared to that in 2010 (2001: 503.4 g/day; 2010: 596.7 g/day; 2019: 588.4 g/day). The daily beverage consumption did not exhibit a significant correlation with the rate of hyperuricemia in Japanese adult women (aged ≥ 20 years) from 2010 to 2019 ($r= 0.169$, $p=0.690$).

Sugar-sweetened beverages

The Ministry of Health, Labour and Welfare in Japan has not investigated the daily consumption of sugar-sweetened beverages among Japanese people.

As stated in the reviews (Choi 2010; Ekpenyong and Daniel 2015; Kakutani-Hatayama et al. 2015; Koguchi 2018; Bouike, Nakata and Moriwaki 2021) and the previous reports (Koguchi 2023), limiting or decreasing the consumption of sugar-sweetened beverages in the Japanese adult population may play an important role in the prevention of hyperuricemia.

Coffee and Cocoa

The daily intake of coffee and cocoa among the Japanese adult population (aged ≥ 20 years) in 2019 was higher compared to that in 2011 (2011: 147.3 g/day; 2019: 164.0 g/day).

The daily intake of coffee and cocoa among Japanese adult men (aged ≥ 20 years) in 2019 was higher compared to that in 2011 (2011: 150.3 g/day; 2019: 170.7 g/day). The daily intake of coffee and cocoa did not exhibit a significant correlation with the rate of hyperuricemia in Japanese adult men (aged ≥ 20 years) from 2011 to 2019 ($r= -0.095$, $p=0.879$).

The daily intake of coffee and cocoa among Japanese adult women (aged ≥ 20 years) in 2019 was higher compared to that in 2011 (2011: 144.8 g/day; 2019: 158.1 g/day). The daily intake of coffee and cocoa did not exhibit a significant correlation with the rate of hyperuricemia in Japanese adult women (aged ≥ 20 years) from 2011 to 2019 ($r= 0.691$, $p=0.086$).

As stated in the reviews (Choi 2010; Ekpenyong and Daniel 2015; Kakutani-Hatayama et al. 2015; Koguchi 2018; Bouike, Nakata and Moriwaki 2021) and in the previous reports (Koguchi 2023), conscious intake of coffee and cocoa seems to be important for the prevention of hyperuricemia through reduced serum uric acid (SUA) concentrations. However, it is imperative to drink coffee, taking into account the daily caffeine intake. Poole et al. (2017) have stated that the daily coffee consumption is three to four cups.

Tea

The daily intake of tea among the Japanese adult population (aged ≥ 20 years) in 2019 was lower compared to that in 2011 (2011: 333.0 g/day; 2019: 262.1 g/day).

The daily intake of tea among Japanese adult men (aged ≥ 20 years) in 2019 was lower compared to that in 2011 (2011: 318.5 g/day; 2019: 253.5 g/day). The daily intake of tea did not exhibit a significant correlation with the rate of hyperuricemia in Japanese adult men (aged ≥ 20 years) from 2011 to 2019 (r= 0.669, p=0.100).

The daily intake of tea among Japanese adult women (aged ≥ 20 years) in 2019 was lower compared to that in 2011 (2011: 345.2 g/day; 2019: 269.7 g/day). The daily intake of tea did not exhibit a significant correlation with the rate of hyperuricemia in Japanese adult women (aged ≥ 20 years) from 2011 to 2019 (r= -0.611, p=0.145).

As stated in the previous reports (Koguchi 2018; Bouike, Nakata and Moriwaki 2021; Koguchi 2023), the conscious intake of tea appears to be important for the prevention of hyperuricemia through reduced serum uric acid (SUA) concentrations. However, it is imperative to drink tea, taking into account the daily caffeine intake.

Alcoholic beverages

The daily consumption of alcoholic beverages among the Japanese adult population (aged ≥ 20 years) in 2019 was higher compared to that in 2011 (2011: 122.4 g/day; 2019: 126.6 g/day).

The daily consumption of alcoholic beverages among Japanese adult men (aged ≥ 20 years) in 2019 was higher compared to that in 2011 (2011: 205.9 g/day; 2019: 212.1 g/day). The daily consumption of alcoholic beverages did not exhibit a significant correlation with the rate of hyperuricemia in Japanese adult men (aged ≥ 20 years) from 2011 to 2019 (r= 0.236, p=0.611).

The daily consumption of alcoholic beverages among Japanese adult women (aged ≥ 20 years) in 2019 was lower compared to that in 2011 (2011: 52.2 g/day; 2019: 51.9 g/day). The daily consumption of alcoholic beverages did not exhibit a significant correlation with the rate of hyperuricemia in Japanese adult women (aged ≥ 20 years) from 2011 to 2019 (r= 0.572, p=0.180).

As stated in the reviews (Choi 2010; Ekpenyong and Daniel 2015; Kakutani-Hatayama et al. 2015; Koguchi 2018; Bouike, Nakata and Moriwaki 2021) and the previous reports (Koguchi 2023), limiting or decreasing the consumption of alcoholic beverages in the Japanese adult population may play an important role in the prevention of hyperuricemia.

Grains

The daily intake of total grains among the Japanese adult population (aged ≥ 20 years) in 2019 was lower compared to that in 2001 and 2010 (2001: 476.2 g/day; 2010: 446.1 g/day; 2019: 410.5 g/day).

The daily intake of total grains among Japanese adult men (aged ≥ 20 years) in 2019 was lower compared to that in 2001 and 2010 (2001: 552.6 g/day; 2010: 523.1 g/day; 2019: 480.6 g/day). The daily intake of total grains did not exhibit a significant correlation with the rate of hyperuricemia in Japanese adult men (aged ≥ 20 years) from 2010 to 2019 (r= 0.328, p=0.428).

The daily intake of total grains among Japanese adult women (aged ≥ 20 years) in 2019 was lower compared to that in 2001 and 2010 (2001: 411.4 g/day; 2010: 380.3 g/day; 2019: 349.3 g/day). The daily intake of total grains was negatively correlated with the rate of hyperuricemia in Japanese adult women (aged ≥ 20 years) from 2010 to 2019 (r= -0.911, p=0.002). These results suggest that the correlation between daily intake of total grains and the rate of hyperuricemia tends to vary with gender and is stronger in Japanese adult women than in Japanese adult men.

Considering the data of mean ratio of energy intake from carbohydrates in total energy intake (carbohydrate/energy) and the daily dietary fiber intake, the daily intake of grains (e.g., cereals, whole grains, high-fiber bread) seems better to increase.

Potatoes

The daily intake of total potatoes among the Japanese adult population (aged ≥ 20 years) in 2019 was lower compared to that in 2001 and 2010 (2001: 62.8 g/day; 2010: 53.7 g/day; 2019: 50.0 g/day).

The daily intake of total potatoes among Japanese adult men (aged ≥ 20 years) in 2019 was lower compared to that in 2001 and 2010 (2001: 64.5 g/day; 2010: 56.0 g/day; 2019: 52.0 g/day). The daily intake of total potatoes did not exhibit a significant correlation with the rate of hyperuricemia in Japanese adult men (aged ≥ 20 years) from 2010 to 2019 (r= -0.125, p=0.768).

The daily intake of total potatoes among Japanese adult women (aged ≥ 20 years) in 2019 was lower compared to that in 2001 and 2010 (2001: 61.5 g/day; 2010: 51.8 g/day; 2019: 48.3 g/day). The daily intake of total potatoes did not exhibit a significant correlation with the rate of hyperuricemia in

Japanese adult women (aged ≥ 20 years) from 2010 to 2019 (r= -0.517, p=0.190).

Considering the data on the mean ratio of energy intake from carbohydrates in total energy intake (carbohydrate/energy) and the daily dietary fiber, vitamin A, vitamin B_6, pantothenic acid, potassium, magnesium, phosphorus, iron intake, the daily potatoes intake seems to be appropriate.

Mushrooms

The daily intake of mushrooms among the Japanese adult population (aged ≥ 20 years) in 2019 was higher compared to that in 2001 and was lower compared to that in 2010 (2001: 16.0 g/day; 2010: 17.8 g/day; 2019: 17.7 g/day).

The daily intake of mushrooms among Japanese adult men (aged ≥ 20 years) in 2019 was higher compared to that in 2001 and was lower compared to that in 2010 (2001: 16.1 g/day; 2010: 18.4 g/day; 2019: 17.6 g/day). The daily intake of mushroom did not exhibit a significant correlation with the rate of hyperuricemia in Japanese adult men (aged ≥ 20 years) from 2010 to 2019 (r= -0.310, p=0.456).

The daily intake of mushrooms among Japanese adult women (aged ≥ 20 years) in 2019 was higher compared to that in 2001 and 2010 (2001: 15.9 g/day; 2010: 17.3 g/day; 2019: 17.8 g/day). The daily intake of mushrooms did not exhibit a significant correlation with the rate of hyperuricemia in Japanese adult women (aged ≥ 20 years) from 2010 to 2019 (r= 0.205, p=0.626).

Considering the daily dietary fiber, vitamin D, vitamin B_1, vitamin B_2, pantothenic acid, folate, potassium, iron, zinc intake, the daily intake of mushroom appears better to increase.

Seaweed

The daily intake of seaweed among the Japanese adult population (aged ≥ 20 years) in 2019 was lower compared to that in 2001 and 2010 (2001: 14.3 g/day; 2010: 11.7 g/day; 2019: 10.6 g/day).

The daily intake of seaweed among Japanese adult men (aged ≥ 20 years) in 2019 was lower compared to that in 2001 and 2010 (2001: 14.0 g/day; 2010: 12.3 g/day; 2019: 11.1 g/day). The daily intake of seaweed did not exhibit a significant correlation with the rate of hyperuricemia in Japanese adult men (aged ≥ 20 years) from 2010 to 2019 (r= 0.443, p=0.272).

The daily intake of seaweed among Japanese adult women (aged ≥ 20 years) in 2019 was lower compared to that in 2001 and 2010 (2001: 14.5 g/day;

2010: 11.3 g/day; 2019: 10.1 g/day). The daily intake of seaweed was negatively correlated with the rate of hyperuricemia in Japanese adult women (aged ≥ 20 years) from 2010 to 2019 (r= -0.728, p=0.041). These results suggest that the correlation between daily seaweed intake and the rate of hyperuricemia tends to vary with gender and is stronger in Japanese adult women than in Japanese adult men.

Considering the daily dietary fiber, vitamin A, vitamin B_2, vitamin B_6, folate, vitamin C, magnesium, iron, zinc intake, the daily intake of seaweed seems better to increase.

Potatoes, Mushrooms and Seaweed

The dietary guidelines for Japanese (the Japanese food guide spinning top) by the Ministry of Health, Labour and Welfare and Ministry of Agriculture, Forestry and Fisheries has recommended that the daily total intake of potatoes, mushrooms and seaweed must be 1-2 servings (approximately 70-140 g), depending on an individual's caloric intake (The Ministry of Health, Labour and Welfare and Ministry of Agriculture, Forestry and Fisheries 2023). The daily total intake of potatoes, mushrooms and seaweed among the Japanese adult population (aged ≥ 20 years) in 2019 was lower compared to that in 2016 (2001: 93.1 g/day; 2019: 88.3 g/day). The daily total intake of potatoes, mushrooms and seaweed among the Japanese adult population (aged ≥ 20 years) seems better to be increased to reach approximately 140 g.

Legumes

The daily intake of total legumes among the Japanese adult population (aged ≥ 20 years) in 2019 was higher compared to that in 2001 and 2010 (2001: 60.4 g/day; 2010: 59.3 g/day; 2019: 64.6 g/day).

The daily intake of total legumes among Japanese adult men (aged ≥ 20 years) in 2019 was higher compared to that in 2001 and 2010 (2001: 62.4 g/day; 2010: 61.2 g/day; 2019: 64.0 g/day). The daily intake of total legumes did not exhibit a significant correlation with the rate of hyperuricemia in Japanese adult men (aged ≥ 20 years) from 2010 to 2019 (r= 0.145, p=0.733).

The daily intake of total legumes among Japanese adult women (aged ≥ 20 years) in 2019 was higher compared to that in 2001 and 2010 (2001: 58.7 g/day; 2010: 57.7 g/day; 2019: 65.1 g/day). The daily intake of total legumes was positively correlated with the rate of hyperuricemia in Japanese adult women (aged ≥ 20 years) from 2010 to 2019 (r= 0.767, p=0.026). These results suggest that the correlation between the daily intake of total legumes and the rate of hyperuricemia is stronger in Japanese adult women than in Japanese adult men.

As stated in the reviews (Ekpenyong and Daniel 2015; Kakutani-Hatayama et al. 2015; Koguchi 2018; Bouike, Nakata and Moriwaki 2021) and the previous reports (Koguchi 2023), increasing the intake of fruit seems to be important for the prevention of hyperuricemia.

The daily intake of total legumes among Japanese adult men (aged ≥ 20 years) in 2019 was 60.4 g. The Ministry of Health, Labour and Welfare in Japan has recommended an intake of legumes of 100 g or more per day (The Ministry of Health, Labour and Welfare, Japan 2023). Considering the results from the balance of the caloric ratio of protein, fat and carbohydrates in the Japanese adult population (aged ≥ 20 years) in 2019 (protein: 15.1%, fat: 28.6%, and carbohydrates: 56.3%), along with the daily intake of dietary fiber, vitamin A, vitamin B_1, vitamin B_2, vitamin B_6, pantothenic acid, folate, potassium, magnesium, phosphorus, zinc intake, it seems better to increase the daily intake of legumes for the prevention of hyperuricemia.

Seeds and Nuts

The daily intake of seeds and nuts among the Japanese adult population (aged ≥ 20 years) in 2019 was higher compared to that in 2001 and 2010 (2001: 2.3 g/day; 2010: 2.2 g/day; 2019: 2.7 g/day).

The daily intake of seeds and nuts among Japanese adult men (aged ≥ 20 years) in 2019 was higher compared to that in 2001 and 2010 (2001: 2.2 g/day; 2010: 2.1 g/day; 2019: 2.6 g/day). The daily intake of seeds and nuts did not exhibit a significant correlation with the rate of hyperuricemia in Japanese adult men (aged ≥ 20 years) from 2010 to 2019 ($r= 0.030$, $p=0.944$).

The daily intake of seeds and nuts of Japanese adult women (aged ≥ 20 years) in 2019 was higher compared to that in 2001 and 2010 (2001: 2.4 g/day; 2010: 2.2 g/day; 2019: 2.8 g/day). The daily intake of seeds and nuts was positively correlated with the rate of hyperuricemia in Japanese adult women (aged ≥ 20 years) from 2010 to 2019 ($r= 0.814$, $p=0.014$). These results suggest that the correlation between the daily intake of seeds and nuts and the rate of hyperuricemia is stronger in Japanese adult women than in Japanese adult men.

Considering the result from the balance of the caloric ratio of protein, fat and carbohydrates in the Japanese adult population (aged ≥ 20 years) in 2019 (protein: 15.1%, fat: 28.6%, and carbohydrates: 56.3%) and the daily dietary fiber, vitamin A, vitamin B_1, vitamin B_2, vitamin B_6, pantothenic acid, folate, potassium, magnesium, phosphorus, zinc intake, it seems that an increase in daily intake of seeds and nuts is needed for the prevention of hyperuricemia.

Fruit

The daily intake of total fruit among the Japanese adult population (aged ≥ 20 years) in 2019 was lower compared to that in 2001 and 2010 (2001: 132.3 g/day; 2010: 103.7 g/day; 2019: 100.2 g/day).

The daily intake of total fruit among Japanese adult men (aged ≥ 20 years) in 2019 was lower compared to that in 2001 and 2010 (2001: 112.8 g/day; 2010: 92.9 g/day; 2019: 87.5 g/day). The daily intake of total fruit did not exhibit a significant correlation with the rate of hyperuricemia in Japanese adult men (aged ≥ 20 years) from 2010 to 2019 (r= -0.130, p=0.760).

The daily intake of total fruit among Japanese adult women (aged ≥ 20 years) in 2019 was lower compared to that in 2001 and 2010 (2001: 148.8 g/day; 2010: 112.9 g/day; 2019: 111.2 g/day). The daily intake of total fruit did not show a significant correlation with the rate of hyperuricemia in Japanese adult women (aged ≥ 20 years) from 2010 to 2019 (r= -0.268, p=0.521).

As stated in the reviews (Ekpenyong and Daniel 2015; Kakutani-Hatayama et al. 2015; Koguchi 2018; Bouike, Nakata and Moriwaki 2021) and the previous reports (Koguchi 2023), an increased intake of fruit seems to be important for the prevention of hyperuricemia through reduced serum uric acid (SUA) concentrations.

The Dietary Guidelines for Americans established by the US Department of Agriculture recommended that the adult population (aged ≥ 19 years) eat 1.5 to 2.5 servings (i.e., cup or ounce equivalents) of fruit per day, depending on an individual's caloric intake (U.S. Department of Agriculture 2023). The Dietary Guidelines for Japanese (the Japanese food guide spinning top) has recommended that daily consumption of fruit must be 2-3 servings (approximately 200-300 g), depending on an individual's caloric intake (The Ministry of Health, Labour and Welfare and Ministry of Agriculture, Forestry and Fisheries 2023). The National Health and Medical Research Council (NHMRC), Australian Government's Australian Guide to Healthy Eating, Eat for Health, Australian Dietary Guidelines, 2013 (2023) has stated that consuming at least two servings of fruit per day (150 g per serve) is recommended for Australian adults (aged ≥ 19 years). Considering the daily dietary fiber, vitamin A, vitamin B_6, vitamin C, folate, potassium, magnesium, phosphorus, iron intake, it appears better to increase the daily intake of fruit (especially less sugary fruit and cherries) for the prevention of hyperuricemia.

Vegetables

The daily intake of total vegetables among the Japanese adult population (aged ≥ 20 years) in 2019 was lower compared to that in 2001 and 2010 (2001: 295.8 g/day; 2010: 281.7 g/day; 2019: 280.5 g/day).

The daily intake of total vegetables among Japanese adult men (aged ≥ 20 years) in 2019 was lower compared to that in 2001 and 2010 (2001: 303.7 g/day; 2010: 289.1 g/day; 2019: 288.3 g/day). The daily intake of total vegetables did not exhibit a significant correlation with the rate of hyperuricemia in Japanese adult men (aged ≥ 20 years) from 2010 to 2019 (r= -0.217, p=0.605).

The daily intake of total vegetables among Japanese adult women (aged ≥ 20 years) in 2019 was lower compared to that in 2001 and 2010 (2001: 289.2 g/day; 2010: 275.3 g/day; 2019: 273.6 g/day). The daily intake of total vegetables did not exhibit a significant correlation with the rate of hyperuricemia in Japanese adult women (aged ≥ 20 years) from 2010 to 2019 (r= 0.371, p=0.366).

As stated in the reviews (Ekpenyong and Daniel 2015; Koguchi 2018; Bouike, Nakata and Moriwaki 2021) and the previous reports (Koguchi 2023), increased intake of vegetables appears to be important for the prevention of hyperuricemia.

The Dietary Guidelines for Americans established by the US Department of Agriculture (2023) recommended that the adult population (aged ≥ 19 years) eat 2.5 to 4 servings (i.e., cup or ounce equivalents) of vegetables per day, depending on an individual's caloric intake. For example, the recommended number of vegetables in the Healthy US-Style Eating Pattern at the 2,000-calorie level is 2.5 cup-equivalents of vegetables per day (US Department of Agriculture 2023). The Ministry of Health, Labour and Welfare in Japan (2023) has recommended that daily consumption of vegetables must be 350 g or more (green-yellow vegetables, 120 g or more). The National Health and Medical Research Council (NHMRC), Australian Government's Australian Guide to Healthy Eating, Eat for Health, Australian Dietary Guidelines, 2013 (2023) has stated that consuming at least five servings of vegetables per day (75 g per serve) is recommended for Australian adults (aged ≥ 19 years). Considering the daily dietary fiber, vitamin A, vitamin B_1, vitamin B_2, vitamin B_6, vitamin C, pantothenic acid, folate, calcium, potassium, magnesium, phosphorus, iron intake, it seems better to increase the daily intake of vegetables for the prevention of hyperuricemia.

Fruit and Vegetables

The daily intake of total fruit and vegetables among the Japanese adult population (aged ≥ 20 years) in 2019 (380.7 g/day) was less than the daily recommended fruit intake by the World Health Organization (World Health Organization 2007; World Health Organization 2023) and the Australian Government (Australian Government 2018). An increase in the daily intake of fruit and vegetables among Japanese people seems to be essential for the prevention of hyperuricemia.

Probiotics

The Ministry of Health, Labour and Welfare in Japan has not investigated the daily intake of probiotics of Japanese people.

As stated in the previous reports (Koguchi 2023), conscious intake of probiotics seems to be important for the prevention of hyperuricemia through reduced serum uric acid (SUA) concentrations.

Table 3. Modification of nutrient intake for the prevention of hyperuricemia in the Japanese adult population in 2019.

Gender	Age	Increased intake	Recognizing encouraged intake	Avoiding overdose	Limiting or decreasing intake
Men	aged ≥ 20 years	Fiber Vitamin A Vitamin E Vitamin B_1 Vitamin B_6 Folate Calcium Potassium Magnesium Zinc	Vitamin B_2 Vitamin C Polyphenol	Total sugars Pantothenic acid Vitamin B_{12} Sodium Phosphorus Copper	Fructose Animal fats, Saturated fatty acids Cholesterol Alcohol Purine Salt
Men	aged 7-49 years			Vitamin D	
Men	aged 15-49 years	Iron			
Men	aged 20-59 years	Vitamin B_2 Vitamin C			
Men	aged ≥ 50 years			Iron	
Men	aged 50-69 years	Vitamin D			
Men	aged ≥ 60 years			Vitamin C	
Men	aged ≥ 75 years	Vitamin D		Vitamin B_2	

Gender	Age	Increased intake	Recognizing encouraged intake	Avoiding overdose	Limiting or decreasing intake
Women	aged ≥ 20 years	Fiber Vitamin A Vitamin E Vitamin B_1 Vitamin B_6 Folate Calcium Potassium Magnesium	Vitamin B_2 Vitamin C Polyphenol	Total sugars Pantothenic acid Vitamin B_{12} Sodium Phosphorus Copper	Fructose Animal fats, Saturated fatty acids Cholesterol Alcohol Purine Salt
Women	aged 20-39 years,	Vitamin D			
Women	aged 20-49 years	Vitamin C			
Women	aged 15-59 years	Iron			
Women	aged 20-59 years,	Vitamin B_2 Zinc			
Women	aged 40-49 years			Vitamin D	
Women	aged ≥ 50 years	Vitamin D		Vitamin C	
	aged 50-69 years	Vitamin D			
Women	aged ≥ 70 years	Zinc			
Women	aged ≥ 60 years			Iron	
Women	aged ≥ 75 years			Vitamin B_2	

Table 4. Modification of food intake for the prevention of hyperuricemia in the Japanese adult population in 2019

Gender	Age	Increased intake	Recognizing encouraged intake	Avoiding overdose	Limiting or decreasing intake
Men	aged ≥ 20 years	Fiber-rich foods (e.g., cereals, whole grains, high-fiber bread) Mushrooms Seaweed Legumes Seeds and Nuts Fruit Vegetables	Vitamin D-rich food Vitamin B_2-rich food Vitamin C-rich food Eggs Dairy products (particularly low-fat dairy products) Coffee Cocoa Tea Probiotics Polyphenol-rich food	Total sugars Vitamin A-rich food Pantothenic acid- rich food Folate-rich food Vitamin B_{12}-rich food Sodium-rich food Phosphorus-rich food Copper-rich food	Purine-rich food (e.g., meat, seafood and organ meats) High-fructose food Sugar-sweetened beverages Alcohol Beverages Confectioneries (sugary foods including desserts and sweets) Animal fats, Saturated fatty acids Cholesterol Salt

Table 4. (Continued)

Gender	Age	Increased intake	Recognizing encouraged intake	Avoiding overdose	Limiting or decreasing intake
Men	aged 7-49 years			Vitamin D-rich food	
Men	aged 15-49 years	Iron-rich food			
Men	aged 20-59 years	Vitamin B_2-rich food Vitamin C-rich food			
Men	aged ≥ 50 years			Iron-rich food	
Men	aged 50-69 years	Vitamin D-rich food			
Men	aged ≥ 60 years			Vitamin C-rich food	
Men	aged ≥ 75 years	Vitamin D-rich food		Vitamin B_2-rich food	
Women	aged ≥ 20 years	Fiber-rich foods (e.g., cereals, whole grains, high-fiber bread) Mushrooms Seaweed Legumes Seeds and Nuts Fruit Vegetables	Vitamin D-rich food Vitamin B_2-rich food Vitamin C-rich food Eggs Dairy products (particularly low-fat dairy products) Coffee Cocoa Tea Probiotics Polyphenol-rich food	Total sugars Vitamin A rich food Pantothenic acid- rich food Folate-rich food Vitamin B_{12}-rich food Sodium-rich food Phosphorus-rich food Copper-rich food	Purine-rich food (e.g., meat, seafood and organ meats) High-fructose food Sugar-sweetened beverages Alcohol Beverages Confectioneries (sugary foods including desserts and sweets) Animal fats, Saturated fatty acids Cholesterol Salt
Women	aged 20-39 years,	Vitamin D-rich food			
Women	aged 20-49 years	Vitamin C-rich food			
Women	aged 15-59 years	Iron-rich food			
Women	aged 20-59 years,	Vitamin B_2-rich food Zinc-rich food			

Gender	Age	Increased intake	Recognizing encouraged intake	Avoiding overdose	Limiting or decreasing intake
Women	aged 40-49 years			Vitamin D-rich food	
Women	aged ≥ 50 years	Vitamin D-rich food		Vitamin C-rich food	
	aged 50-69 years	Vitamin D-rich food			
Women	aged ≥ 70 years	Zinc-rich food			
Women	aged ≥ 60 years			Iron-rich food	
Women	aged ≥ 75 years			Vitamin B_2-rich food	

The Japanese Diet

The basic form of Japanese food is a menu consisting of "one soup and three dishes", that is, rice, soup stock, and three side dishes (one main dish and two side dishes). The form of this menu is changing with the times (The Ministry of Agriculture, Forestry and Fisheries 2020). There are various cooking methods for side dishes for a Japanese-styled diet such as stewing, grilling, steaming, boiling, dressing, and deep-frying (The Ministry of Agriculture, Forestry and Fisheries 2020). By combining these methods with seasonal foods such as vegetables, edible wild plants, seafood, and seaweed, a wide variety of side dishes can be prepared (The Ministry of Agriculture, Forestry and Fisheries 2020). Foods used in the Japanese-styled diet include grains (mainly rice), vegetables, mushrooms, fish, shellfish, seaweed, and wagyu beef (The Ministry of Agriculture, Forestry and Fisheries 2020). The dishes were prepared mainly using vegetables and seafood (The Ministry of Agriculture, Forestry and Fisheries 2020).

The Japanese economy revived to pre-World War II levels around 1955 (The Ministry of Agriculture, Forestry and Fisheries 2020). In Japan, the 1960s was a time when the post-war chaos calmed down, and the eating habits became stable (The Ministry of Agriculture, Forestry and Fisheries 2020). Therefore, it is thought that the menu of Japanese food rapidly expanded with a variety of dishes due to the Westernization of meals from 1955 to 1965 (The Ministry of Agriculture, Forestry and Fisheries 2020). For example, as potato dishes, Japanese people ate mainly miso soup and floured potatoes in 1960. The GNP of Japan grew to the second-largest capitalist country in the world in 1968. Along with this economic growth, Japanese people's dietary habits started to change rapidly, and the protein among the Japanese people, namely meat, eggs, milk and dairy products, and seafood, increased rapidly, whereas consumption of rice and potatoes has fallen to less than half of what it was in the 1910s (The Ministry of Agriculture, Forestry and Fisheries 2020). During the period of high economic growth in Japan from 1955 to 1973, the storage period of foods became longer due to the spread of refrigerators, and it became possible to cook fried foods, stir-fried foods, Chinese dishes, and Western dishes at home with the spread of city gas. The Ministry of Health, Labour and Welfare and Ministry of Agriculture, Forestry and Fisheries in Japan (The Ministry of Health, Labour and Welfare and Ministry of Agriculture, Forestry and Fisheries 2010) regard eating habits around 1970-1980 as "Japanese eating habits". The Japanese-styled diet is a balanced diet that consists of the staple food (e.g., rice), main dish, side dishes, fruit, and a moderate amount of milk and dairy products. Compared to the Japanese diet in 1965, the Japanese diet in 1980, consumption of rice decreased 20%, intakes of meat, milk, vegetable oils, fruit, and seafood increased 2-fold, 1.5-fold, 2.33-fold, 1.38-fold, and 1.25-fold, respectively, and the intake of vegetables remained about the same (The Ministry of Health, Labour and Welfare. Health Service Bureau 2020). This phenomenon indicates that the Westernization of eating habits has progressed. The basic style of the Japanese-style diet was preserved in each household until about the 1980s. Although the balance of a main dish and side dishes struck an ideal balance by around the 1980s, the consumption of meat, fat, milk and dairy products also increased, and the food self-sufficiency ratio declined (The Ministry of Agriculture, Forestry and Fisheries 2020). Eating out with family became an everyday affair, and meals at home were also Westernized (The Ministry of Agriculture, Forestry and Fisheries 2020). The number of main dishes decreased slightly, and side dishes increased, particularly showing the growth of the ratio of milk and dairy foods and meat (The Ministry of Agriculture, Forestry and Fisheries 2020). Since 1986, changes in eating habits due to diversified lifestyles have included changes in home cooking, decline in traditional food culture, loneliness of families, advances in food simplification by increased sales of retort pouch foods and increased penetration of microwave ovens (90%), and a decrease in the food self-sufficiency rate. After the 1980s, occasions for eating out with family increased and the Westernization of home cooking progressed (The Ministry of Agriculture, Forestry and Fisheries 2020). Compared to the

Japanese food in 1960, 1990, and 2005, the Japanese food in 1975 used more sugar and sweeteners, legumes, fruit, seaweed, seafood, eggs, seasonings and spices, and there were many kinds of ingredients, whereas consumption of preferred beverages (e.g., soft drinks, coffee, tea, and cocoa) was small (The Ministry of Health, Labour and Welfare. Health Service Bureau 2020; Tsuduki 2019). For example, Japanese people ate clam chowder, croquettes, and potato salad in addition to the above dishes in 2005. The Ministry of Agriculture, Forestry and Fisheries (The Ministry of Agriculture, Forestry and Fisheries 2020) has stated that the ideal balance of the caloric ratio of protein, fat and carbohydrate for healthy life is protein: 15%, fat: 25%, and carbohydrates: 60%, and the caloric ratio of the three macronutrients (protein, fat, and carbohydrate) in Japanese people was well balanced in 1980. However, the dietary life of Japanese people thereafter tended to have too much meat and fat, with a decreased amount of rice, and the balance of the caloric ratio of protein, fat, and carbohydrate in Japanese people in 2010 became closer to a Western type of diet (the caloric ratio of protein, fat and carbohydrates in the US and France from 2005 to 2007) (The Ministry of Agriculture, Forestry and Fisheries 2020). Compared to the Japanese diet in 1980, in the Japanese diet in 2013, consumption of rice, vegetables, fruit, and seafood decreased 25%, 19.4%, 9.1%, and 25%, respectively, while the intake of meat and vegetable oils increased 1.5-fold and 1.29-fold, respectively, and the intake of milk was the same amount (The Ministry of Health, Labour and Welfare. Health Service Bureau 2020). Compared to the caloric ratio of protein, fat, and carbohydrates of the Japanese adult population (aged ≥ 20 years) in 2013, the caloric ratio of protein and fat in the Japanese adult population (aged ≥ 20 years) in 2019 increased 0.3% and 2.7%, respectively and the caloric ratio of carbohydrates in the Japanese adult population (aged ≥ 20 years) in 2019 decreased 3.0%. Yamanaka et al. (1994) stated that the nutritional intake among the Japanese people has changed dramatically due to the Westernization of life since around 1965, resulting in primary gout may have increased accordingly by the increase in the number of patients with diabetes mellitus and obesity.

The Dietary guidelines for Japanese (the Japanese food guide spinning top) proposed by the Ministry of Health, Labour and Welfare and Ministry of Agriculture, Forestry and Fisheries in Japan (2023) are as follows:

1) the daily consumption of staple food must be 4-8 servings (1 serving: the amount of carbohydrates contained in the material is approximately 40 g), depending on an individual's caloric intake;
2) (the daily consumption of side dishes (vegetables, mushrooms, potatoes and seaweed) must be 5-7 servings (approximately 350-490 g), depending on an individual's caloric intake;
3) the daily consumption of main dishes must be 3-6 servings (1 serving: the amount of proteins contained in the material is approximately 6 g), depending on an individual's caloric intake;
4) the daily consumption of milk and milk products must be 2-3 servings (milk: approximately 100 g/serving; yogurt: approximately 83 g/serving; cheese: approximately 20 g/serving), depending on an individual's caloric intake;
5) the daily consumption of fruit must be 2-3 servings (approximately 200-300 g), depending on an individual's caloric intake; and
6) the daily total consumption of confectionery (rice crackers: 3-4) and beverages (Japanese rice wine: 180 mL; beer: 500mL; wine: 260mL; distilled spirits: 100mL) must be at approximately 200 kcal. Among Japanese adults, individuals with higher adherence to Japanese dietary guidelines (the Japanese food guide spinning top) was associated with a lower risk of total mortality (cancer, cardiovascular disease, heart disease, cerebrovascular disease) and mortality from cardiovascular disease, particularly from cerebrovascular disease, in Japanese adults (Kurotani et al. 2016).

Conclusion

A high serum uric acid (SUA) concentration (hyperuricemia) is frequently associated with gout (Khanna et al. 2012) and is a risk factor for gout (as uratosis) (Saag and Choi 2006; Hisatome et al. 2018; Cabău et al. 2020; Li, Zhang and Zeng 2020). The prevalence of gout in Japan has increased markedly since the 1960s (Mikanagi 1963; The Ministry of Health, Labour and Welfare; Household Statistics Office 2023; Kawasaki and Shichikawa 2006; Oshima 1965; Hakoda and Kasagi 2018) and has been increasing (1986: 0.255 million; 2016: 1.105 million; 2019: 1.254 million; 2022: 1.305 million) (The Ministry of Health, Labour and Welfare. Household Statistics Office 2023). The Westernization in the Japanese diet starting in 1955 is thought to be one factor in the increase in the prevalence of gout. The introduction of the

Western lifestyle to Japanese people, such as a diet containing greater amounts of meat and saturated fatty acids, has been associated with the increases in SUA levels and the incidence of hyperuricemia and gout (Kagan et al. 1974). The prevalence of hyperuricemia is influenced by multiple factors, such as genetics, gender, age, lifestyle, food, eating habits, and economic development (Liu et al. 2013). Therefore, hyperuricemia is recognized as a lifestyle-related disease.

The previous chapters (Koguchi 2023) summarize the results of reported clinical research (clinical trials and epidemiological studies) describing associations between SUA concentration or hyperuricemia and dietary factors; that is to say, intake of α-linolenic acid, fiber, vitamin D, vitamin E, vitamin B_1, vitamin B_2, folate, vitamin B_{12}, vitamin C, calcium, magnesium, iron, zinc, and polyphenol may play an effective role in the prevention and management of hyperuricemia. Modification of nutrient intake for the prevention of hyperuricemia in the Japanese adult population (aged $\geq$ 20 years) in 2019 was shown in Table 3. The daily intakes of vitamin A, vitamin E, vitamin B_1, vitamin B_6, folate, magnesium, zinc, total fiber, calcium, and potassium in the Japanese adult population (aged $\geq$ 20 years) were below the Recommended Dietary Allowances (RDAs) or the Adequate Intakes (AIs) established by the Institute of Medicine of the National Academy of Sciences in the US (2021). It seems that the Japanese adult population (aged $\geq$ 20 years) should take in more fiber, vitamin A, vitamin E, vitamin B_1, vitamin B_6, folate, calcium, potassium, magnesium, and zinc to reach the Recommended Dietary Allowances (RDAs) or the Adequate Intakes (AIs) established by the Institute of Medicine of the National Academy of Sciences in the US (2021). Modification of food intake for the prevention of hyperuricemia in the Japanese adult population (aged $\geq$ 20 years) in 2019 was shown in Table 4. Recognizing the intake of foods rich in the above nutrients (i.e., α-linolenic acid, fiber, vitamin A, vitamin D, vitamin E, vitamin B_1, vitamin B_2, vitamin B_6, folate, vitamin B_{12}, vitamin C, calcium, potassium, magnesium, iron, zinc, and polyphenol is important).

To properly choose and consume the following foods that contain the above-mentioned nutrients may play a helpful role in the prevention of hyperuricemia for the Japanese adult population (aged $\geq$ 20 years); that is to say, meat (poultry), seafood (eel, herring, salmon, sardines, anchovy, tuna, trout, mackerel), fish oil (cod liver oil), seeds and nuts (broad bean seed, pumpkin seeds, chia seeds, sunflower seeds, almonds, sesame seeds, pistachio nuts, hazelnuts, peanuts, pecan nuts, walnuts, flaxseeds, pine nuts), grains (white rice, buckwheat, bread, wheat germ), whole grains (brown rice, brown cereal, breakfast cereals, oatmeal, ready-to-eat cereal, fortified with 10% of the daily value for vitamin D), potatoes (konjac), mushrooms (maitake mushrooms, shiitake mushrooms, wood ear), legumes (black-eyed peas, common beans, edamame, green peas, kidney beans, soybeans, chickpeas, lentils), seaweed, fruit (acerolas, apples, apricots, avocados, bananas, blackberries, black currants, black elderberries, cherries, European cranberries, kiwifruit, mangos, nectarines, oranges, papayas, peaches, pears, plums, raisins, red raspberries, strawberries, watermelons), vegetables (asparaguses, black olives, broad bean pods, broccoli, chicory, kales, garlic, brussels sprouts, carrots, ginger, globe artichokes, Jew's mallows, lettuces, mustard greens, okra, onions, spinach, parsley, tomatoes, peppers, radishes, cucumbers, zucchinis, pumpkins, leafy greens, Chinese cabbages, pickles), soy products (soy milk, tofu, soy meat), dairy products (low-fat milk, low-fat yogurt, milk, cheese, yogurt), eggs, spices (capers, caraways, cloves, cumin, curry, turmeric), oils (olive oil), coffee, tea (black tea, green tea), and chocolates and cocoa powders (The Council for Science and Technology, Ministry of Education, Culture, Sports, Science and Technology in Japan 2023; US Department of Health & Human Services; National Institutes of Health; Office of Dietary Supplements 2023). Furthermore, it should be considered to reduce the intake of one serving of high-pantothenic acid foods [e.g., beef liver, pork liver, chicken liver, chicken breast, beef kidney, pork kidney, tuna, anchovy, shitake mushrooms, potatoes, breakfast cereals, sunflower seeds, natto, avocados, milk, Greek yogurt, eggs, green tea, baker's yeast (The Council for Science and Technology, Ministry of Education, Culture, Sports, Science and Technology in Japan 2023; US Department of Health & Human Services; National Institutes of Health; Office of Dietary Supplements 2023), high-vitamin B_{12} foods (e.g., beef, turkey, beef liver, chicken liver, clams, tuna, salmon, anchovy, sweetfish, lamprey, breakfast cereals, tempeh, seaweed, milk, yogurt, cheese, eggs, nutritional yeast) (The Council for Science and Technology, Ministry of Education, Culture, Sports, Science and Technology in Japan 2023; US Department of Health & Human Services; National Institutes of Health; Office of Dietary Supplements 2023), high-phosphorus foods [e.g., yogurt, milk, cheese, salmon, scallops, sardines, flying fish, dried squid, chicken, lentils, cashew nuts, potatoes] (The Council for Science and Technology, Ministry of Education, Culture, Sports, Science and Technology in Japan 2023; US Department of Health & Human Services; National Institutes of Health; Office of Dietary Supplements 2023). High-copper foods [e.g., beef liver, oysters, baking chocolate, potatoes, shiitake mushrooms, cashew nuts, crab, sunflower seeds, turkey giblets, squid, mantis shrimp, Sakura shrimp, octopus (The Council for Science and Technology, Ministry of Education, Culture, Sports, Science and Technology in Japan 2023; US Department of Health & Human Services; National Institutes of Health; Office of Dietary Supplements 2023), and decrease the intake of animal fat [e.g., beef, beef tallow, pork, margarine, butter (The Council for Science and Technology, Ministry of Education, Culture, Sports, Science and Technology in Japan 2023)], saturated fatty acids [e.g., coconut oil, coconut powder, butter, shortening, beef, beef tallow, pork, margarine, whipped cream, cheese (The Council for Science and Technology, Ministry of Education, Culture, Sports, Science and Technology in Japan 2023)], cholesterol [e.g., eggs, herring roe, dried squid, anchovy, anchovy liver, foie gras, Sakura shrimp, dried shrimp, sand lance, caviar, lamprey, salmon roe (The Council for Science and Technology, Ministry of Education, Culture, Sports, Science and Technology in Japan 2023), and salt and limit the intake of one serving of purine-rich foods (e.g., beef, pork, lamb, organ meats, and meat extracts, seafood, yeast extracts, peas, beans, lentils, asparaguses, cauliflowers, spinach, mushrooms, bamboo shoots, nori, wakame, soup stock, oyster sauce, consommé, Chinese soup) (Koguchi 2021; Koguchi 2022; Kaneko et al. 2014; Hisatome et al. 2018).

Modification of food intake for the prevention of hyperuricemia in Japanese adult population (aged $\geq$ 20 years) in 2019 is suggested as follows: limiting or decreasing alcohol beverage consumption; limiting or decreasing intake of purine-rich food (e.g., meat, seafood and organ meats), animal fats, saturated fatty acids, cholesterol, high-fructose food, sugar-sweetened beverages, confectioneries (sugary foods including desserts and sweets), salt, oils and fats; avoiding overdose of total sugars, foods rich in vitamin A, vitamin B_5 (pantothenic acid), folate, vitamin B_{12}, sodium, phosphorus, and copper; replacement of saturated fatty acids (e.g., dairy fats, meat fat) with mono- and polyunsaturated fatty acids (particularly n-3 polyunsaturated fatty acids) (e.g., macadamia nuts, almonds, peanuts and peanut butter, olive oil, canola oil, avocados); increasing the intake of fiber-rich foods (e.g., cereals, whole grains, high-fiber bread), milk and dairy products (particularly low-fat dairy products), mushrooms, seaweed, legumes, seeds and nuts, fruit, vegetables, which contain rich in carbohydrates (particularly dietary fiber), vitamin A, vitamin E, vitamin B_1, vitamin B_2, vitamin B_6, folate, vitamin B_{12}, vitamin C, calcium, potassium, magnesium, zinc, and polyphenol; recognizing the intake of eggs, milk and dairy products (particularly low-fat dairy products), coffee, cocoa, tea, and probiotics; and maintenance of good hydration (Table 4). The guidelines for management of hyperuricemia and gout conducted by Hisatome et al. (2018) has stated dietary counseling as follows: prevent excessive purine intake; prevent excessive fructose intake; limit alcohol drinking; and drink sufficient water. Koike et al. (2023) observed that thirty-three subjects with asymptomatic hyperuricemia underwent the above dietary counseling in line with the guideline for 6 months. When compared to baseline, SUA and urinary uric acid (UA) excretion levels were significantly decreased, and renal fractional excretion of UA was significantly increased at 6 months (Koike et al. 2023). These results revealed the effectiveness of dietary counseling in line with the guideline in subjects with asymptomatic hyperuricemia. The guidelines have recommended weight loss for overweight and obese people (Khanna et al. 2012; Richette et al. 2017; Hisatome et al. 2018; FitzGerald et al. 2020; Khanna et al. 2020), vigorous intensity aerobic physical activity (Hisatome et al. 2018) and smoking cessation (Khanna et al. 2012) for the management of gout. Furthermore, the important points of behavior for the prevention and management of hyperuricemia in Japanese adult population (aged $\geq$ 20 years) is suggested as follows: weight management including proper calorie intake; weight loss for overweight and obese people; adequate physical exercise (e.g., moderate intensity aerobic exercise for 30 minutes on 5-7 days per week, vigorous intensity aerobic physical activity for 75 minutes per week); and smoking cessation. The above behavior seems to be a beneficial strategy both for prevention and management of hyperuricemia in Japanese adult population (aged $\geq$ 20 years) in 2019.

Prevention of hyperuricemia and/or gout should consider the effects of chronic kidney disease (CKD), urolithiasis, obesity, diabetes mellitus, hypertension, and cardiovascular disease (CVD), which are comorbidities of hyperuricemia and/or gout. Hypertension, diabetes mellitus, dyslipidemia, and CKD are major health issues in Japan today. The previous reports summarize the beneficial effects of dietary patterns [i.e., the Mediterranean diet, the Dietary Approaches to Stop Hypertension (DASH) diet, and vegetarian diets] for the prevention of hyperuricemia, gout, and some hyperuricemia and gout-associated comorbidities [e.g., CKD, obesity, diabetes mellitus, and CVD] (Koguchi 2021; Koguchi 2022; Koguchi 2023). The National Health and Medical Research Council (NHMRC), Australian Government's Australian Guide to Healthy Eating, Eat for Health, Australian Dietary Guidelines, 2013 (2023) and Australian's health 2018 (2023) emphasize the importance of limiting the intake of foods and drinks high in saturated fat, added salt, added sugars and alcohol, based on evidence that these foods are associated with increased risk of obesity and/or chronic diseases, including CVD and type 2 diabetes mellitus. Limiting intake of foods containing saturated fat, added salt, added sugars and alcohol seems to apply to the prevention and management of hyperuricemia (Koguchi 2018). Furthermore, choosing and eating SUA-lowering foods containing nutrients and phytochemicals in the Mediterranean diet, the DASH diet, and vegetarian diets may also lead to preventing not only hyperuricemia, but also gout and some hyperuricemia and gout-associated comorbidities [e.g., CKD (Krishnamurthy et al. 2012), obesity (Yahfoufi et al. 2018), diabetes mellitus (Forouhi et al. 2018; Yahfoufi et al. 2018), and CVD (Yahfoufi et al. 2018) caused by inflammation from elevated SUA concentrations, as described in the previous reports (Koguchi 2021; Koguchi 2022; Koguchi 2023). The author wishes to emphasize that dietary habits of Japanese adult population (aged $\geq$ 20 years) should refer or adopt dietary patterns such as the Mediterranean diet, the DASH diet, and vegetarian diets. However, taking into consideration the choices and intake of proper foods for prevention of each comorbidity of hyperuricemia is essential. Large-scale prospective cohort studies and randomized controlled trials are needed to examine the effects of the Mediterranean diet, the DASH diet, and vegetarian diets with SUA-lowering foods choices on individuals with or without comorbidities of hyperuricemia in the Japanese adult population.

Disclaimer

None

References

Australian Government. 2023. "*Australian's health 2018*." Accessed July 15. https://www.aihw.gov.au/reports/australias-health/australias-health-2018/contents/indicators-of-australias-health/fruit-and-vegetable-intake

Australian Government National Health and Medical Research Council (NHMRC) Department of Health and Ageing. 2023. "Australian Dietary Guidelines- providing the scientific evidence for healthier Australian diets (2013)." Accessed July 28. https://www.eatforhealth.gov.au/sites/default/files/2022-09/n55_australian_dietary_guidelines.pdf

Bouike Y, Nakata E, Moriwaki Y. 2021. "Gout friendly foods that reduce urate-review." *J Nutr Health Sci* 8:105.

Cabău G, Crişan TO, Klück V, PoppRA, Joosten LAB. 2020. "Urate-induced immune programming: Consequences for gouty arthritis and hyperuricemia." *Immunol Rev* 294:92-105.

Caliceti C, Calabria D, Roda A, Cicero A. 2017. "Fructose intake, serum uric acid, and cardiometabolic disorders: A critical review." *Nutrients* 9:395.

Chang WC. 2011. "Dietary intake and the risk of hyperuricemia, gout and chronic kidney disease in elderly Taiwanese men." *Aging Male* 14:195-202.

Choi HK. 2010. "A prescription for lifestyle change in patients with hyperuricemia and gout." *Curr Opin Rheumatol* 22:165-172.

Choi HK, Mount DB, Reginato AM. 2005. "Pathogenesis of gout." *Ann Intern Med* 143:499-516.

Chuang SY, Lee SC, Hsieh YT, Pan WH. 2011. "Trends in hyperuricemia and gout prevalence: Nutrition and Health Survey in Taiwan from 1993-1996 to 2005-2008." *Asia Pac J Clin Nutr* 20:301-308.

Dornas WC, de Lima WG, Pedrosa ML, Silva ME. 2015. "Health implications of high-fructose intake and current research." *Adv Nutr* 6:729-737.

Ekpenyong CE, Daniel N. 2015. "Roles of diets and dietary factors in the pathogenesis, management and prevention of abnormal serum uric acid levels." *PharmaNutrition* 3:29-45.

Feig DI, Kang D-H, Johnson RJ. 2008. "Uric acid and cardiovascular risk." *N Engl J Med* 359:1811-1821.

FitzGerald JD, Dalbeth N, Mikuls T, Brignardello-Petersen R, Guyatt G, Abeles AM, Gelber AC, Harrold LR,

Ford ES, Choi HK. 2013. "Associations between concentrations of uric acid with concentrations of vitamin A and beta-carotene among adults in the United States." *Nutr Res* 33:995-1002.

Forouhi NG, Misra A, Mohan V, Taylor R, Yancy W. 2018. "Dietary and nutritional approaches for prevention and management of type 2 diabetes." *BMJ* 361: k2234.

Fujimori S, Ito H, Kato K, Watanabe H, Matsuura H, Ogata N, Yamonouchi J. 2006. "Hyperuricemia/gout is not increasing in Japan." *Gout Nucleic Acid Metabol* 30:13-19.

Gao X, Curhan G, Forman JP, Ascherio A, Choi HK. 2008. "Vitamin C intake and serum uric acid concentration in men." *J Rheumatol* 35:1853-1858.

Hakoda M, Kasagi F. 2018. "Trends in gout and hyperuricemia in Japan." *Gout and nucleic acid metabolism* 42:110.

Hisatome I, Ichida K, Mineo I, Ohtahara A, Ogino K, Kuwabara M, Ishizaka N, Uchida S, Kurajoh M, Kohagura K, Sato Y, Taniguchi A, Tsuchihashi T, Terai C, Nakamura T, Hamaguchi T, Hamada T, Fujimori S, Masuda I, Moriwaki Y, Yamamoto T. on behalf of guideline development group. 2018. *Japanese Society of Gout and Uric & Nucleic Acids Guidelines for Management of Hyperuricemia and Gout: 3 rd edition*. Tokyo: SHINDAN TO CHIRYO SHA, Inc.

Hosojima M, Kaseda R, Kondo H, Fujii M, Kubota M, Watanabe R, Tanabe N, Kadowaki M, Suzuki Y, Saito A. 2016. "Beneficial effects of rice endosperm protein intake in

Japanese men with risk factors for metabolic syndrome: a randomized, crossover clinical trial." *BMC Nutr* 2:25.

Huang HY, Appel LJ, Choi MJ, Gelber AC, Charleston J, Norkus EP, Miller ER 3 rd. 2005. "The effects of vitamin C supplementation on serum concentrations of uric acid: results of a randomized controlled trial." *Arthritis Rheum* 52:1843-1847.

INRA. 2023. "Phenol-Explorer database." Accessed April 27. http://phenol-explorer.eu/compounds.

Institute of Medicine of the National Academy of Sciences. 2021. "*Food and Nutrition Board. Dietary Reference Intakes: The essential guide to nutrient requirements.*" Accessed July 10. Washington, D.C.: The National Academy Press. https://www.nap.edu/catalog/11537.html

Institute of Medicine. Food and Nutrition Board. 2011. "*Dietary Reference Intakes: Recommended Dietary Allowances and Adequate Intakes, Total Water and Macronutrients.*" Accessed July 10. Washington, D.C.: The National Academy Press. https://www.ncbi.nlm.nih.gov/books/NBK56068/table/summarytables.t4/?report=objectonly

Institute of Medicine. Food and Nutrition Board. 2011. "*Dietary Reference Intakes for Calcium and Vitamin D.*" Washington, D.C.: The National Academy Press.

Institute of Medicine. National Academies of Sciences, Engineering, and Medicine, Health and Medicine Division, Food and Nutrition Board. 2019. "*Committee to review the Dietary Reference Intakes for Sodium and Potassium.*" Washington, D.C.: The National Academy Press.

Japan Preventive Association of Life-style related Disease. 2023. "Hyperuricemia/Gout." Accessed July 7. https://seikatsusyukanbyo.com/statistics/disease/hyperuricemia/

Japanese Society of Gout and Nucleic Acid Metabolism. 2002. *Guidelines for Management of Hyperuricemia and Gout: 1 st edition.* Tokyo:Dentsu, Sudler & Hennessey, Inc.

Jenkins DJ, Kendall CW, Vidgen E, Augustin LS, van Erk M, Geelen A, Parker T, Faulkner D, Vuksan V, Josse RG, Leiter LA, Connelly PW. 2001. "High-protein diets in hyperlipidemia: effect of wheat gluten on serum lipids, uric acid, and renal function." *Am J Clin Nutr* 74:57-63.

Joosten LAB, Crişan TO, Bjornstad P, Johnson RJ. 2020. "Asymptomatic hyperuricaemia: a silent activation of the innate immune system." *Nat Rev Rheumatol* 16:75-86.

Kagan A, Harris BR, Winkelstein W Jr, Johnson KG, Kato H, Syme SL, Rhoads GG, Gay ML, Nichaman MZ, Hamilton HB, Tillotson J. 1974. "Epidemiologic studies on coronary heart disease and stroke in Japanese men living in Japan, Hawaii and California: demographic, physical, dietary and biochemical characteristics." *J Chronic Dis* 27:345-364.

Kaneko K, Aoyagi Y, Fukuuchi T, Inazawa K, Yamaoka N. 2014. "Total purine and purine base content of common foodstuffs for facilitating nutritional therapy for gout and hyperuricemia." *Biol Pharm Bull* 37:709-721.

Kakutani-Hatayama M, Kadoya M, Okazaki H, Kurajoh M, Shoji T, Koyama H, Tsutsumi Z, Moriwaki Y, Namba M, Yamamoto T. 2015. "Nonpharmacological management of gout and hyperuricemia: Hints for better lifestyle." *Am J of Lifestyle Med* 11:321-329.

Kawasaki T, Shichikawa K. 2006. "Epidemiological survey of gout by resident examination." *Gout and nucleic acid metabolism* 30:66.

Khanna D, Fitzgerald JD, Khanna PP, Bae S, Singh MK, Neogi T, Pillinger MH, Merill J, Lee S, Prakash S, Kaldas M, Gogia M, Perez-Ruiz F, Taylor W, Lioté F, Choi H, Singh JA, Dalbeth N, Kaplan S, Niyyar V, Jones D, Yarows SA, Roessler B, Kerr G, King C, Levy G, Furst DE, Edwards NL, Mandell B, Schumacher HR, Robbins M, Wenger N, Terkeltaub R. 2012. "2012 American College of Rheumatology guidelines for management of gout. Part 1: systematic nonpharmacologic and pharmacologic therapeutic approaches to hyperuricemia." *Arthritis Care Research* 64:1431-1446.

Khanna D, King C, Levy G, Libbey C, Mount D, Pillinger MH, Rosenthal A, Singh JA, Sims JE, Smith BJ,
Wenger NS, Bae SS, Danve A, Khanna PP, Kim SC, Lenert A, Poon S, Qasim A, Sehra ST, Sharma TSK, Toprover M, Turgunbaev M, Zeng L, Zhang MA, Turner AS, Neogi T. 2020. "2020 American College of Rheumatology guideline for the management of gout." *Arthritis Care Research* 72:744-760.

Kim Y, Choi JH, Kang J, Kim G-T, Lee S-G. 2020. "Associations serum retinol and α-tocopherol levels with uric acid concentrations: analysis of a population-based, nationally representative sample." *Nutrients* 12:1797.

Koguchi T. 2018. "Essentials of dietary habits for prevention and suppression of hyperuricemia." *Curr Top Pharmacol* 22:77-133.

Koguchi T. 2021. "Modification of dietary habits for prevention of gout in Japanese people: Gout and the Japanese diet." *Am J Health Res* 9:117-127.

Koguchi T. 2021. "Modification of dietary habits for prevention of gout in Japanese people; Gout and diet." *Am J Health Res* 9:176-189.

Koguchi T. 2022. "Modification of macronutrient intake for prevention of gout in Japanese people in 2019: 2022 update." *Am J Health Res* 10: 83-106.

Koguchi T. 2022. "Modification of micronutrient intake for prevention of gout in Japanese people in 2019: 2022 update." *Am J Health Res* 10:107-131.

Koguchi T. 2022. "Modification of animal product intake for prevention of gout in Japanese people in 2019: 2022 update." *Am J Health Res* 10:140-153.

Koguchi T. 2022. "Modification of plant-based food intake for prevention of gout in Japanese people in 2019: 2022 update." *Am J Health Res* 10:154-168.

Koguchi T. 2023. "Dietary nutrients for prevention and management of hyperuricemia." *Hyperuricemia: Symptoms, Diagnosis and Treatment*. New York: Nova Science Publishers, Inc.

Koguchi T. 2023. "Foods and dietary patterns for prevention and management of hyperuricemia." *Hyperuricemia: Symptoms, Diagnosis and Treatment.* New York: Nova Science Publishers, Inc.

Koike R, Kawakami Y, Kondo R, Onishi M, Akiyama M, Asai T, Arai H. 2023. "Effect of dietary counselling on patients with asymptomatic hyperuricemia." *J Med Invest* 70: 34-40.

Krishnamurthy VMR, Wei G, Baird BC, Murtaugh M, Chonchol MB, Raphael KL, Greene T, Beddhu S. 2012. "High dietary fiber intake associated with decreased inflammation and all-cause mortality in patients with chronic kidney disease." *Kidney Int* 81:300-306.

Kuhnau J. 1976. "The flavonoids. A class of semi-essential food components: their role in human nutrition." *World* Rev *Nutr Diet* 24:117-191.

Kuo CF, Grainge MJ, Zhang W, Doherty M. 2015. "Global epidemiology of gout: prevalence, incidence and risk factors." *Nat Rev Rheumatol* 11:649-662.

Kurotani K, Akter S, Kashino I, Goto A, Mizoue T, Noda M, Sasazuki S, Sawada N, Tsugane S, Japan Public Health Center based Prospective Study Group. 2016. "Quality of diet and mortality among Japanese men and women: Japan Public Health Center based prospective study." *BMJ* 352: i1209.

Li L, Zhang Y, Zeng C. 2020. "Update on the epidemiology, genetics, and therapeutic options of hyperuricemia." *Am J Transl Res* 12:3167-3181.

Liu L, Lou S, Xu K, Meng Z, Zhang Q, Song K. 2013. "Relationship between lifestyle choice and hyperuricemia in Chinese men and women." *Clin Rheumatol* 32:233-239.

Liu Y, Xia Y, Wu Q, Chang Q, Zhao Y. 2021. "Associations between serum vitamins and serum uric acid in a population of Shenyang, China." *J Nutr Sci Vitaminol* 67:77-83.

Major TJ, Topless RK, Dalbeth N, Merriman TR. 2018. "Evaluation of the diet wide contribution to serum urate levels: meta-analysis of population based cohorts." *BMJ* 363: k3951.

Mikanagi K. 1963. "Gout in Japan." T*he Kyosai Medical Journal* 12:14-37.

National Institute of Health and Nutrition. 2023. "Nutrient intake survey." Accessed July 9. www.nibiohn.go.jp/eiken/kenkounippon21/eiyouchousa/keinen_henka_time.html.

Nishioka K, Mikanagi K, Hirose K. 1974. "Clinical study of gout and hyperuricemia: Epidemiology and pathogenesis." *Rheum* 14:95-105.

Oshima Y. 1965. "Clinical studies on Japanese gout." *J Jpn Soc Int Med* 54:291-310.

Poole R, Kennedy OJ, Roderick P, Fallowfield JA, Hayes PC, Parkes J. 2017. "Coffee consumption and health: umbrella review of meta-analyses of multiple health outcomes." *BMJ* 359: j5024.

Richette P, Doherty M, Pascual E, Barskova V, Becce F, Castaneda-Sanabria J, Coyfish M, Guillo S, Jansen TL, Jansens H, Lioté F, Mallen C, Nuki G, Perez-Ruiz F, Pimentao J, Punzi L, Pywell T, So A, Tausche AK, Uhlig T, Zavada J, Zhang W, Tubach F, Bardin T. 2017. "2016 updated EULAR evidence-based recommendations for the management of gout." *Ann Rheum Dis* 76:29-42.

Roman YM. 2019. "Perspectives on the epidemiology of gout and hyperuricemia." *Hawaii J Med Public Health* 78:71-76.

Saag KG, Choi HK. 2006. "Epidemiology, risk factors, and lifestyle modifications for gout." *Arthritis Res Ther* 8 (suppl 1): S2.

Sun SZ, Empie MW. 2012. "Fructose metabolism in humans-what isotopic tracer studies tell us." *Nutr Metab* 9:89.

Tani Y, Asakura K, Sasaki S, Hirota N, Notsu A, Todoriki H, Miura A, Fukui M, Date C. 2015. "The influence of season and air temperature on water intake by food groups in a sample of free-living Japanese adults." *Eur J Clin Nutr* 69:907-913.

Tappy L, Morio B, Azzout-Mamiche D, Champ M, Gerber M, Houdart S, Mas E, Rizkalia S, Slama G, Mariotti F, Margaritis I. 2018. "French recommendations for sugar intake in adults: a novel approach chosen by ANSES." *Nutrients* 10:989.

Terkeltaub R, Edwards NL. 2013. *Gout; Diagnosis and management of gouty arthritis and hyperuricemia.* (Terkeltaub R, Edwards NL., eds.) vol.3. NY: Professional Communications, Inc.

The Council for Science and Technology, Ministry of Education, Culture, Sports, Science and Technology in Japan. 2023. "Standard tables of food composition in Japan -2020- (Eighth Revised Edition), Report of the Subdivision Resources." Accessed April 28. https://www.mext.go.jp/content/20201225-mxt_kagsei-mext_01110_011.pdf.

The Ministry of Agriculture, Forestry and Fisheries. 2020. "Japanese food culture textbook." Accessed July 8. https://www.maff.go.jp/j/keikaku/syokubunka/culture/eiyo.html.

The Ministry of Agriculture, Forestry and Fisheries. 2020. "WASHOKU, traditional dietary cultures of the Japanese." Accessed July 8. https://www.maff.go.jp/e/japan_food/washoku/pdf/wasyoku_english.pdf.

The Ministry of Health, Labour and Welfare. Health Service Bureau. 2020. "National Health and Nutrition Survey Japan, 1946-2017." Accessed July 8. https://www.mhlw.go.jp/bunya/kenkou/kenkou_eiyou_chousa.html.

The Ministry of Health, Labour and Welfare. Household Statistics Office. 2023. "Comprehensive Survey of Living Conditions, 2022." Accessed July 8. https://www.e-stat.go.jp/stat-search/files?page=1&layout=datalist&toukei=00450061&tstat=000001206248&cycle=7&tclass1=000001206254&tclass2val=0&metadata=1&data=1

The Ministry of Health, Labour and Welfare and Ministry of Agriculture, Forestry and Fisheries. 2023. "Japanese Food Guide Spinning Top, Tokyo." Accessed July 8. http://www.maff.go.jp/j/balance_guide/b_sizai/attach/pdf/index-56.pdf.

The Ministry of Health, Labour and Welfare, Japan. 2023. "Dietary Reference Intakes for Japanese, 2020." Accessed July 15. https://www.mhlw.go.jp/file/06-Seisakujouhou-10900000-Kenkoukyoku/Overview.pdf.

Tomita M, Mizuno M. 2006. "Is hyperuricemia increasing? Focusing on gender difference." *Gout Nucleic Acid Metabol* 30:1-5.

Tsuduki T. 2019. "The Japanese diet that is effective for health maintenance." *J Integr Stud Diet Habits* 30:71-78 (in Japanese).

U.S. Department of Agriculture. 2023. "Dietary Guidelines for Americans 2015-2020, eighth edition." Accessed April 28. https://health.gov/sites/default/files/2019-09/2015-2020_Dietary_Guidelines.pdf

U.S. Department of Health & Human Services. National Institutes of Health. Office of Dietary Supplements. 2023. "Dietary Supplement Fact Sheets." Accessed April 28. https://ods.od.nih.gov/factsheets/list-all/

World Health Organization, Food and Agriculture Organization, and United Nations University. 2007. "Protein and amino acid requirements in human nutrition." *Tech Rep Ser* 935.

World Health Organization. 2007. "*Prevention of cardiovascular disease. Guidelines for assessment and management of cardiovascular risk.*" Geneva, Switzerland: WHO Press.

World Health Organization. 2015. *Guideline: Sugars intake for adults and children.* Geneva, Switzerland: WHO Press.

World Health Organization 2023. "Healthy diet." Accessed April 28. https://www.who.int/news-room/fact-sheets/detail/healthy-diet

Yahfoufi N, Alsadi N, Jambi M, Matar C. 2018. "The immunomodulatory and anti-inflammatory role of polyphenols." *Nutrients* 10:1618.

Yamanaka H, Sakuyama R, Watanabe J, Kamatani N, Kashiwazaki S. 1994. "Gout in females and in younger ages-current view-." *Hyperuricemia and gout* 2:23-30 (in Japanese).

Yanagimoto M. 2004. "Statistical analysis of the direction in which the food consumption pattern in Japan was advancing." *Nippon Shokuhin Kagaku Kogaku Kaishi* 51:524-530 (in Japanese).

Yoon J-H, Baek SJ. 2005. "Molecular targets of dietary polyphenols with anti-inflammatory properties." *Yonsei Med J* 46:585-596.

Zhang M, Ye C, Wang R., Zhang Z, Huang X, Halimulati M, Sun M, Ma Y, Zhang Z. 2023. "Association between dietary acid load and hyperuricemia in Chinese adults: Analysis of the China Health and Nutrition Survey (2009)." *Nutrients* 15:1806.

Zhu JN, Qi XY, Tan Y, Lyu XH. 2016. "Dietary factors associated with hyperuricemia and glycolipid metabolism disorder in middle-aged and elderly people." *Sichuan Da Xue Xue Bao Yi Xue Ban* 47:68-72.

Zykova SN, Storhaug HM, Toft I, Chadban SJ, Jenssen TG, White SL. 2015. "Cross-sectional analysis of nutrition and serum uric acid in two Caucasian cohorts: the AusDiab Study and the Tromsø study." *Nutr J* 14:49.

Chapter 2

Foods and Dietary Patterns for the Prevention and Management of Hyperuricemia

Takashi Koguchi*, **PhD**

Department of Human Education, Kokugakuin Tochigi Junior College, Tochigi-shi, Tochigi, Japan

Abstract

A high serum uric acid (SUA) concentration (hyperuricemia) is frequently associated with gout. Hyperuricemia is associated with a higher prevalence of comorbidities (e.g., chronic kidney disease, obesity, hypertension, diabetes mellitus and cardiovascular disease) compared to subjects with a normal serum uric acid (SUA) level. Taking into account the Acceptable Macronutrient Distribution Ranges (AMDRs), the Adequate Intakes (AIs), the Recommended Dietary Allowances (RDAs), the Tolerable Upper Intake Level (UL) of dietary reference intakes for nutrients set by the Institute of Medicine of the National Academy of Sciences in the U.S., diet and dietary patterns for the prevention of hyperuricemia referencing the results of clinical research reported are suggested as follows: choice and intake foods containing nutrients which decrease SUA concentration; avoidance of purine-rich diet, a dietary urate index dietary pattern, uric acid-prone dietary pattern, animal foods dietary pattern, and the Western diet; encourage low-fat diet or low-carbohydrate diet in individuals with hyperuricemia, high-protein diet in individuals with hyperlipidemia, calorie restricted diet (40% carbohydrate including whole grains, 30% protein, and 30% fat) in gout patients, purine-low diet, high-protein, low-carbohydrate without calorie restriction (Atkins diet) in overweight or obese participants, high fruit and soybean products diet in individuals with hyperuricemia, less

* Corresponding Author's Email: echo130@nifty.com.

In: Hyperuricemia
Editor: Warren Y. Salinas
ISBN: 979-8-89113-239-9

protein-rich and more vegetable/fruit-rich materials diet, soybean products and fruit dietary pattern, polyphenol-rich dietary pattern, higher adherence to the Mediterranean diet (the traditional Mediterranean diet) and its dietary pattern, higher adherence to the Dietary Approaches to Stop Hypertension (DASH) diet and its dietary pattern, and plant-based diet. The healthy dietary patterns (e.g., the Mediterranean diet, the DASH diet, plant-based diet) are associated with a significantly lower risk for gout and hyperuricemia-associated comorbidities. This review describes the importance of diet and proper choice of foods to control serum uric acid concentration for the prevention and management of hyperuricemia.

Keywords: cardiovascular disease, chronic kidney disease, DASH diet, diabetes mellitus, food, gout, hypertension, hyperuricemia, hyperuricemia-associated comorbidities, Mediterranean diet, obesity, plant-based diet, purine, uric acid

Introduction

A high serum uric acid (SUA) concentration (hyperuricemia) is frequently associated with gout (Khanna et al. 2012) and is a risk factor for gout (as uratosis) (Saag and Choi 2006; Hisatome et al. 2018; Cabău et al. 2020; Li, Zhang and Zeng 2020). Hyperuricemia is considered the precursor of gout (Choi, Mount and Reginato 2005; Saag and Choi 2006). Hyperuricemia is the main factor that leads to long-term systemic inflammation in patients with gout (Cabău et al. 2020). High SUA levels and joint pain are caused by problems with the body's immune response (Cabău et al. 2020; Joosten et al. 2020). Asymptomatic hyperuricemia induced by urate can contribute to the development of obesity, chronic kidney disease (CKD), diabetes mellitus, and hypertension by stimulating inflammation (Joosten et al. 2020). The prevalence of hyperuricemia and its complications has caused a heavy economic burden on society and families (Joosten et al. 2020).

The incidence of hyperuricemia and gout may be related to changes in lifestyle, such as the prevalence of a high-purine diet, fructose beverages, and alcohol consumption (Jakše et al. 2019; Yokose, McCormick and Choi 2021). The Japanese Society of Gout and Uric & Nucleic Acids has stated that hyperuricemia is recognized as a lifestyle-related disease and an increase in hyperuricemia and gout patients is attributed to changes in environmental factors (e.g., purine intake, fructose intake, meat and visceral intake, alcohol consumption, strenuous muscle exercise, stress, obesity) rather than genetic factors (Hisatome et al. 2018). Compared to people who do not have hyperuricemia, the diet of individuals with hyperuricemia included a higher intake of meat, seafood (fish and shellfish), beer and wine and a lower intake of carbohydrates (Miao et al. 2008). Higher fiber intakes are usually associated with healthier diets (higher fruit and vegetable intake) and lifestyle (Sun et al. 2010). The following dietary changes could explain the decrease in the prevalence of hyperuricemia in Taiwan (Pan et al. 2011): an increased avoidance of products made from animal fats; increased use of vegetable oil; increase in the intake of fruit and vegetables, soy products, fish, whole grains, nuts and seeds; and decrease in the intake of red meat, carbohydrates and sodium-containing foods.

Choosing and eating foods containing nutrients which decrease SUA concentration can lead to the prevention and management of hyperuricemia. In the previous chapter, dietary nutrient intake for the prevention and management of hyperuricemia in the general population (especially adults) is suggested as follows: the percentage of carbohydrate, protein, fat, and n-3 polyunsaturated fatty acids and n-6 polyunsaturated fatty acids in total energy intake should be within the range of the Acceptable Macronutrient Distribution Ranges (AMDRs) set by the Institute of Medicine of the National Academy of Sciences in the U.S. They include: paying attention to the intake of total sugars [maximum limit to the intake of 100 g/day (Tappy et al., 2018)]; limiting or decreasing intake of fructose, animal fats, saturated fatty acids, cholesterol, and salt; replacement of saturated fatty acids (e.g., dairy fats, meat fat) with mono- and polyunsaturated fatty acids (particularly n-3 polyunsaturated fatty acids) (e.g., macadamia nuts, almonds, peanuts and peanut butter, olive oil, canola oil, avocados); maintenance of good hydration; limiting or decreasing alcohol consumption; limiting intake of purine; paying attention to the intake of vitamin A, vitamin B_5 (pantothenic acid), and folate to avoid high serum vitamin A, vitamin B_5 (pantothenic acid), and vitamin B_9 levels, respectively; paying attention to vitamin D intake to avoid vitamin D deficiency; and recognizing encouraged intake of fiber, animal sources of protein (e.g., casein, lactalbumin), vegetable sources of protein (e.g., wheat gluten, rice endosperm protein), polyphenol, vitamin E, vitamin B_1;, vitamin B_2, folate, vitamin B_{12}, vitamin C, calcium, magnesium, iron, and zinc. It is necessary to recognize what food intake is important as potential dietary habits are critical in preventing hyperuricemia in the general population (especially adults).

This article describes what foods should be chosen in a proper diet or dietary pattern to control SUA concentrations for the prevention and management of hyperuricemia in the general population (especially adults) referencing the results of reported clinical research.

Hyperuricemia-Associated Comorbidities

Hyperuricemia is a risk factor for chronic kidney disease (CKD) (Japanese Society of Nephrology 2012, 145; Hisatome et al. 2018). Asymptomatic hyperuricemia is a biomarker of both increased risk for and presence of vascular disease (e.g., hypertension, coronary artery disease, kidney disease). It may also have certain causal effects on vascular disease, hypertension, and the progression of CKD (Feig, Kang and Johnson 2008). In the U.S. National Health and Nutrition Examination Survey (NHANES) 2007-2008, the comorbidities of individuals with hyperuricemia, gout, or both hyperuricemia and gout were hypertension, CKD, obesity (body mass index: BMI $\geq$ 30 kg/m^2), diabetes mellitus, nephrolithiasis, and cardiovascular disease (CVD)(i.e., myocardial infarction, heart failure, stroke), though the prevalence of the comorbidities of gout are different from those of hyperuricemia or both hyperuricemia and gout (Zhu, Pandya and Choi 2012). Prevention of hyperuricemia and/or gout should consider the effects of CKD, urolithiasis, obesity, diabetes mellitus, hypertension, and CVD, which are comorbidities of hyperuricemia and/or gout. Li et al. (Li, Zhang and Zeng 2020) have stated that it is currently unclear that there is a causal relationship between hyperuricemia and multiple comorbidities such as acute and chronic kidney disease, diabetes mellitus, metabolic syndrome, CVD, hypertension, and dyslipidemia. Some studies have reported that hyperuricemia has been associated with an increased risk of some diseases related to oxidative stress, such as obesity (Ogura et al. 2004), metabolic syndrome (Yoo et al. 2005), and CVD (Okura et al. 2009).

Sattui et al. (Sattui, Singh and Gaffo 2014) have summarized an update on evidence, experimental, epidemiological and clinical intervention trials, describing associations between hyperuricemia and several comorbidities. To discuss evidence on the association and causality with hyperuricemia, they (Sattui, Singh and Gaffo 2014) took up hypertension, coronary heart disease (CHD), congestive heart failure, stroke, CKD, insulin resistance and metabolic syndrome, type 2 diabetes mellitus, neuro-degenerative disorders as comorbidities. Hyperuricemia often precedes the development of obesity, diabetes, and hypertension (Richette and Bardin 2010). The role of diet which decreases SUA concentration may provide a strategy to treat hyperuricemia associated diseases, such as gout, CKD, hyperlipidemia, hypertension, CHD, and diabetes mellitus. Therefore, it is thought that the prevention and management of hyperuricemia by dietary control are very important for healthy subjects and for individuals with or without comorbidities of hyperuricemia.

Association between Foods and Plasma Uric Acid Concentrations, Serum Uric Acid Concentrations or Hyperuricemia Risk

The Institute of Medicine of the National Academy of Sciences in the U.S. (2021) has set Dietary Reference Intakes values: the Estimated Average Requirement (EAR), the Recommended Dietary Allowance (RDA), the Adequate Intake (AI), the Tolerable Upper Intake Level (UL), the Acceptable Macronutrient Distribution Ranges (AMDRs) for vitamins, minerals, macronutrients, and energy in life stage and gender groups.

Recognizing dietary patterns, adopting choice and moderate intakes of serum uric acid (SUA)-lowering foods is important for the prevention and management of hyperuricemia. Based on the results of clinical research (clinical trials and epidemiological studies), the association between dietary nutrients, foods or dietary patterns and hyperuricemia were reviewed in detail by Koguchi (2018; 2021; 2022).

Meat

Meat intake increased plasma uric acid (PUA) or serum uric acid (SUA) concentrations in normal human subjects (Brulé, Sarwar and Savoie 1992). Consumption of red meat should be low, because limiting the intake of red meat would reduce SUA levels (Zhu, Pandya and Choi 2011).

In epidemiological studies, increased meat intake was associated with increased SUA concentrations (Loenen et al. 1990; Choi, Liu and Curhan 2005; Haldar et al. 2007; Williams 2008; Chuang et al. 2011; Kontogianni et al. 2012; Zgaga et al. 2012; Zykova et al. 2015; Major et al. 2018; Xia et al. 2020;) and hyperuricemia risk (Choi, Liu and Curhan 2005; Sigie et al. 2005; Yu et al. 2008; Guasch-Ferré et al. 2013; Desideri, Puig and Richette 2015; Zhu et al. 2016; Li, Yu and Li 2018; Han et al. 2019).

Red meat, which is the main source of saturated fatty acids, was positively associated with insulin resistance (Feskens and Kromhout 1990) and reduced renal UA excretion (Facchini et al. 1991; Muscelli et al. 1996; Ter Maaten et al. 1997). It is speculated that an increase in SUA levels is attributed to the amounts of purines and saturated fatty acids.

The PREvención con DIeta MEDiterránea (PREDIMED) study in elderly participants at high cardiovascular risk in Spain revealed that the consumption of less than 1 serving a day of red meat or processed meat compared with higher intake was associated with a 23% reduced risk of hyperuricemia and the results showed a positive association between the high consumption of red meat or processed meat and the risk of hyperuricemia (Guasch-Ferré et al. 2013).

In epidemiological studies, increased intake of organ meats was associated with increased SUA concentration (Chuang et al. 2011) and hyperuricemia risk (Yu et al. 2008). Poultry intake has been associated with hyperuricemia risk in two epidemiological studies (Chang 2011; Zhu et al. 2016). Whereas one epidemiological study has found no association of poultry intake with hyperuricemia risk (Villegas et al. 2012). The difference in the results for the frequency of hyperuricemia may be due to the type and location of meat, the content of nutrients contained in the meat (especially fatty acids and purines).

The National Health and Medical Research Council (NHMRC), the Australian Government's Australian Guide to Healthy Eating, Eat for Health, Australian Dietary Guidelines, 2013 (2023) all have stated that a maximum of 455 g per week [one serve (65 g) per day] of lean meats is recommended for Australian adults aged $\geq$ 19 years.

Hisatome et al. (2018) have recommended that the intake of meat (beef, pork, chicken, sheep meat) and giblets for one meal (serving) are 80 g and 40 g, respectively. Terkeltaub and Edwards (2013, 143-156) have stated that meat (beef, pork, and lamb) consumption for hyperuricemia and gout patients is $\leq$6 oz (170.10 g) per day as a starting point.

Seafood

Fish intake increased plasma uric acid (PUA) or serum uric acid (SUA) concentrations in normal human subjects (Brulé, Sarwar and Savoie 1992). In epidemiological studies, increased intake of seafood (including fish and shellfish) was associated with increased SUA concentrations (Loenen et al. 1990; Choi, Liu and Curhan 2005; Haldar et al. 2007; Xia et al. 2020) and hyperuricemia risk (Choi, Liu and Curhan 2005; Yu et al. 2010; Chang 2011; Villegas et al. 2012; Guasch-Ferré et al. 2013; Xiong et al. 2013; Desideri, Puig and Richette 2015; Ren et al. 2016; Li, Yu and Li 2018; Han et al. 2019;).

Hisatome et al. (2018) have recommended that the intake of fish, shellfish, prawn and shrimp, and crab per one serving should be 80 g, ≤60 g, ≤50 g, and 100g, respectively. Terkeltaub and Edwards (2013, 143-156) have recommended that seafood (especially, shellfish and crustaceans) consumption for hyperuricemia and gout patients should be ≤6 oz (170.10 g) per day as a starting point.

Eggs

Eggs contain vitamin A, vitamin D, vitamin B_1, pantothenic acid, folate, phosphorus, and iron (The Council for Science and Technology, Ministry of Education, Culture, Sports, Science and Technology in Japan 2023; U.S. Department of Health & Human Services. National Institutes of Health. Office of Dietary Supplements 2023).

In epidemiological studies, increased egg intake was associated with decreased serum uric acid (SUA) concentrations (Chuang et al. 2011; Major et al. 2018) and hyperuricemia risk (Chang 2011).

Dairy Products

Dairy products (i.e., milk, cheese, yogurt, ice cream) contain vitamin A, vitamin D, vitamin B_1, vitamin B_2, vitamin B_6, pantothenic acid, folic acid, calcium, magnesium, phosphorus, iron, and zinc (The Council for Science and Technology, Ministry of Education, Culture, Sports, Science and Technology in Japan 2023; U.S. Department of Health & Human Services. National Institutes of Health. Office of Dietary Supplements 2023). Dairy products are low in purine (Kaneko et al. 2014; Hisatome et al. 2018).

In clinical trials, milk (Dalbeth et al. 2010) and dairy products (Ghadirian et al. 1995; Carabin et al. 2009; Dalbeth et al. 2010; Dalbeth and Palmano 2011; Hunter et al. 2012) decreased serum uric acid (SUA) concentrations. In a randomized controlled trial, ingestion of a dairy-free diet for 4 weeks markedly increased SUA concentrations (Ghadirian et al. 1995).

In epidemiological studies, increased intake of dairy products was associated with decreased SUA concentrations (Loenen et al. 1990; Choi, Liu and Curhan 2005; Chuang et al. 2011; Dalbeth and Palmano 2011;

Kontogianni et al. 2012; Zgaga et al. 2012; Zykova et al. 2015; Beydoun et al. 2018; Major et al. 2018) and hyperuricemia risk (Choi, Liu and Curhan 2005; Chuang et al. 2011; Nickolai and Kiss 2016; Beydoun et al. 2018; Li, Yu and Li 2018; Mena-Sánchez et al. 2020). The cross-sectional and short-term intervention studies of healthy subjects have demonstrated that the intake of low-fat dairy products has a moderate urate-lowering effect (Dalbeth and Palmano 2011).

The ingestion of milk proteins (casein, lactalbumin) and orotic acid has been shown to exert a uricosuric effect in healthy subjects (Moi et al. 2014). Ingested milk promotes renal oxypurine excretion, thereby reducing the availability of precursor substrates necessary for urate production (Garrel et al. 1991; Ghadirian et al. 1995; Dalbeth et al. 2010).

Terkeltaub and Edwards (2013, 143-156) recommend consuming 2 servings per day of nonfat or low-fat yogurt or milk. Choi (2010) recommends consuming skim milk or other low-fat dairy products up to two servings daily. The Ministry of Health, Labour and Welfare in Japan (2023) has recommended that the daily dairy product intake must be 130 g or more. The Dietary guidelines for Japanese (The Japanese food guide spinning top) has recommended that the daily consumption of milk and milk products must be 2-3 servings (milk: approximately 100 g/serving; yogurt: approximately 83 g/serving; cheese: approximately 20 g/serving), depending on an individual's caloric intake (The Ministry of Health, Labour and Welfare and Ministry of Agriculture, Forestry and Fisheries 2023). The recommended amount of dairy in the Healthy U.S.-Style Eating Pattern at 2,000-calorie level is 3 cup-equivalents of dairy per day for adults (U.S. Department of Agriculture 2023). National Health and Medical Research Council (NHMRC), Australian Government's Australian Guide to Healthy Eating, Eat for Health, Australian Dietary Guidelines, 2013 (2023) have stated that consuming at least two and a half servings of milk, cheese, yogurt and/or alternatives, mostly reduced fat, is recommended for Australian adults aged $\geq$ 19 years.

Beverages

Sugar-Sweetened Beverages

Consumption of sugar-sweetened beverages, a major source of fructose, has risen sharply in recent decades all over the world (Basu et al. 2013). The predominant sources of fructose in the diet are nonalcoholic beverages, which occupy 46% of total fructose intake (Marriott, Cole and Lee 2009).

In a randomized controlled trial, consumption of soft drinks (600 mL) increased plasma UA (PUA) concentrations by 17 μmol/L at 60 min compared with the glucose control beverages (600 mL) (Carran et al. 2016). A randomized controlled trial in overweight and obese subjects for 6 months showed that consumption of sucrose-sweetened soft drinks increased PUA concentrations compared with isocaloric milk, diet cola and water (Bruun et al. 2015). A pilot study in healthy, overweight women for 2 weeks revealed that the area under the curve (AUC) within 16 h (16h-AUC) for PUA concentrations was increased in subjects consuming sucrose-sweetened beverages compared with the baseline (before consuming sucrose-sweetened beverages) (Price et al. 2021). A pilot study in patients with chronic kidney disease (CKD), type 2 diabetes without CKD, and in healthy subjects indicated that fructose drink (35 g fructose) increased postprandial serum uric acid (SUA) concentrations compared with the baseline (before consuming fructose drink) (Olfsson et al. 2019).

In epidemiological studies, increased intake of sugar-sweetened beverages was associated with increased SUA concentrations (Choi et al. 2008; Nguyen et al. 2009; Chuang et al. 2011; Kontogianni et al. 2012; Zgaga et al. 2012; Merriman, Dalbeth N, Johnson 2014; Major et al. 2018; Xia et al. 2020; Ebrahimpour-Koujan et al. 2021; Siqueira et al. 2021) and hyperuricemia risk (Choi et al. 2008; Desideri, Puig JG, Richette 2015; Ebrahimpour-Koujan et al. 2020; Siqueira et al. 2021). Consumption of sugary beverages is low, because limiting the intake of sugary beverages would reduce SUA levels (Zhu et al., 2011). The meta-analysis conducted by Ebrahimpour-koujan et al. (2020) have found that sugar-sweetened beverages consumption is significantly associated with an increased risk of hyperuricemia in adult population.

Coffee and Tea

In epidemiological studies, increased intake of coffee was associated with decreased serum uric acid (SUA) concentrations (Kiyohara et al. 1999; Choi and Curhan 2007; Pham et al. 2010; Chuang et al. 2011) and hyperuricemia risk (Kiyohara et al. 1999; Choi and Curhan 2007; Pham et al. 2010; Nickolai and Kiss 2016; Li, Yu and Li 2018). Choi and Curhan (2007) have stated the view that it is important to note that daily intake of at least 4 cups of coffee was linked with mean SUA level reduction of only 0.18-0.22 mg/dL. From the viewpoint of the prevention and suppression of hyperuricemia, drinking 1-4 cups of coffee or decaffeinated coffee per day appear to be beneficial. Poole et al. (2017) have stated that the daily coffee consumption is three to four cups.

The intake of green tea (Panza et al. 2008) and black tea (Bahorun et al. 2010) decreased serum uric acid (SUA) concentrations. In epidemiological studies, an increased intake of green tea was associated with increased SUA concentrations (Teng et al. 2013) but an increased intake of tea drunk by Chinese adults was associated with decreased hyperuricemia risk (Yu et al. 2010; Li et al. 2015). However, a systematic review and meta-analysis conducted by Zhang et al. (2017) have found that tea consumption does not seem to be associated with SUA levels and hyperuricemia risk. It seems that the effect of tea on SUA concentration and hyperuricemia risk varies depending on the type of tea and needs to be evaluated in the future.

The proposed mechanisms of higher coffee and tea intake associated with lower SUA levels and reduced hyperuricemia risk are presumed to involve the following three factors: (1) soluble dietary fiber suppresses the digestion and/or absorption of dietary purines in rats (Koguchi et al. 2002; Koguchi et al. 2003; Koguchi et al. 2004; Koguchi 2018; Koguchi and Tadokoro 2019); (2) antioxidants, such as the phenol chlorogenic acid in coffee, the catechin in green tea, and the theaflavin in black tea, may reduce SUA concentrations by inhibition of xanthine oxidase activity (Pérez-Jiménez 2010; Chen et al. 2015); (3) caffeine (1,3,7-trimethyl xanthine) may inhibit xanthine oxidase activity (Kela, Vijayvargiya and Trivedi 1980) and enhance renal uric acid (UA) excretion (Tsai et al. 2012). The European Food Safety Authority (EFSA) (2015) has recommended that the maximum daily intake of caffeine in healthy adults, except pregnant women, is 400 mg. It is imperative to drink coffee and/or tea, taking into account the daily caffeine intake.

Alcoholic Beverages

Alcoholic beverage consumption increased plasma uric acid (PUA) or serum uric acid (SUA) concentrations (van der Gaag et al. 2000; Choi et al. 2004; Choi and Curhan 2004; Yamamoto et al. 2004). In epidemiological studies, increased consumption of alcoholic beverages was associated with increased SUA concentrations (Choi et al. 2004; Choi and Curhan 2004; Williams 2008; Zykova et al. 2015; Major et al. 2018) and hyperuricemia risk (Yu et al. 2008; Villegas et al. 2012).

The above clinical research (clinical trials and epidemiological studies) showed that the degree of increase in SUA concentrations and hyperuricemia risk varied according to the type of alcohol beverage. In the epidemiological studies, Choi and Curhan (2004) found that SUA levels significantly increased with increasing beer or liquor intake, but not with wine, and SUA levels decreased with increasing wine intake except for the top category (≥ 1 serving per day). Zykova et al. (2015) observed that the highest consumers of beer and spirits had significantly higher SUA levels in both the AusDiab Study and the Tromsø study cohorts, however the highest consumers of wine in the AusDiab Study cohort had significantly lower SUA levels (> 10 g alcohol per day versus non-drinkers). Clinical studies showed that the degree of increase in SUA concentration by the same amount of alcohol intake was beer (15%) > red wine (9%) > spirits (8%) (van der Gaag et al. 2000). The amounts of purines contained in the alcoholic beverages was beer > wine > spirits (Kaneko et al. 2014; Hisatome et al. 2018). Purines contained in alcoholic beverages contribute to an increase in plasma UA concentration (Yamamoto et al. 2005). It is assumed that SUA concentrations are associated with the amounts of purines in alcoholic beverages.

Villegas et al. (2012) found that the consumption of alcoholic drinks (wine, beer, and liquor) was associated with a higher prevalence of hyperuricemia in Shanghai men and the prevalence of hyperuricemia was beer > wine (grape and rice) > liquor, in the case of consumption of greater than 3 drink a day [ethanol: beer, ≥ 37.8g; wine ≥ 36.9g; liquir, ≥ 38.7g]. In a cross-sectional and prospective analysis in 4,449 elderly participants at high cardiovascular risk from the PREvención con DIeta MEDiterránea (PREDIMED) study in Spain, consumption of greater than or equal to 7 glasses a week of wine was associated with a 21% increased risk of hyperuricemia (Guasch-Ferré et al. 2013).

In the case of men who consumed 10 g alcohol a day, the increase in SUA concentration was higher with beer than wine (Williams 2008). In the case of moderate wine consumption, polyphenols in wine confer a protective effect against hyperuricemia, apart from its antioxidant effect. Chrysohoou et al. (2003) reported that the most beneficial values of biochemical and clinical parameters were found with alcohol intake of 100-200 mL (12% alcohol), even after adjustment for various potential cofounders. Terkeltaub and Edwards (2013, 143-156) have stated that all forms of alcohol promote hyperuricemia and an ideal amount of alcohol intake for patients with hyperuricemia and gout is one drink per day and ≤ 2 servings in a 24-hour period.

Grains

A novel rice-derived peptide which was isolated and identified from the extract of shelled fruits of the Oryza sativa, it suppressed SUA concentrations via suppressing xanthine oxidase activity and alleviated renal damage through inhibiting the activation of the nucleotide-binding and oligomerization domain-like receptor, leucine-rich repeat and pyrin domain-containing 3 (NLRP3) inflammasome in hyperuricemic mice (Liu et al. 2020).

In a randomized, crossover clinical trial in adult male subjects with risk factors for metabolic syndrome for 4 weeks, the intake of rice endosperm protein (10 g/day) significantly decreased SUA concentrations compared with the casein group or the baseline (Hosojima et al. 2016). An increase in the intake of rice is important for a decrease in SUA concentrations.

In epidemiological studies, increased intake of bread and/or margarine (including low-fat margarine, i.e., 40% fat) (Loenen et al. 1990; Major et al. 2018), high-fiber bread (Zykova et al. 2015; Major et al. 2018), and cereals (Zykova et al. 2015; Major et al. 2018) were associated with decreased SUA concentrations.

The Australian Dietary Guidelines (2023) have proposed that the general recommended minimal intake of grain foods is 6 servings per day for a healthy 70-kg man. The recommended amount of grains in the Healthy U.S.-Style Eating Pattern at the 2,000 calorie level is 6 oz equivalents of grains per day (U.S. Department of Agriculture 2023). National Health and Medical Research Council (NHMRC), the Australian Government's Australian Guide to Healthy Eating, Eat for Health, Australian Dietary Guidelines, 2013 (2023) have stated that consuming at least four to six servings of grain (cereal) foods, mostly wholegrain and/or cereal fiber varieties per day is recommended for Australian adults aged ≥ 19 years.

Mushrooms

In a review reported by Kozarski et al. (2016), they have stated that edible mushrooms have been related to significant antioxidant properties due to their bioactive compounds, such as polyphenols, polysaccharides, vitamins (vitamin C, E, A), carotenoids and minerals (zinc, copper, manganese, iron, selenium). Anti-inflammatory and antioxidant properties of edible mushrooms were highlighted by Muszyńska et al. (2018).

Though mushrooms, excluding shiitake mushrooms, king trumpet mushrooms, and nameko mushrooms are high in purine, increased mushroom intake was associated with reduced serum uric acid (SUA) concentrations (Chuang et al. 2011) and decreased hyperuricemia risk (Yu et al. 2008; Zhang et al. 2021).

Seaweed

Seaweed contains dietary fiber, vitamin A, vitamin B_2, vitamin B_6, folate, vitamin C, magnesium, iron, zinc, and purines.

Though seaweed (e.g., nori, wakame) are high in purine, increased seaweed intake was associated with decreased serum uric acid (SUA) concentrations in the Nutrition and Health Survey in Taiwan (NAHSIT) study (Chuang et al. 2011).

Legumes

Common beans, broad bean seeds, soybeans and soy products (soy paste, soy bacon, soy flour, soy meat, soy tempe, tofu) contain polyphenols that suppress uric acid (UA) production by the inhibition of xanthine oxidase activity (Lin et al. 2002; INRA 2023) (Table 1).

Legumes are rich in protein, complex carbohydrates, dietary fiber, folate, flavonoids, and various micronutrients (e.g., phytochemicals) (Mozaffarian, Appel and Van Horn 2011). In epidemiological studies, increased intake of legumes was associated with decreased serum uric acid (SUA) concentrations (Chuang et al. 2011; Kontogianni et al. 2012) and hyperuricemia risk (Guasch-Ferré et al. 2013). It is speculated that legumes lower SUA levels through both the suppression of purine absorption by dietary fiber (DF) (Koguchi et al. 2002; Koguchi et al. 2003; Koguchi et al. 2004; Koguchi and Tadokoro 2019) and the inhibition of xanthine oxidase by genistein (Lin et al. 2002). Legume intake was inversely associated with serum concentrations of inflammatory biomarkers [high sensitive C-reactive protein (hs-CRP), tumor necrosis factor-alpha (TNF-α), and interleukin-6 (IL-6)] in a cross-sectional study among Iranian women (Esmaillzadeh and Azadbakht 2012). It seems that intake of legumes has a beneficial effect for SUA concentrations through anti-inflammation effect.

In a review by Messina et al. (Messina, Messina and Chan 2011), clinical studies indicated that soy foods did not markedly affect SUA levels. In a pooled analysis from two 6-month randomized controlled trials, Liu et al. (2015) found that soy intake did not increase SUA levels among Chinese postmenopausal women with prediabetes or prehypertension. In epidemiological studies, the increased intake of soy and soy products were associated with decreased hyperuricemia risk (Yu et al. 2008; Yu et al. 2010; Villegas et al. 2012; Liu et al. 2014; Li, Yu and Li 2018). Soy promotes renal oxypurine excretion, thereby reducing the availability of precursor substrates necessary for urate production (Garrel et al. 1991). Bitzer et al. (2017) have stated that soy may prevent hyperuricemia and gout through the anti-inflammatory pathway. A mouse study found that soy protein concentrates lower the nucleotide-binding and oligomerization domain-like receptor, leucine-rich repeat and pyrin domain-containing 3 (NLRP3) inflammasome and caspase-1 enzyme activity in dextran sulfate sodium-induced inflammation mice.

The recommended amount of legumes in the Healthy U.S.-Style Eating Pattern at the 2,000 calorie level is 1.5 cup-equivalents of legumes per day (U.S. Department of Agriculture 2023). The Ministry of Health, Labour and Welfare in Japan (2023) has recommended an intake of legumes of 100 g or more per day. Hisatome et al. (2018) have recommended that the intake of dried soybeans, dried adzuki beans, green soybeans, fermented soybeans, broad beans, tofu, soybean fiber, and soybean milk per one serving should be 35 g, 40 g, 40 g, 40 g, 50 g, 100 g, 100 g, and 200 g, respectively. As legumes are purine-rich foods, it is necessary to elucidate the association between the intake of legumes and SUA concentration or hyperuricemia risk by means of many large-scale prospective cohort studies and long term randomized controlled trials in the future.

Seeds and Nuts

Generally speaking, nuts are rich in unsaturated fatty acids, plant protein, dietary fiber, antioxidant vitamins (e.g., folate, vitamin E), minerals (e.g., magnesium and potassium), and phytochemicals (e.g., phenolic compounds) (Mozaffarian, Appel and Van Horn 2011).

Almonds, hazelnuts, pecan nuts, and pistachio nuts contain polyphenols that suppress uric acid (UA) production by the inhibition of xanthine oxidase activity (INRA 2023).

Walnut meal hydrolysates and dephenolized walnut meal hydrolysates decreased SUA levels and protected the renal function in potassium oxonate-induced hyperuricemic rats and inhibited xanthine oxidase activity *in vitro* (Li et al. 2018). Flaxseed suppressed the elevation of serum urea nitrogen, creatinine, and UA concentrations in rats with renal dysfunction induced by glycerol (El-Sayed et al. 2014).

Meta-analysis of cross-sectional data has found that increased intake of peanuts is associated with decreased serum uric acid (SUA) concentrations

(Major et al. 2018). In a cross-sectional study, increased intake of walnuts and pine nuts were inversely associated with decreased hyperuricemia risk (Wang et al. 2021), whereas no significant association was found between hyperuricemia risk and the intake of peanuts, melon seeds, cashews, or total nuts (Wang et al. 2021). In a cross-sectional study, nut consumption was associated with lower concentrations of circulating inflammatory molecules and adiponectin, a potent anti-inflammatory adipokine (Ros 2009). Since SUA concentrations have been associated with several inflammatory markers [neutrophil count, C-reactive protein, interleukin-1 receptor antagonist (IL-1ra), interleukin-6 (IL-6), interleukin-18 (IL-18), tumor necrosis factor-alpha (TNF-α)] in individuals with or without hyperuricemia [SUA concentration > 7.5 mg/ dL (450 μmol/L) in men and > 6.2 mg/dL (372 μmol/L) in women] (Ruggiero et al. 2006), further animal experiments, long-term follow-up studies, and randomized controlled trials will be required to evaluate the efficacy of nut intake for individuals with or without hyperuricemia.

Celery seed, aqueous extract and celery seed oil extract suppressed the elevation of SUA, xanthine oxidase, reactive oxygen species (ROS) levels and increased serum superoxide dismutase (SOD) and glutathione peroxidase (GSH-Px) in mice with hyperuricemia induced by potassium oxonate and yeast extract (Li et al. 2019). These results suggest that celery seed extracts may have anti-hyperuricemic properties, partially through an antioxidative effect.

Saag and Choi (2006) have recommended that the daily intake of nuts and legumes should be 1 to 3 servings. Schlesinger (2005) has recommended intake of nuts 1-3 times per day (13-15 g per once). The serving of almonds for human is 30g/person/day (Reagan-Shaw, Nihal and Ahmad 2008). Hisatome et al. (2018) has recommended that the intake of peanuts and almonds per one meal are 20 g and 15 g, respectively.

Fruit and Vegetables

Fruit and vegetables are a rich source of carbohydrates, dietary fiber, vitamin A (β-carotene), vitamin C, vitamin E, potassium, and magnesium (Saura-Calixto and Goñi 2009; The Council for Science and Technology, Ministry of Education, Culture, Sports, Science and Technology in Japan 2023; U.S. Department of Health & Human Services. National Institutes of Health. Office of Dietary Supplements 2023). Other important constituents are phytochemicals such as antioxidants, flavones, flavonoids, and polyphenols (Saura-Calixto and Goñi 2009).

In epidemiological studies, increased intake of fruit and vegetables was associated with decreased serum uric acid (SUA) concentrations (Chuang et al. 2011) and hyperuricemia risk (Zhu et al. 2016). In a cross-sectional study, a greater variety in fruit and vegetables intake was associated with lower inflammation (serum C-reactive protein concentration) in Puerto Rican adults (Bhupathiraju and Tucker 2011). The intake of fruit and vegetables has a beneficial effect for SUA concentrations from a point of view of an anti-inflammation effect.

The World Health Organization (2007) has recommended increasing fruits and vegetables (to 400-500 g daily) for the prevention of cardiovascular disease (CVD) in healthy adults. The World Health Organization's recommendations for a healthy diet (World Health Organization 2023) has also stated that eating at least 400 g, or five portions, of fruit and vegetables per day reduces the risk of noncommunicable diseases (NCDs), including diabetes, heart disease, stroke and cancer, and helps to ensure an adequate daily intake of dietary fiber. The Australian government (2023) has proposed that the minimum recommended number of servings of fruit per day is 2 for people aged ≥ 9 years and the minimum recommended number of servings of vegetables per day is 5-6 for people: males aged 19-50 years, 6; males aged 51-70 years, 5.5; males aged > 70 years, 5; females aged ≥ 12 years, 5. The dietary guideline in the U.S. calls for 5 to 13 servings of fruits and vegetables a day, depending on an individual's caloric intake (U.S. Department of Agriculture, 2005).

Fruit

Blackberries, black currants, black elderberries, European cranberries, apricots, grapes, fox grapes, nectarines, peaches, plums, red raspberries, sour cherries, strawberries, sweet cherries, quinces, loquats, apples, pears, and custard apples contain polyphenols that suppress uric acid (UA) production by inhibition of xanthine oxidase activity (INRA 2023).

Tart cherry (*prunus cerasus*) juice decreased serum uric acid (SUA) concentrations in rats with hyperuricemia by inhibiting the xanthine oxidase (EC 1.17.3.2)/xanthine oxidoreductase (EC1.17.1.4) activity in the liver (Haidari et al. 2009). In clinical trials, cherries and cherry products decreased SUA concentrations (Blau 1950; Martin et al. 2011; Jacob et al. 2003). In epidemiological studies, increased intake of fruit (Williams 2008;

Kontogianni et al. 2012; Zykova et al. 2015) and noncitrus fruit (Major et al. 2018) were associated with decreased SUA concentrations.

Plasma UA (PUA) concentrations in ten healthy females who consume 2 servings (280g) of Bing sweet cherries, grapes or strawberries decreased by 14.5%, 6.5% or 8.4% at 5 hours postdose, as compared with the predose baseline, respectively (Jacob et al. 2003). This result reveals that the lowering effect of cherries on PUA concentration is stronger than that of grapes or strawberries. This report suggests that cherries exert their urate-lowering effect by increasing the rate of renal glomerular filtration and/or reducing tubular reabsorption (Jacob et al. 2003). Cherries contain vitamins A, C, E, and phenolic compounds (e.g., anthocyanins and quercetin) and have antioxidant and anti-inflammatory properties (Collins, Saag and Singh 2019; Santos et al. 2021). Eating 280 g of cherries in healthy adults for 1 month had a significant reduction in blood levels of substances associated with inflammation and immune cell activity [C-reactive protein, nitric oxide, regulated upon activation, normal T-cell expressed, and secreted (RANTES)]. The anti-inflammatory effects of substances in cherries may be beneficial for the management and prevention of hyperuricemia (Kelly et al. 2006). Since the cherries have antioxidant and anti-inflammatory properties, it may play an important role in the decrease in SUA levels.

In a randomized, double-blind, placebo- and positive-controlled clinical pilot study in subjects with hyperuricemia for 24 weeks, *Terminalia chebula* or *Terminalia bellerica* significantly reduced SUA concentrations compared to the placebo group (Usharani et al. 2016). *Terminalia chebula* and *Terminalia bellerica* have antioxidant property and the probable mechanism of action of the antioxidant property is the inhibition of xanthine oxidase (Hazra et al. 2010).

There is a relatively small amount of fructose in an individual fruit and the presence of other nutrients in the fruit (e.g., fiber, vitamin C, and many important secondary metabolites) may slow fructose absorption or partially block the fructose metabolic effect of uric acid (UA) formation and inhibit superoxide generation (Jakše et al. 2019). Zou et al. (Zou, Zhao and Wang 2021) have stated that the effects of fruit components (fructose, purine, polyphenols, vitamin C, dietary fiber, and minerals) on SUA concentration and their underlying mechanisms are as follows: (1) UA synthesized by fructose and purine metabolism; (2) inhibiting xanthine oxidase; (3) reducing reabsorption of UA; and (4) improving the excretion of UA.

The Dietary Guidelines for Americans established by the U.S. Department of Agriculture (2023) recommended that the adult population aged ≥ 19 years eat fruit of 1.5 to 2.5 servings (i.e., cup or ounce equivalents) per day, depending on an individual's caloric intake. For example, the recommended amount of fruits in the Healthy U.S.-Style Eating Pattern at the 2,000-calorie level is 2 cup-equivalents of fruits per day (U.S. Department of Agriculture 2023). The Dietary Guidelines for Japanese (the Japanese food guide spinning top) has recommended that daily consumption of fruit must be 2-3 servings (approximately 200-300 g), depending on an individual's caloric intake (The Ministry of Health, Labour and Welfare and Ministry of Agriculture, Forestry and Fisheries 2023). Willett and Stampfer (2003) have stated that the intake of fruit is 2 to 3 servings among patients with hyperuricemia or gout. The healthy eating pyramid created by Saag and Choi (2006) recommends 2-3 servings of fruit daily among patients with gout and hyperuricemia. The National Health and Medical Research Council (NHMRC), Australian Government's Australian Guide to Healthy Eating, Eat for Health, Australian Dietary Guidelines, 2013 (2023) has stated that consuming at least two servings of fruit per day (150 g per serve) is recommended for Australian adults aged ≥ 19 years.

Purine-Rich Vegetables

Bamboo shoots are high in dietary fiber, 3.3 g/100 g; protein, 3.5 g/100 g; potassium, 470 mg/100 g (The Council for Science and Technology, Ministry of Education, Culture, Sports, Science and Technology in Japan 2023). Bamboo shoots are also purine-rich foods (30.8-63.3 mg/100 g) (Kaneko et al. 2014). In an epidemiological study, increased intake of bamboo shoots was associated with increased SUA concentrations (Chuang et al. 2011).

Intake of purine-rich vegetables (peas, beans, lentils, cauliflowers, and spinach) was not associated with plasma UA (PUA) concentrations in a population-based case-control study conducted in Scotland (1999-2006) (Zgaga et al. 2012). In epidemiological studies, there was no association between the intake of purine-rich vegetables (peas, beans, lentils, spinach, mushrooms, and cauliflowers) and hyperuricemia risk (Choi, Liu and Curhan 2005; Villegas et al. 2012; Li, Yu and Li 2018). This phenomenon can probably explain that the increased intake of vegetable protein and dietary fiber (DF) protect against the risk of hyperuricemia (Sun et al. 2010; Villegas et al. 2012). Hisatome et al. (2018) have recommended that intake of cauliflower, bamboo shoots, spinach and mushroom per serving should be 50 g, 50 g, 40 g, and 50 g, respectively.

Vegetables

Black olives, broad bean pods, broccoli, and globe artichokes contain polyphenols that suppress uric acid (UA) production by the inhibition of xanthine oxidase activity (INRA 2023). It seems important to choose these vegetables in order to maintain SUA concentrations at normal levels in healthy people.

In epidemiological studies, increased intake of tomatoes and tomato juice were associated with increased serum uric acid (SUA) concentrations (Flynn et al. 2015; Major et al. 2018). However, a prospective clinical trial in 35 young women showed that raw ripe tomato intake (90 g) before lunch for 4 weeks has been significantly associated with a decrease in SUA concentration with 0.16 mg/dL (Vinha et al. 2014). In a crossover study, consumption of tomato sauce (150 g) increased plasma UA (PUA) concentration by 46 μmol/L at 48 h compared with the baseline (before consuming tomato sauce) (Lee et al. 2009). The intervention study showed no significant difference in PUA or SUA concentrations after consumption of tomato sauce (Abete et al. 2013), tomato extract (Engelhard, Gazer and Paran 2006) or tomato juice (Jacob et al. 2008). These differences in outcomes may be attributed to the amount of tomato intake per week and the method of tomato preparation, which can influence the contents of chemicals that affect SUA levels.

In an epidemiological study, the increased intake of carrots was associated with decreased SUA concentrations (Chuang et al. 2011).

The increased intake of vegetables was associated with decreased hyperuricemia risk (Yu et al. 2008; Han et al. 2019). This phenomenon can probably explain why an increased intake of vegetable protein (Choi et al. 2004) and dietary fiber (Lyu et al. 2003) decreased hyperuricemia risk.

The Dietary Guidelines for Americans established by the U.S. Department of Agriculture (2023) recommended that the adult population aged ≥ 19 years eat 2.5 to 4 servings (i.e., cup or ounce equivalents) of vegetables per day, depending on an individual's caloric intake. For example, the recommended amount of vegetables in the Healthy U.S.-Style Eating Pattern at the 2,000-calorie level is 2.5 cup-equivalents of vegetables per day (U.S. Department of Agriculture 2023). The Ministry of Health, Labour and Welfare in Japan (2023) has recommended that daily consumption of vegetables must be 350 g or more (green-yellow vegetables, 120 g or more). National Health and Medical Research Council (NHMRC), Australian Government's Australian Guide to Healthy Eating, Eat for Health, Australian Dietary Guidelines, 2013 (2023) has stated that consuming at least five servings of vegetables per day (75 g per serve) is recommended for Australian adults aged ≥ 19 years.

Probiotics

DM-2918-A, which is a lactic acid bacteria isolated from Chinese sauerkraut, had the ability to degrade nucleosides (inosine and guanosine) in *in vitro* and oral administration of DM-2918-A. It suppressed elevation of serum uric acid (SUA) concentration in potassium oxonate combined with a high-purine dietinduced hyperuricemic rats (Li et al. 2014).

In UA-induced hyperuricemic mice, *Limosilactobacillus fermentum* JL-3 strain, isolated from 'Jiangshui' (a fermented Chinese food), significantly decreased serum UA, creatinine, BUN, malondialdehyde (MDA), interleukin-1β (IL-1β) levels and the amount of urinary UA excretion and interleukin-1β (IL-1β) and xanthine oxidase levels in the liver and interleukin-1β (IL-1β) levels in the kidney compared with the control group (Wu et al. 2021). *Limosilactobacillus fermentum* JL-3 strain significantly decreased relative abundance of *Bacteroidetes* in the feces and increased butyric acid concentration in the feces compared with the control group (Wu et al. 2021). These results suggest that *Limosilactobacillus fermentum* JL-3 strain has UA-lowering effect and attenuates oxidative stress and inflammation and regulates gut microbiota dysbiosis in UA-induced hyperuricemic mice (Wu et al. 2021).

Probiotic bacteria of the *Lactobacillus* and *Bifidobacterium* genera reduced inflammation and hyperuricemia in murine models (Bai, Jiang and Jiang 2014; Li et al. 2014; Chen et al. 2017).

A randomized placebo-controlled, parallel group, double-blinded study showed that SUA concentration on the dose of 2 g fermented barley extract per day for 12 weeks was lower than that on placebo group in subjects with SUA levels of 6.0-7.9 mg/dL (Hokazono et al. 2010).

The mechanism by which probiotics reduce hyperuricemia is still being studied, and is not completely understood.

Association between Diets or Dietary Patterns and Plasma Uric Acid Concentrations, Serum Uric Acid Concentrations or Hyperuricemia Risk

Diets

Low-fat Diet or Low-carbohydrate Diet

The mean SUA concentration reductions at 24 months from the baseline among individuals with hyperuricemia [SUA $\geq$ 7.0 mg/dL (416 μmol/L)] were

65 and 77 µmol/L for low-fat and low-carbohydrate diets, respectively (Yokose et al. 2020).

High-Protein Diet

High in vegetable protein (specifically, wheat gluten) protein diet (27% of total energy from protein) lowered SUA concentrations in hyperlipidemia in a randomized, crossover trial (Jenkins et al. 2001).

Purine Rich Diet and Purine Free Diet

A purine rich diet will produce a transient elevation in SUA levels by 1.0-2.0 mg/dL (59-118 µmol/L) and conversely, a purine free diet, containing the same amount of calories, taken for seven to ten days decreases SUA level by the same amount (Emmerson 1996).

A purine free diet results in an average reduction of the plasma UA concentaration of from 1.0 to 1.2 mg/dL (Gutman and Yu 1952; Seegmiller et al. 1961).

High Fruit and Soybean Products Diet

In an open randomized controlled trial in Chinese asymptomatic hyperuricemia adults for 3 months, Zhang et al. (2016) found that the standard diet (dietary guidelines for hyperuricemia) and high fruit and soybean products diet significantly decreased serum uric acid (SUA) concentrations compared with each baseline, respectively. However, no differences were observed in SUA concentrations between the standard diet and high fruit and soybean products diet (Zhang et al. 2016).

Less Protein-Rich and More Vegetable/Fruit-Rich Materials Diet

In a clinical trials, the less protein-rich and more vegetable/fruit-rich materials diet significantly decreased serum uric acid (SUA) concentrations and significantly increased urinary uric acid (UUA) excretion and uric acid (UA) clearance, compared with the protein-rich and less vegetable/fruit materials diet (Kanbara and Seyama 2011; Kanbara et al. 2012). These reports suggest that urine alkalization by eating a less protein-rich and more vegetable/fruits-rich materials diet is important and effective for promoting UA excretion (Kanbara and Seyama 2011; Kanbara et al. 2012).

Calorie Restricted Diet Composed of 40% Carbohydrate Including Whole Grains, 30% Protein, and 30% Fat

In an observational study performed by Dessein et al. (2000), thirteen non-diabetic men with gout (median age 50, range 38-62) ingested a calorie restricted diet (1,600 kcal a day) composed of 40% carbohydrate [replacement of refined carbohydrates (e.g., white flour, white rice) with complex ones (e.g., whole wheat flour, brown rice)], 30% protein, and 30% fat [replacement of saturated fats (e.g., dairy fats, meat fat) with mono- and polyunsaturated fats (e.g., macadamia nuts, almonds, peanuts and peanut butter, olive oil, canola oil, avocados)] for 16 weeks. The mean serum uric acid (SUA) concentration decreased by 18% in gout patients after four months of dietary intervention.

High-Protein, Low-Carbohydrate without Calorie Restriction (Atkins Diet)

In the dietary intervention randomized controlled trial of overweight or obese participants (body mass index (BMI) $\geq$ 27) for six months, consumption of the "Atkins diet" (i.e., high-protein diet without calorie restriction) reduced SUA levels despite substantial purine loading (Lu et al. 2014).

A Dietary Urate Index Dietary Pattern

In a large prospective cohort study, a dietary urate index was positively associated with serum uric acid (SUA) concentrations in the total population of whites and African Americans (Beydoun et al. 2018). A dietary urate index was as follows: (1) added sugars (teaspoons/d or approximately 4.2g/day); (2) alcoholic beverages (drinks/d, with one drink defined as 12 fl oz of beer, 5fl oz of wine or 1.5 fl oz of eighty-proof distilled spirits; 1 g = approximately 0.03 fl oz); (3) ounce equivalents/d of red meats (1oz = 28.3 g); (4) ounce equivalents/d of fish (sum of fish high and low in n-3 fatty acids); (5) cup equivalents/d of legumes; (6) cup equivalents/d of dairy products (milk, cheese and yogurt); (7) dietary vitamin C from foods in mg/day; and (8) caffeine from all sources (g/day) (Beydoun et al., 2018).

Uric Acid-prone Dietary Pattern

In a cross-sectional study of 266 ethnic Chinese adults in Taiwan, there was a positive association between the "uric acid-prone" (composes of meat, seafood, organ meat, eggs and beverages) dietary pattern and plasma uric acid (PUA) concentrations after adjusted for age, gender, and body mass index (BMI) (Tsai et al. 2012).

Soybean Products and Fruit Dietary Pattern

In a case-control study in Chinese adults, there was a negative association between the "soybean products and fruit" (high in soybean products, fruit, vegetables and starchy tubers) dietary pattern and the risk of asymptomatic hyperuricemia [serum uric acid (SUA) level > 7.0 mg/ dL (416.4 µmol/L) among men and > 6.0 mg/dL (356.9 µmol/L) among women], independent of blood lipids (Zhang et al. 2012).

Animal Foods Dietary Pattern

In a case-control study in Chinese adults, there was a positive association between the "animal products and fried food" (high in pork, eggs, animal giblets, poultry and fried wheat products while low in fruit and vegetables) dietary pattern and the risk of asymptomatic hyperuricemia [serum uric acid (SUA) level > 7.0 mg/ dL (416.4 µmol/L) among men and > 6.0 mg/dL (356.9 µmol/L) among women] (Zhang et al. 2012). In a case-control study in a Chinese population, the animal foods dietary pattern characterized by higher intake of an animal organ, seafood and processed meat products was associated with higher prevalence of newly diagnosed hyperuricemia (Xia et al. 2018).

The Western Diet and the Western Dietary Pattern

The Western Diet

The Western diet is characterized by high intake of red and processed meats, animal fat, beverages sweetened with sugar, sweets, desserts, french fries, and refined grains contains many foods and low intake of fresh fruit and vegetables and low-fat dairy products (Kuo et al. 2015; Kramer 2017; Rai et al. 2017).

The Western diet was associated with increased risk of gout (Kuo et al. 2015; Rai et al. 2017) and chronic kidney disease (CKD) (Hariharan, Vellanki and Kramer 2015; Kramer 2017).

The Western Dietary Pattern

The "Western" (high in beef, lamb, cake, and beverages including juice and alcoholic beverages) dietary pattern was not associated with the risk of asymptomatic hyperuricemia in a case-control study in China (Zhang et al. 2012). The increased intake of fried foods was associated with increased hyperuricemia risk (Chang 2011).

The Western dietary pattern was associated with increased risk of type 2 diabetes mellitus (van Dam et al. 2002) and coronary heart disease (CHD) (Hu et al. 2000).

The Mediterranean Diet and the Mediterranean Dietary Pattern

Higher Adherence to the Mediterranean Diet (the Traditional Mediterranean Diet)

The traditional Mediterranean diet is characterized by a high intake of fruit, vegetables, legumes, olive oil, nuts, and whole grain. There is moderate consumption of wine, dairy products, and poultry, and a low consumption of red meat, sweet beverages, creams, and pastries (Guasch-Ferré et al. 2013). Briefly, olive oil is a key component of the Mediterranean diet, being the main source of vegetable fat, especially monounsaturated fatty acids, high in whole-grain foods and fiber, and rich in fruit, vegetables, legumes, and nuts. Small portions of cheese and yogurt are eaten daily. Fish is consumed in varying amounts. Red meat, poultry, eggs, and sweets are consumed sparingly, modest amounts of red wine complement meals and regular physical activity is a part of daily life (Skerret and Willett 2010). Daily products, especially yogurt and cheese, are taken on a daily basis, while consumption of fish and poultry is recommended up to twice a week, while 4-7 eggs per week can be eaten (Stamostergiou et al. 2018; Barnaba et al. 2020).

Plasma uric acid (PUA) concentration on the consumption of the vegetable-soup "gazpacho" (500 mL/day) for 14 days was significantly lower than that at baseline (before drinking the soup) in healthy men (Sánchez-Moreno et al. 2004).

In an intervention study in patients with hyperuricemia [mean serum uric acid (SUA) concentration: 9.12 mg/dL (542.46 μmol/L)] for 6 months, the Mediterranean diet provoked a 20% reduction in serum uric acid (SUA) concentration [mean SUA concentration 6.92 mg/dL (411.6 μmol/L)] after the first month and SUA concentrations remained constant for five months [mean SUA concentration 6.1-6.4 mg/dL (362.8-380.7 μmol/L)] in patients with hyperuricemia [mean SUA concentration 9.12 mg/dL (542.5 μmol/L)] (Chatzipavlou et al. 2014). The mean SUA concentration reductions at 24 months from baseline among individuals with hyperuricemia [SUA $\geq$ 7.0 mg/dL (416 μmol/L)] was 83 μmol/L for the Mediterranean diet (Yokose et al. 2020). Higher adherence to the Mediterranean diet was associated with decreased SUA concentrations (Chrysohoou et al. 2011; Kontogianni et al. 2012;

Alkerwi et al. 2015) and a lower likelihood of hyperuricemia (Chrysohoou et al. 2011; Kontogianni et al. 2012). The Mediterranean diet has antioxidant (Bulló, Lamuela-Raventós and Salas-Salvadó 2011) and anti-inflammatory properties (Estruch et al. 2006). It is speculated that the Mediterranean diet plays a potential role for prevention and suppression of hyperuricemia.

Greater adherence to the Mediterranean diet was associated with decreased risk of renal function (Smyth et al. 2016), chronic kidney disease (CKD) (Huang et al. 2013; Hu et al. 2019), kidney stone (Rodriguez et al. 2020), obesity (Tyrovolas et al. 2009), cardiovascular disease (CVD) (Gopinath et al. 2011; Psaltopoulou et al. 2013; Kontogianni and Panagiotakos 2014; Tektonidis et al. 2015; Badimon, Chagas and Chiva-Blanch 2019), cancer (Sofi et al. 2008; Ríos-Hoyo et al. 2014), Parkinson's disease (Sofi et al. 2008), Alzheimer's disease (Sofi et al. 2008), dementia and dementia progression (Solfrizzi et al. 2017), noncontrolled asthma (Barros et al. 2008), and renal-cause mortality (Smyth et al. 2016).

The Mediterranean diet is encouraged for the prevention and/or management of type 2 diabetes mellitus (Forouhi et al. 2018; American Diabetes Association 2019).

The Mediterranean Dietary Pattern

The Mediterranean dietary pattern has health benefits. The Mediterranean dietary pattern can be characterized by the following four essential dietary indicators: (1) monounsaturated to saturated fatty acid ratio (range: 1.6 to 2.0); (2) intake of dietary fiber (41 to 62 g/person/day); (3) antioxidant capacity of the whole diet (3500 to 5300 trolox equivalent/person/day); and (4) phytosterols intake (370 to 555 mg/person/day) (Saura-Calixto and Goñi 2009).

A systematic review reported by Vedder et al. (2019) concluded that diet interventions, including low-calorie diet (but not fasting), purine-low diets, and different variations of the Mediterranean diet, were able to decrease serum uric acid (SUA) concentrations in patients with asymptomatic hyperuricemia or gout.

The Mediterranean dietary pattern was associated with a decreased risk of being overweight or obesity (Romaguera et al. 2010), all-cause mortality (Mitrou et al. 2007), and cancer-cause mortality (Mitrou et al. 2007).

The Dietary Approaches to Stop Hypertension (DASH) Diet and the DASH Dietary Pattern

Higher Adherence to the Dietary Approaches to Stop Hypertension (DASH) Diet

The Dietary Approaches to Stop Hypertension (DASH) diet emphasizes a high intake of fruit, vegetables, nuts and legumes, low fat dairy foods, and whole grains; low intake of sodium, sweets including sweetened beverages, red meat, processed meat, saturated fats, and total fats (Appel et al. 1997; Karanja et al. 1999; Campbell 2017). The composition of macronutrients and minerals of the DASH diet are as follows: total fat, 27% of calories; saturated fat, 6% of calories; cholesterol, 150 mg; protein, 18% of calories; carbohydrate, 55% of calories; fiber, 30 g; sodium, 2,300 mg; potassium, 4,700 mg; calcium, 1,250 mg; magnesium, 500 mg (Skerret and Willett 2010; Campbell 2017).

In a randomized, crossover feeding trial with 103 adults with prehypertension or stage 1 hypertension, the DASH diet reduced serum uric acid (SUA) concentration compared with the control diet, and this effect was greater among participants with hyperuricemia (Juraschek et al. 2016). In a randomized-controlled 90 day trial with 103 pre-hypertensive or hypertensive adults (SUA concentration $\geq$ 6 mg/dL), the DASH diet lowered SUA concentrations compared to the typical American diet (Tang et al. 2017). In a randomized trial of African Americans with controlled hypertension from an urban clinic, partial replacement of diet with DASH foods lowered SUA concentrations compared with higher baseline SUA concentrations (SUA concentration > 8 mg/dL) (Juraschek et al. 2018). Feng et al. (2023) have stated that adopting the DASH diet might be helpful in reducing SUA level, and the effect might be partly mediated by BMI.

Higher adherence to the DASH diet was associated with decreased SUA concentrations (Gao et al. 2021; Feng et al. 2023; Zhu et al. 2023) and a lower hyperuricemia risk (Gao et al. 2021; Yi et al. 2022; Zhu et al. 2023). In cross-sectional population-based study, the DASH diet was correlated negatively with the SUA levels among non-smoking, non-hypertension, and non-hyperuricemia participants (Feng et al. 2023). There was a strong positive relationship between insulin resistance and hyperuricemia (Fam 2002; Choi, Mount and Reginato 2005; Krishnan et al. 2012). Insulin resistance was associated with subclinical vascular injury and early kidney damage (Adeva-Andany et al. 2020). Hyperuricemia reduces endothelial nitric oxide (NO) bioavailability (Hayden and Tyagi 2004; Sattui, Singh and Gaffo 2014).

Experimental animal models have shown that hyperuricemia-induced vascular dysfunction, inflammation and increased oxidative stress leads to insulin resistance (Gustafsson and Unwin 2013). Yi et al. (2022) have stated that the effect of improving insulin resistance and regulating renin-angiotensin in the DASH diet may play a cooperate role in reducing the SUA concentration and thereby reducing hyperuricemia risk.

A meta-analysis by Soltani et al. (Soltani, Chitsazi and Salehi-Abargouei 2018) found that adherence to the DASH diet significantly decreased serum sensitive C-reactive protein (CRP) levels in adults.

Higher adherence to the DASH diet was associated with decreased risk of gout (Rai et al. 2017), kidney disease (Rebholz et al. 2016), overweight/obesity (Campbell 2017), type 2 diabetes mellitus (Barros et al. 2008; Liese et al. 2009; Campbell 2017), coronary heart disease (CHD) (Fung et al. 2008), stroke (Fung et al. 2008), kidney stones (Taylor, Fung and Curhan 2009), dementia and dementia progression (Soltani et al. 2020), all-cause mortality (Reedy et al. 2014; Soltani et al. 2020), renal-cause mortality (Smyth et al. 2016), cardiovascular disease (CVD)-cause mortality (Reedy et al. 2014; Soltani et al. 2020), stroke-cause mortality (Soltani et al. 2020), and cancer-cause mortality (Reedy et al. 2014; Soltani et al. 2020).

The guidelines have encouraged the DASH diet for patients with type 2 diabetes mellitus (American Diabetes Association 2019) and hypertension (Unger et al. 2020). The National Kidney Foundation-Kidney Disease Outcomes Quality Initiative Guidelines on Hypertension and Antihypertensive Agents in CKD recommended a modified version of the DASH diet (protein intake: 0.6-0.8 g/kg/day; phosphorus intake: 0.8-1.0 g/day; potassium intake: 2-4 g/day) for persons with CKD stages 3 and 4 (eGFR between 15 and 59 mL/min/1.73 m^2) (Kidney Disease Outcomes Quality Initiative (K/DOQI) 2004).

The Dietary Approaches to Stop Hypertension (DASH) Dietary Pattern

The DASH dietary pattern is characterized by a diet rich in fruit, vegetables, nuts and legumes, low-fat dairy products and whole grains, and with low intake of sodium, sugar-sweetened beverages, and red and processed meats. The DASH dietary pattern was associated with a lower risk of gout, suggesting that its effect of lowering serum uric acid (SUA) levels in individuals with hyperuricemia translates to a lower risk of gout (Rai et al. 2017).

In a randomized controlled trial, a DASH-style diet emphasizing plant-based protein reduced SUA levels by 0.12 mg/dL compared with baseline at the end of the 6-week feeding period (Belanger et al. 2021). The DASH-style diet emphasizing plant-based protein also lowered SUA levels compared with those emphasizing carbohydrates or unsaturated fat (Belanger et al. 2021).

Vegetarian Diet (Plant-Based Diet)

Vegetarians avoid purine-rich meat and seafood, while consuming more vegetables, whole grains, seeds and nuts (Chiu et al. 2014; Orlich et al. 2014). Taiwanese vegetarians had a lower intake of dairy, eggs, coffee, tea, sugar sweetened beverages, and higher intakes of soybeans, fruit, vegetables, dietary fiber, vitamin C, and avoiding meat and fish, compared with Taiwanese nonvegetarians (Chiu et al. 2019).

In the EPIC-Oxford cohort study, SUA concentrations in vegetarians or fish eaters were lower than those in meat eaters and vegans (Schmidt et al. 2013). Individuals consuming a vegan diet had higher SUA concentrations compared to vegetarians (Schmidt et al. 2013). This result seems to be attributed to the lack of consumption of dairy products.

In a randomized, open, crossover trial in low-to-moderate cardiovascular profile for 3 months, compared with baseline, a lacto-ovo-vegetarian diet reduced serum creatinine, SUA, blood urea nitrogen (BUN) levels, BUN/creatinine ratio and increased estimated glomerular filtration rate (eGFR)(Dinu et al. 2021). Compared with omnivores, vegetarians had lower BUN, serum creatinine, and SUA levels and higher estimated glomerular filtration rate (eGFR) (Xu et al. 2020). Xu et al. (2020) have stated that healthy adult vegetarians have better renal function than omnivores, and the higher dietary fiber intake associated with vegetarian diets may contribute to the protective effect on renal function.

Two cohort studies showed that a vegetarian diet was associated with a lower plasma or serum UA concentration (Szeto, Kwok and Benzie 2004; Yang et al. 2011). The plant-based dietary pattern was inversely associated with blood uric acid concentrations (Zhou et al. 2022).

Vegetarian diets have been shown to reduce hyperuricemia-associated comorbidities, such as hypertension (Yokoyama et al. 2014; Chuang et al. 2016), diabetes mellitus (Tonstad et al. 2013; Chiu et al. 2018), and cardiovascular diseases (CVD) (Crowe et al. 2013; Kahleova, Levin and Barnard 2018). Vegetarian dietary patterns reduce CVD mortality and the risk of coronary heart disease (CHD) (Kahleova, Levin and Barnard 2018).

Effect of Diet and Dietary Pattern on Plasma Uric Acid Concentrations, Serum Uric Acid Concentrations, and Hyperuricemia Risk

Recent studies have found that an animal-based dietary pattern is associated with blood uric acid concentrations (Zhou et al. 2022) and animal foods dietary patterns are characterized by higher intake of an animal organ, seafood and processed meat products is associated with a higher prevalence of newly diagnosed hyperuricemia (Xia et al. 2018). An observational study found that a strict purine-free diet reduced the serum uric acid (SUA) level by 15-20% (Nicholls and Scott 1972). The dietary measure for the prevention of hyperuricemia recommended at the present time is the restriction of intake of purines (Choi 2010; Terkeltaub. and Edwards 2013, 143-156; Ekpenyong and Daniel 2015; Hisatome et al. 2018). Many researchers (Vuorinen-Markkola and Yki-Järvinen 1994; Fam 2002; Schlesinger 2005; Underwood 2006; Terkeltaub and Edwards 2013, 143-156) have announced that traditional low purine diets are generally unpalatable and nutritionally poor, and are not usually recommended. Because a decreasing intake of purine-rich foods generally leads to refraining from foods with high nutritional value, there are many practical problems with this strategy. Havlik et al. (2010) have found that protein-rich vegetable-based meat substitutes are more suitable for dietary considerations in a low-purine diet for hyperuricemic subjects. An increased level of dietary acid load, which is low fruit and vegetables, was linked to an elevated hyperuricemia risk (Shao et al. 2022). Epidemiological studies have found that vegetarian diets (Yang et al. 2011) and higher adherence to the Mediterranean diet (Chrysohoou et al. 2011; Kontogianni et al. 2012; Alkerwi et al. 2015) are associated with decreased SUA concentrations. The Mediterranean diet (Chatzipavlou et al. 2014; Yokose et al. 2020) and the Dietary Approaches to Stop Hypertension (DASH) diet (Juraschek et al. 2016) reduced SUA concentrations in patients with hyperuricemia. Greater adherence to the Mediterranean diet was associated with decreased risk of hyperuricemia (Chrysohoou et al. 2011; Kontogianni et al. 2012), chronic kidney disease (CKD) (Huang et al. 2013; Hu et al. 2019), obesity (Tyrovolas et al. 2009), and cardiovascular disease (CVD) (Gopinath et al. 2011; Psaltopoulou et al. 2013; Kontogianni and Panagiotakos 2014; Tektonidis et al. 2015; Badimon, Chagas and Chiva-Blanch 2019). Higher adherence to the Dietary Approaches to Stop Hypertension (DASH) diet was associated with a decreased risk of gout (Rai et al. 2017), kidney disease (Rebholz et al. 2016), overweight/obesity (Campbell 2017), type 2 diabetes mellitus (Barros et al. 2008; Liese et al. 2009; Campbell 2017), and CVD [chronic heart disease, coronary heart disease (CHD), stroke] (Fung et al. 2008). Recognizing the dietary habits for the prevention and management of hyperuricemia with proper choices of foods and dietary patterns seem to play a helpful role in the prevention of gout and some comorbidities of hyperuricemia.

Fruits, vegetables, and various herbs consist of many phytochemicals, and other micronutrient compounds that have been shown to inhibit uric acid (UA) synthesis (Hafez, Abdel-Rahman and Naguib 2017). Phytochemicals, which are found in fruit, vegetables, grains, beans, and other plants, have potent antioxidant activity and may attenuate the nucleotide-binding and oligomerization domain-like receptor, leucine-rich repeat and pyrin domain-containing 3 (NLRP3) pathway (Joseph, Edirisingle and Burton-Freeman 2016; Tozser and Benko 2016), suggesting exert inhibitory effects on the NLRP3 inflammasome-mediated diseases (Jhang, Lin and Yen 2018). Both the Mediterranean diet and the DASH diet include a high intake of fruit, vegetables, whole-grain cereals, legumes and nuts, together with a moderate consumption of fish and low-fat dairy products, and a low consumption of meat, meat products, and sweets and commercial pastries. The DASH diet is a moderate form of a plant-rich diet and is described as being similar to a "lacto-ovo vegetarian" diet (Jakše et al. 2019).

The review reported by Sun et al. (2022) has stated that the Mediterranean and DASH diets help reduce SUA concentrations and thus prevent hyperuricemia; that is to say, probiotics alleviate hyperuricemia by ways of absorbing purine, restoring gut microbiota dysbiosis and inhibiting xanthine oxidase activity and polyphenols. Peptides and alkaloids exert various anti-hyperuricemic effects, by regulating urate transporters, blocking the active sites of xanthine oxidase and inhibiting the toll-like receptor 4 (TLR4)/ nuclear factor kappa B (NF-κB) signaling pathway and NLRP3 signaling pathway.

In the category of a Mediterranean-style diet, the DASH diet is most probably best defined and evidence based regarding cardiovascular risk factors (Vedder et al. 2019). The American Diabetes Association (ADA) (2019) has encouraged the Mediterranean diet, the DASH diet, and plant-based diets for the management of type 2 diabetes and prediabetes. Therefore, the Mediterranean diet and the DASH diet would possibly play a role in the prevention of hyperuricemia and its comorbidities including various lifestyle-related diseases.

Conclusion

To properly choose and consume the foods that contain the serum uric acid (SUA)-lowering nutrients which are important for the prevention and management of hyperuricemia in the general population (especially adults). Foods rich in α-linolenic acid, fiber, vitamin D, vitamin E, vitamin B_1, vitamin B_2, folate, vitamin B_{12}, vitamin C, calcium, magnesium, iron, zinc, and polyphenol for the prevention and management of hyperuricemia are shown in Table 1.

Hyperuricemia is a risk factor for gout (as uratosis) (Saag and Choi 2006; Hisatome et al. 2018; Cabău et al. 2020; Li, Zhang and Zeng 2020). The guidelines for the management of gout highlight the importance of limiting or avoiding the intake of purines (Hisatome et al. 2018; FitzGerald et al. 2020), purine-rich foods (meat, seafood, organ meats, yeast extract) (Jordan et al. 2007; Khanna et al. 2012), high-fructose (FitzGerald et al. 2020), sugar-sweetened drinks (Richette et al. 2017), desserts (Khanna et al. 2012), table sugar (Khanna et al. 2012), sauces and gravies (Khanna et al. 2012), alcohol (especially beer and spirits) (Richette et al. 2017; Hisatome et al. 2018; FitzGerald et al. 2020), and heavy meals (Richette et al. 2017). The Centers for Disease Control and Prevention (CDC) (2023) has recommended avoiding foods that may trigger a gout flare, including foods high in purines (like a diet rich in red meat, organ meat, and seafood), and limiting alcohol intake (particularly beer and hard liquor). As this article describes, the above nutrients and foods increase SUA concentrations. Furthermore, the guidelines have stated that important lifestyle changes in gout patients include weight control (Khanna et al. 2012; Richette et al. 2017; Hisatome et al. 2018; FitzGerald et al. 2020), physical activity (Khanna et al. 2012; Richette et al. 2017; Hisatome et al. 2018), smoking cessation (Khanna et al. 2012), and proper hydration (Khanna et al. 2012; Hisatome et al. 2018). General health, diet and lifestyle measures for gout patients recommended by the guidelines (Khanna et al. 2012; Richette et al. 2017; Hisatome et al. 2018; FitzGerald et al. 2020) seem to fit also for the prevention of hyperuricemia.

Dietary habits for the prevention and management of hyperuricemia prevention and management of hyperuricemia in the general population (especially adults) described in this article are shown in Table 2. Diet and dietary patterns for the prevention of hyperuricemia referencing the results of clinical research are suggested as follows: choice and intake of foods containing nutrients which decrease SUA concentration; avoidance of purine-rich diet, a dietary urate index dietary pattern, uric acid-prone dietary pattern, animal foods dietary pattern, and the Western diet. They encourage a low-fat or low-carbohydrate diet in individuals with hyperuricemia, a high-protein diet in individuals with hyperlipidemia, a calorie restricted diet (40% carbohydrate including whole grains, 30% protein, and 30% fat) in gout patients, a purine-low diet, high-protein, low-carbohydrate without calorie restriction (Atkins diet) in overweight or obese participants, a high fruit and soybean products diet in individuals with hyperuricemia, less protein-rich and more vegetable/fruit-rich materials diet, soybean products and fruit dietary pattern, polyphenol-rich dietary pattern, higher adherence to the Mediterranean diet (the traditional Mediterranean diet) and its dietary pattern, higher adherence to the Dietary Approaches to Stop Hypertension (DASH) diet and its dietary pattern, and plant-based diet. The healthy dietary patterns (e.g., the Mediterranean diet, the DASH diet, plant-based diet) are associated with significantly lower risk for gout and hyperuricemia-associated comorbidities. However, it must take into account the Acceptable Macronutrient Distribution Ranges (AMDRs), the Adequate Intakes (AIs), the Recommended Dietary Allowances (RDAs), and the Tolerable Upper Intake Level (UL) of dietary reference intakes for nutrients set by the Institute of Medicine of the National Academy of Sciences in the U.S., though there is limited information on the exact content of purines and nutrients contained in foods mainly because several factors, such as food processing procedures, can affect its content.

Table 1. Foods rich in α-linolenic acid, fiber, vitamin D, vitamin E, vitamin B_1, vitamin B_2, folate, vitamin B_{12}, vitamin C, calcium, magnesium, iron, zinc, and polyphenol for prevention and management of hyperuricemia*,**

Food classification	Food items
Meats	rotisserie chicken, turkey
Seafood	abalone, anchovy, blue crab, clams, cuttlefish, herring, lamprey, mackerel, oysters, salmon, salmon roe, sardines, shrimp, sweetfish, trout, tuna
Eggs	
Dairy products	cheese, cottage cheese, frozen yogurt, Greek yogurt, low-fat milk, low-fat yogurt, milk, Mozzarella part skim, parmesan cheese, yogurt
Beverages	chocolate dark beverage, chocolate milk beverage, cocoa, whole milk, whole chocolate milk, soy milk, almond milk, coffee, black tea, green tea, oolong tea, peppermint tea
Grains	barley, bread, egg noodles, macaroni, quinoa, wheat germ, white rice
Whole grains	breakfast cereals, brown rice, oatmeal, oats cereals, high fiber-bran ready-to-eat cereals, Iron-fortified ready-to-eat cereals and breads, Vitamin D (10% of the daily value)-ready-to-eat cereals, shredded wheat ready-to-eat cereals
Potatoes	konjac, potato with skin

Food classification	Food items
Mushrooms	maitake mushrooms, shitake mushrooms, wood ear
Seaweed	
Legumes	adzuki beans, black beans, broad bean seed, chickpeas, common beans, cranberry beans, edamame, french beans, kidney beans, navy beans, soybeans, lentils, peas, pinto beans, soybeans, white beans, yellow beans
Soy products	soy bacon, soy flour, soy paste, soy meat, soy milk, tempe, tofu
Seeds and Nuts	almonds, Brazil nuts, broad bean seeds, cashew nuts, chestnuts, chia seeds, hazelnuts, peanuts, pecan nuts, pine nuts, pistachio nuts, pumpkin seeds, sesame seeds, sunflower seeds, walnuts
Fruit	acerolas, apples, apricots, avocados, bananas, blackberries, black currants, black elderberries, cantaloupes, cherries, citrons, European cranberries, grapefruit, grapes, guavas, kiwifruit, mangos, nectarine, oranges, peaches, pears, plums, prunes, raspberries, strawberries
Vegetables	acorn squash, artichokes, black olives, broad bean pods, broccoli, brussels sprouts, cabbages, carrots, cauliflowers, chicory, Chinese cabbages, garlic, globe artichoke, green olives, green pepper, kales, onions, red pepper, parsley, pumpkins, spinach, tomatoes, turnip greens
Confectioneries	chocolate dark, chocolate milk
Oils	olive oil, cod liver oil, flaxseed oil, perilla oil
Herbs	basil, common sage, common thyme, lemon verbena, Italian oregano, marjoram, Mexican oregano, oregano, rosemary, spearmint
Spices	caper, caraway, cinnamon, clove, cumin, curry, ginger, nutmeg, turmeric

*The Council for Science and Technology, Ministry of Education, Culture, Sports, Science and Technology in Japan (2023).

**U.S. Department of Health & Human Services. National Institutes of Health. Office of Dietary Supplements (2023).

Table 2. Dietary habits for prevention and management of hyperuricemia in the general population (especially adults)

Food or Diet	Behaviour
Purine-rich food (e.g., meat, seafood and organ meats)	Limiting intake.
Fish oil	Consume at least 250 mg/day of long-chain n-3 polyunsaturated fatty acid or at least 2 servings/week of oily fish (Mozaffarian and Wu 2011).
Eggs	Recognizing encouraged intake.
Dairy products (particularly low-fat dairy products)	Recognizing encouraged intake.
Sugar-sweetened beverages	Limiting or decreasing intake.
Coffee and Tea	Recognizing encouraged intake.
Alcohol Beverages	Limiting or decreasing consumption. Sensible moderate drinking for overall health benefits is 1-2 drinks/day for men and ≤1 drink/day for women (Choi 2005). An ideal amount of alcohol intake for patients with hyperuricemia and gout is one drink per day and ≤ 2 servings in a 24-hour period (Terkeltaub and Edwards 2013).

Table 2. (Continued)

Food or Diet	Behaviour
Fiber-rich foods (e.g., cereals, whole grains, high-fiber bread)	Recognizing encouraged intake.
Mushrooms	Recognizing encouraged intake.
Seaweed	Recognizing encouraged intake.
Legumes and Soy products	Recognizing encouraged intake.
Seeds and Nuts	Recognizing encouraged intake.
Fruit and Vegetables	Recognizing encouraged intake.
Confectioneries (sugary foods including desserts and sweets)	Limiting or decreasing intake.
Probiotics	Recognizing encouraged intake.
Diet	
The Western diet	Avoid intake.
Purine-rich diet	Avoid intake.
A dietary urate index dietary pattern	Avoid intake.
Uric acid-prone dietary pattern	Avoid intake.
Animal foods dietary pattern	Avoid intake.
Low-fat diet or Low-carbohydrate diet	Recognizing encouraged intake for individuals with hyperuricemia.
High-protein diet	Recognizing encouraged intake for individuals with hyperlipidemia.
Calorie restricted diet (40% carbohydrate including whole grains, 30% protein, and 30% fat)	Recognizing encouraged intake for gout patients.
Purine-low diets	Recognizing encouraged intake.
High-protein, low-carbohydrate without calorie restriction (Atkins diet)	Recognizing encouraged intake for overweight or obese participants.
Less protein-rich and more vegetable/fruit-rich materials diet	Recognizing encouraged intake.
High fruit and soybean products diet	Recognizing encouraged intake for individuals with hyperuricemia.
Soybean products and fruit dietary pattern	Recognizing encouraged intake.
Polyphenol-rich dietary pattern	Recognizing encouraged intake.
The Mediterranean diet	Recognizing encouraged intake.
The DASH diet	Recognizing encouraged intake.
Plant-based diet	Recognizing encouraged intake.
Meal strategies	It is essential to maintain a moderate amount of one serving, which is composed of staple food, side dishes, main dishes, milk and dairy products, fruit, and vegetables. Consumption of meals and drinks should be done generally about 80% of satiety.

Food or Diet	Behaviour
Weight management	Weight management including proper calorie intake and adequate exercise.
Exercise	Adequate physical exercise (e.g., moderate intensity aerobic exercise for 30 minutes on 5-7 days per week, vigorous intensity aerobic physical activity for 75 minutes per week).
Smoking cessation	Encouraged.

Referring to or adopting dietary patterns such as the Mediterranean diet, the DASH diet, and vegetarian diet (plant-based diet), the author wishes to emphasize the following five dietary indicators for the prevention and management of hyperuricemia in the general population (especially adults): (1) limiting intake of salt and purine-rich foods (e.g., beef, pork, lamb, organ meats, and meat extracts, seafood, yeast extracts, peas, beans, lentils, asparaguses, cauliflowers, spinach, mushrooms, bamboo shoots, nori, wakame, soup stock, oyster sauce, consommé, Chinese soup) (Kaneko et al. 2014; Hisatome et al. 2018); (2) limiting or decreasing alcohol beverage consumption; (3) limiting or decreasing intake of one serving of animal fat (e.g., beef, beef tallow, pork, margarine, butter), saturated fatty acids (e.g., coconut oil, coconut powder, butter, shortening, beef, beef tallow, pork, margarine, whipped cream, cheese), cholesterol (e.g., eggs, herring roe, dried squid, anchovy, anchovy liver, foie gras, sakura shrimp, dried shrimp, sand lance, caviar, lamprey, salmon roe (The Council for Science and Technology, Ministry of Education, Culture, Sports, Science and Technology in Japan 2023); (4) limiting or decreasing intake of confectioneries (sugary foods including desserts and sweets) and sugar-sweetened beverages; (5) recognizing the intake of probiotics and foods rich in α-linolenic acid, fiber, milk protein (casein and lactalbumin), vegetable protein (especially wheat gluten, rice endosperm protein, and soy protein), vitamin D, vitamin E, vitamin B_1, vitamin B_2, folate, vitamin B_{12}, vitamin C, calcium, magnesium, iron, zinc, and polyphenol (Table 1); (6) considering the intakes of high-vitamin A foods (e.g., beef liver, sweet potato, spinach, pumpkin pie), and high-vitamin B_5 (pantothenic acid) foods (e.g., beef liver, breakfast cereals), and high-folate (e.g., beef liver, spinach, black-eyed peas, breakfast cereals)(U.S. Department of Health & Human Services. National Institutes of Health. Office of Dietary Supplements 2023) so as not to increase serum vitamin A, vitamin B_5 (pantothenic acid), and vitamin B_9 concentrations.

Uric acid (UA) is the primary antioxidant in human plasma and accounts for more than 60% of the capacity to scavenge free oxidative radicals in the serum (Fabbrini et al. 2014). Maintaining SUA concentrations within the normal physiological range may lead to the prevention of somehyperuricemia-associated comorbidities [e.g., CVD (e.g., atherosclerosis, heart failure, stroke), diabetes mellitus] through the beneficial effects of the antioxidant properties of UA. Choosing and eating SUA-lowering foods containing nutrients and phytochemicals in the Mediterranean diet, the DASH diet, and vegetarian diet (plant-based diet) may also lead to preventing not only hyperuricemia, but also gout and some hyperuricemia-associated comorbidities [e.g., chronic kidney disease (CKD) (Krishnamurthy et al. 2012), obesity (Yahfoufi et al. 2018), diabetes mellitus (Forouhi et al. 2018; Yahfoufi et al. 2018), and cardiovascular disease (CVD) (Yahfoufi et al. 2018)] caused by inflammation from elevated SUA concentrations. For example, the National Health and Medical Research Council (NHMRC), Australian Government's Australian Guide to Healthy Eating, Eat for Health, Australian Dietary Guidelines, 2013 (2023) emphasizes the importance of limiting the intake of foods and drinks high in saturated fat, added salt, added sugars and alcohol, based on evidence that these foods are associated with increased risk of obesity and/or chronic diseases, including CVD and type 2 diabetes mellitus. The American College of Cardiology and the American Heart Association (Arnett et al. 2019), with respect to the prevention of CVD, have encouraged the intake of fruits, vegetables, legumes, nuts, whole grains, and fish, and have proposed minimizing the consumption of trans fats, added sugars (including sugar-sweetened beverages), red meats, sodium, and saturated fats. It is speculated that consuming these foods corresponds to the prevention of hyperuricemia, but excessive intake of fish should be avoided. It is also necessary to decide on appropriate alcohol consumption. Therefore, taking into consideration the choices and intake of proper foods for the prevention of each comorbidity of hyperuricemia is essential. Large-scale prospective cohort studies, and randomized controlled trials are needed to examine the effects of the Mediterranean diet, the DASH diet, and vegetarian diets (plant-based diets) with SUA-lowering foods choices on patients with comorbidities of hyperuricemia.

Disclaimer

None.

References

Abete I, Perez-Cornago A, Navas-Carretero S, Bondia-Pons I, Zulet MA, Martinez JA. 2013. "A regular lycopene enriched tomato sauce consumption influences antioxidant status of healthy young subjects: A crossover study." *J Funct Foods* 5:28-35.

Adeva-Andany MM, Fernández-Fernández C, Carneiro-Freire N, Castro-Quintela E, Pedre-Piñeiro A, Seco-Filgueira M. 2020. "Insulin resistance underlies the elevated cardiovascular risk associated with kidney disease and glomerular hyperfiltration." *Rev Cardiovasc Med* 21:41-56.

Alkerwi A, Vernier C, Crichton GE, Sauvageot N, Shivappa N, Hébert JR. 2015. "Cross-comparison of diet quality indices for predicting chronic disease risk: findings from the Observation of Cardiovascular Risk actors in Luxembourg (ORISCAV-LUX) study." *Br J Nutr* 113:259-269.

American Diabetes Association. 2019. "Lifestyle management: standards of medical care in diabetes-2019." *Diabetes Care* 42: S46-S60.

Appel LJ, Moore TJ, Obarzanek E, Vollmer WM, Svetkey LP, Sacks FM, Bray GA, Vogt TM, Cutler JA, Windhauser MM, Lin PH, Karanja N. 1997. "A clinical trial of the effects of dietary patterns on blood pressure. DASH Collaborative Research Group." *N Engl J Med* 336:1117-1124.

Arnett DK, Blumenthal RS, Albert MA, Buroker AB, Goldberger ZD, Hahn EJ, Himmelfarb CD, Khera A, Lloyd-Jones D, McEvoy JW, Michos ED, Miedema MD, Muñoz D, Smith Jr SC, Virani SS, Williams KA, Yeboah J, Ziaeian B. 2019. "2019 ACC/AHA Guideline on the primary prevention of cardiovascular disease." *Circulation* 140: e596-e646.

Australian Government. 2023. "Australian's health 2018." Accessed April 26. https://www.aihw.gov.au/reports/australias-health/australias-health-2018/contents/indicators-of-australias-health/fruit-and-vegetable-intake.

Badimon L, Chagas P, Chiva-Blanch G. 2019. "Diet and cardiovascular disease: Effects of foods and nutrients in classical and emerging cardiovascular risk factors." *Curr Med Chem* 26:3639-3651.

Bahorun T, Luximon-Ramma A, Gunness TK, Sookar D, Bhoyroo S, Jugessur R, Reebye D, Googoolye K, Crozier A, Aruoma OI. 2010. "Black tea reduces uric acid and C-reactive protein levels in humans susceptible to cardiovascular diseases." *Toxicology* 278:68-74.

Bai Y, Jiang Y, Jiang Y. 2014. "*Lactobacillus bulgaricus* mutants decompose uremic toxins." *Renal Failure* 36:790-794.

Barnaba L, Intorre F, Azzini E, Ciarapica D, Venneria E, Foddai MS, Maiani F, Raguzzini A, Polito A. 2020. "Evaluation of adherence to Mediterranean diet and association with clinical and biological markers in an Italian population." *Nutrition* 77:110813.

Barros R, Moreira A, Fonseca J, de Oliveira JF, Delgado L, Castel-Branco MG, Haahtela T, Lopes C, Moreira P. 2008. "Adherence to the Mediterranean diet and fresh fruit intake are associated with improved asthma control." *Allergy* 63:917-923.

Basu S, McKee M, Galea G, Stuckler D. 2013. "Relationship of soft drink consumption to global overweight, obesity, and diabetes: a cross-national analysis of 75 countries." *Am J Public Health* 103:2071-2077.

Belanger MJ, Wee CC, Mukamal KJ, Miller ER, Sacks FM, Appel LJ, Shmerling RH, Choi HK, Juraschek S P. 2021. "Effects of dietary macronutrients on serum urate: results from the OmniHeart trial." *Am J Clin Nutr* 113:1593-1599.

Beydoun MA, Fanelli-Kuczmarski MT, Canas J-A, Beydoun HA, Evans MK, Zonderman AB. 2018. "Dietary factors are associated with serum uric acid trajectory differentially by race among urban adults." *Br J Nutr* 120:935-945.

Bhupathiraju SN, Tucker KL. 2011. "Greater variety in fruit and vegetable intake is associated with lower inflammation in Puerto Rican adults." *Am J Clin Nutr* 93:37-46.

Bitzer ZT, Wopperer AL, Chrisfield BJ, Tao L, Cooper TK, Vanamala J, Elias R, Hayes JE, Lambert JD. 2017. "Soy protein concentrate mitigates markers of colonic inflammation and loss of gut barrier function in vitro and in vivo." *J Nutr Biochem* 40:201-208.

Blau LW. 1950. "Cherry diet control for gout and arthritis." *Tex Rep Biol Med* 8:309-311.

Brulé D, Sarwar G, Savoie L. 1992. "Changes in serum and urinary uric acid levels in normal human subjects fed purine-rich foods containing different amounts of adenine and hypoxanthine." *J Am Coll Nutr* 11: 353-358.

Bruun JM, Maersk M, Belza A, Astrup A, Richelsen B. 2015. "Consumption of sucrose-sweetened soft drinks increases plasma levels of uric acid in overweight and obese subjects: a 6-month randomised controlled trial." *Eur J Clin Nutr* 69:949-953.

Bulló M, Lamuela-Raventós R, Salas-Salvadó J. 2011, "Mediterranean diet and oxidation: nuts and olive oil as important sources of fat and antioxidants." *Curr Top Med Chem* 11:1797-1810.

Cabău G, Crişan TO, Klück V, PoppRA, Joosten LAB. 2020. "Urate-induced immune programming: Consequences for gouty arthritis and hyperuricemia." *Immunol Rev* 294:92-105.

Campbell AP. 2017. "DASH eating plan: an eating pattern for diabetes management." *Diabetes Spectr* 30:76-81.

Carabin IG, Lyon MR, Wood S, Pelletier X, Donazzolo Y, Burdock GA. 2009. "Supplementation of the diet with the functional fiber PolyGlycoplex is well tolerated by healthy subjects in a clinical trial." *Nutr J* 8:9.

Carran EL, White SJ, Reynolds AN, Haszard JJ, Venn BJ. 2016. "Acute effect of fructose intake from sugar-sweetened beverages on plasma uric acid: a randomised controlled trial." *Eur J Clin Nutr* 70:1034-1038.

Centers for Disease Control and Prevention. 2023. "Gout." Accessed April 27. https://www.cdc.gov/arthritis/basics/gout.html.

Chang WC. 2011. "Dietary intake and the risk of hyperuricemia, gout and chronic kidney disease in elderly Taiwanese men." *Aging Male* 14:195-202.

Chatzipavlou M, Magiorkinis G, Koutsogeorgopoulou L, Kassimos D. 2014. "Mediterranean diet intervention for patients with hyperuricemia: a pilot study." *Rheumatol Int* 34:759-762.

Chen G, Tan M-L, Li K-K, Leung P-C, Ko C-H. 2015. "Green tea polyphenols decreases uric acid level through xanthine oxidase and renal urate transporters in hyperuricemic mice." *J Ethnopharmacol* 175:14-20.

Chen R, Chen M, Chen Y, Hsiao C, Chen H, Chen S, Wu M, Yech Y, Yuan G, Wang Y. 2017. "Evaluating the urate-lowering effects of different microbial fermented extracts in hyperuricemic models accompanied with a safty study." *J Food Drug Anal* 25:597-606.

Chiu THT, Huang H-Y, Chiu Y-F, Pan W-H, Kao H-Y, Chiu JPC, Lin M-N, Lin C-L. 2014. "Taiwanese vegetarians and omnivores: dietary composition, prevalence of diabetes and IFG." *PLoS One* 9: e88547.

Chiu THT, Liu CH, Chang CC, Lin MN, Lin CL. 2019. "Vegetarian diet and risk of gout in two separate prospective cohort studies." *Clin Nutr* 39:837-844.

Chiu THT, Pan W-H, Lin M-N, Lin C-L. 2018. "Vegetarian diet, change in dietary patterns and diabetes risk: a prospective study." *Nutr Diabates* 8:12.

Choi HK. 2010. "A prescription for lifestyle change in patients with hyperuricemia and gout." *Curr Opin Rheumatol* 22:165-172.

Choi HK, Atkinson K, Karlson EW, Willett W, Curhan G. 2004. "Purine-rich foods, dairy and protein intake, and the risk of gout in men." *N Engl J Med* 350:1093-1103.

Choi HK. Atkinson K, Karlson EW, Willett W, Curhan G. 2004. "Alcohol intake and risk of incident gout in men: a prospective study." *Lancet* 363:1277-1281.

Choi HK, Curhan G. 2004. "Beer, liquor, and wine consumption and serum uric acid level; The Third National Health and Nutrition Examination Survey." *Arthritis Rheum* 51:1023-1029.

Choi HK, Curhan G. 2007. "Coffee, tea, and caffeine consumption and serum uric acid level: The third national health and nutrition examination survey." *Arthritis Rheum* 57:816-821.

Choi HK, Liu S, Curhan G. 2005. "Intake of purine-rich foods, protein, and dairy products and relationship to serum levels of uric acid: The Third National Health and Nutrition Examination Survey." *Arthritis Rheum* 52:283-289.

Choi HK, Mount DB, Reginato AM. 2005. "Pathogenesis of gout." *Ann Intern Med* 143:499-516.

Choi JWJ, Ford ES, Gao X, Choi HK. 2008. "Sugar-sweetened soft drinks, diet soft drinks, and serum uric acid level: The third national health and nutrition examination survey." *Arthritis. Rheum* 59:109-116.

Chrysohoou C, Panagiotakos DB, Pitsavos C, Skoumas J, Toutouza M, Papaioannou I, Toutouzas PK, Stefanadis C. 2003. "Effects of chronic alcohol consumption on lipid levels, inflammatory and haemostatic factors in the general population: the "ATTICA" Study." *Eur J Cardiovasc Prev Rehabil* 10:355-361.

Chrysohoou C, Skoumas J, Pitsavos C, Masoura C, Siasos G, Galiatsatos N, Psaltopoulou T, Mylonakis C, Margazas A, Kyvelou S, Mamatas S, Panagiotakos DB, Stefanadis C. 2011. "Long-term adherence to the Mediterranean diet reduces the prevalence of hyperuricemia in elderly individuals, without known cardiovascular disease: the Ikaria study." *Maturitas* 70:58-64.

Chuang S-Y, Chiu THT, Lee C-Y, Liu T-T, Tsao CK, Hsiung CA, Chiu Y-F. 2016. "Vegetarian diet reduces the risk of hypertension independent of abdominal obesity and inflammation: a prospective study." *J Hypertens* 34: 2164-2171.

Chuang SY, Lee SC, Hsieh YT, Pan WH. 2011. "Trends in hyperuricemia and gout prevalence: Nutrition and Health Survey in Taiwan from 1993-1996 to 2005-2008." *Asia Pac J Clin Nutr* 20:301-308.

Collins MW, Saag KG, Singh, JA. 2019. "Is there role for cherries in the management of gout?" *Ther Adv Musculoskeletal Dis* 11:1-16.

Crowe FL, Appleby PN, Travis RC, Key TJ. 2013. "Risk of hospitalization or death from ischemic heart disease among British vegetarians and nonvegetarians: results from the EPIC-Oxford cohort study." *Am J Clin Nutr* 97:597-603.

Dalbeth N, Palmano K. 2011. "Effects of dairy intake on hyperuricemia and gout." *Curr Rheumatol Rep* 13: 132-137.

Dalbeth N, Wong S, Gamble GD, Horne A, Mason B, Pool B, Fairbanks L, McQueen FM, Cornish J, Reid I R, Palmano K. 2010. "Acute effect of milk on serum urate concentrations: a randomized controlled crossover trial." *Ann Rheum Dis* 69:1677-1682.

Desideri G, Puig JG, Richette P. 2015. "The management of hyperuricemia with urate deposition." *Curr Med Res Opin* 31 (Suppl 2):27-32.

Dessein PH, Shipton EA, Stanwix AE, Joffe BI, Ramokgadi J. 2000. "Beneficial effects of weight loss associated with moderate calorie/carbohydrate restriction, and increased proportional intake of protein and unsaturated fat on serum urate and lipoprotein levels in gout: a pilot study." *Ann Rheum Dis* 59:539-543.

Dinu M, Colombini B, Pagliai G, Giangrandi I, Cesari F, Gori A, Giusti B, Marcucci R, Sofi F. 2021. "Effects of vegetarian versus Mediterranean diet on kidney function: Finding from the CARDIVEG study." *Eur J Clin Invest* 51: e13576.

Ebrahimpour-Koujan S, Saneei P, Larijani B, Esmaillzadeh A. 2020. "Consumption of sugar sweetened beverages and dietary fructose in relation to risk of gout and hyperuricemia: a systematic review and meta-analysis." *Crit Rev Food Sci Nutr* 60:1-10.

Ebrahimpour-Koujan S, Saneei P, Larijani B, Esmaillzadeh A. 2021. "Consumption of sugar-sweetened beverages and serum uric acid concentrations: a systematic review and meta-analysis." *J Hum Nutr Diet* 34: 305-313.

Ekpenyong CE, Daniel N. 2015. "Roles of diets and dietary factors in the pathogenesis, management and prevention of abnormal serum uric acid levels." *PharmaNutrition* 3:29-45.

El-Sayed HH, El-Moneim A, Darwish H, Ysein EM, Zehairy GD. 2014. "Biochemical and biological study on the effect of flaxseed on rats suffer from nephropathy." *IOSR Journal of Environmental Science, Toxicology, and Food Technology (IOSR-JESTFT)* 8:59-66.

Emmerson BT. 1996. "The management of gout." *N Engl J Med* 334:445-451.

Engelhard YN, Gazer B, Paran E. 2006. "Natural antioxidants from tomato extract reduce blood pressure in patients with grade-1-hypertenaion: A double-blind, placebo-controlled pilot study." *Am Heart J* 151:100.

Esmaillzadeh A, Azadbakht L. 2012. "Legume consumption is inversely associated with serum concentrations of adhesion molecules and inflammatory biomarkers among Iranian women." *J Nutr* 142:334-339.

Estruch R, Martínez-González MA, Corella D, Salas-Salvadó J, Ruiz-Gutiérrez V, Covas MI, Fiol M, Gómez-Gracia E, López-Sabater MC, Vinyoles E, Arós F, Conde M, Lahoz C, Lapetra J, Sáez G, Ros E, PREDIMED Study Investigators. 2006. "Effects of a Mediterranean-style diet on cardiovascular risk factors: a randomized trial." *Ann Intern Med* 145:1-11.

European Food Safety Authority (EFSA). 2015. "Scientific opinion on the safety of caffeine. EFSA Panel on Dietetic Products, Nutrition and Allergies (NDA)." *EFSA Journal* 13:4102.

Fabbrini E, Serafini, M, Colic Baric C, Hazen SL, Klein S. 2014. "Effect of plasma uric acid on antioxidant capacity, oxidative stress, and insulin sensitivity in obese subjects." *Diabetes* 63:976-981.

Facchini F, Chen TD, Hollenbeck CB, Reaven GM. 1991. "Relationship between resistance to insulin-mediated glucose uptake, urinary uric acid clearance, and plasma uric acid concentration." *JAMA* 266:3008-3011.

Fam AG. 2002. "Gout, diet, and the insulin resistance syndrome." *J Rheumatol* 29:1350-1355.

Feig DI, Kang D-H, Johnson RJ. 2008. "Uric acid and cardiovascular risk." *N Engl J Med* 359:1811-1821.

Feng J, Huang Y, Wang H, Wang C, Xu H, Ke P, He Y, Tian Q, Cao S, Lu Z. 2023. "Association between adherence to the Dietary Approaches to Stop Hypertension diet and serum uric acid." *Sci Rep* 13:6347.

Feskens EJ, Kromhout D. 1990. "Habitual dietary intake and glucose tolerance in euglycaemic men: the Zutphen Study." *Int J Epidemiol* 19:953-959.

FitzGerald JD, Dalbeth N, Mikuls T, Brignardello-Petersen R, Guyatt G, Abeles AM, Gelber AC, Harrold L R, Khanna D, King C, Levy G, Libbey C, Mount D, Pillinger MH, Rosenthal A, Singh JA, Sims JE, Smith BJ, Wenger NS, Bae SS, Danve A, Khanna PP, Kim SC, Lenert A, Poon S, Qasim A, Sehra ST, Sharma TSK, Toprover M, Turgunbaev M, Zeng L, Zhang MA, Turner AS, Neogi T. 2020. "2020 American College of Rheumatology guideline for the management of gout." *Arthritis Care Research* 72:744-760.

Flynn TJ, Cadzow M, Dalbeth N, Jones DB, Stamp LK, Hindmarsh JH, Todd AS, Walker RJ, Topless R, Merriman TR. 2015. "Positive association of tomato consumption with serum urate: support for tomato consumption as an anecdotal trigger of gout flares." *BMC Musculoskelet Disord* 16: 196.

Forouhi NG, Misra A, Mohan V, Taylor R, Yancy W. 2018. "Dietary and nutritional approaches for prevention and management of type 2 diabetes." *BMJ* 361: k2234.

Fung TT, Chiuve SE, McCullough ML, Rexrode KM, Logroscino G, Hu FB. 2008. "Adherence to a DASH-style diet and risk of coronary heart disease and stroke in women." *Arch Intern Med* 168: 713-720.

Gao Y, Cui LF, Sun YY, Yang WH, Wang JR, Wu SL, Gao X. 2021. "Adherence to the Dietary Approaches to Stop Hypertension (DASH) diet and hyperuricemia: a cross-sectional study." *Arthritis Care Res* 73:603-611.

Garrel DR, Verdy M, PetitClerc C, Martin C, Brulé D, Hamet P. 1991. "Milk-and soy-protein ingestion; Acute effect on serum uric acid concentration." *Am J Clin Nutr* 53:665-669.

Ghadirian P, Shatenstein B, Verdy M, Hamet P. 1995. "The influence of dairy products on plasma uric acid in women." *Eur J Epidemiol* 11:275-281.

Gopinath B, Harris DC, Flood VM, Burlutsky G, Brand-Miller J, Mitchell P. 2011. "Carbohydrate nutrition is associated with the 5-year incidence of chronic kidney disease." *J Nutr* 141:433-439.

Guasch-Ferré M, Bulló M, Babio N, Martínez-González MA, Estruch R, Covas M-I, Wärnberg J, Arós F, Lapetra J, Serra-Majem L, Basora J, Salas-Salvadó J. 2013. "Mediterranean diet and risk of hyperuricemia in elderly participants at high cardiovascular risk." *J Gerontol A Biol Sci Med Sci* 68:1263-1270.

Gustafsson D, Unwin R. 2013. "The pathophysiology of hyperuricaemia and its possible relationship to cardiovascular disease, morbidity and mortality." *BMC nephrology* 14:164.

Gutman AB, Yu TF. 1952. "Gout, a derangement of purine metabolism." *Advan Int Med* 5:227-302.

Hafez RM, Abdel-Rahman TM, Naguib RM. 2017. "Uric acid in plants and microorganisms: Biological applications and genetics-A review." *J Adv Res* 8:475-486.

Haidari F, Mohammad Shahi M, Keshavarz SA, Rashidi MR. 2009. "Inhibitory effects of tart cherry (*prunus cerasus*) juice on xanthine oxidoreductase activity and its hypouricemic and antioxidant effects on rats." *Mal J Nutr* 15:53-64.

Haldar S, Rowland IR, Barnett YA, Bradbury I, Robson PJ, Powell J, Fletcher J. 2007. "Influence of habitual diet on antioxidant status: a study in a population of vegetarians and omnivores." *Eur J Clin Nutr* 61:1011-1022.

Han Q-X, Zhang D, Zhao Y-L, Liu L, Li J, Zhang F, Luan F-X, Liu D-W, Liu Z-S, Cai G-Y, Chen X-M, Zhu H-Y. 2019. "Risk factors for hyperuricemia in Chinese centenarians and near- centenarians." *Clinical Interventions in Aging* 14:2239-2247.

Hariharan D, Vellanki K, Kramer H. 2015. "The western diet and chronic kidney disease." *Curr Hypertens Rep* 17:16.

Hazra B, Sarkar R, Biswas S, Mandal N. 2010. "Comparative study of the antioxidant and reactive oxygen species scavenging properties in the extracts of the fruits of *Terminalia chebula*, *Terminalia bellerica* and *Emblica officinalis*." *BMC Complement Altern Med* 10:20.

Havlik J, Plachy V, Fernandez J, Rada V. 2010. "Dietary purines in vegetarian meat analogues." *J Sci Food Agric* 90: 2352-2357.

Hayden MR, Tyagi SC. 2004. "Uric acid: A new look at an old risk marker for cardiovascular disease, metabolic syndrome, and type 2 diabetes mellitus: The urate redox shuttle." *Nutr Metab* 1:10.

Hisatome I, Ichida K, Mineo I, Ohtahara A, Ogino K, Kuwabara M, Ishizaka N, Uchida S, Kurajoh M, Kohagura K, Sato Y, Taniguchi A, Tsuchihashi T, Terai C, Nakamura T, Hamaguchi T, Hamada T, Fujimori S, Masuda I, Moriwaki Y, Yamamoto T. on behalf of guideline development group. 2018. *Japanese Society of Gout and Uric & Nucleic Acids Guidelines for Management of Hyperuricemia and Gout: 3 rd edition*. Tokyo: SHINDAN TO CHIRYO SHA, Inc.

Hokazono H, Omori T, Yamamoto T, Akaoka I, Ono K. 2010. "Effects of a fermented barley extract on subjects with slightly high serum uric acid or mild hyperuricemia." *Biosci Biotechnol Biochem* 74:828-834.

Hosojima M, Kaseda R, Kondo H, Fujii M, Kubota M, Watanabe R, Tanabe N, Kadowaki M, Suzuki Y, Saito A. 2016. "Beneficial effects of rice endosperm protein intake in Japanese men with risk factors for metabolic syndrome: a randomized, crossover clinical trial." *BMC Nutr* 2:25.

Hu EA, Steffen LM, Grams ME, Crews DC, Coresh J, Appel LJ, Rebholz CM. 2019. "Dietary patterns and risk of incident chronic kidney disease: the Atherosclerosis Risk in Communities study." *Am J Clin Nutr* 110:713-721.

Hu FB, Rimm EB, Stampfer MJ, Ascherio A, Spiegelman D, Willett WC. 2000. "Prospective study of major dietary patterns and risk of coronary heart disease in men." *Am J Clin Nutr* 72:912-921.

Huang X, Jiménez-Moleón JJ, Lindholm B, Cederholm T, Arnlöv J, Risérus U, Sjögren O, Carrero JJ. 2013. "Mediterranean diet, kidney function, and mortality in men with CKD." *Clin J Am Soc Nephrol* 8: 1548-1555.

Hunter DC, Brown R, Green T, Thomson C, Skeaff M, Williams S, Todd JM, Lister CE, McGhie T, Zhang J, Martin H, Rippon P, Stanley R, Skinner MA. 2012. "Changes in markers of inflammation, antioxidant capacity and oxidative stress in smokers following consumption of milk, and milk supplemented with fruit and vegetable extracts and vitamin C." *Int J Food Sci Nutr* 63:90-102.

INRA. 2023. "Phenol-Explorer database." Accessed April 27. http://phenol-explorer.eu/compounds.

Institute of Medicine of the National Academy of Sciences. 2021. *Food and Nutrition Board. Dietary Reference Intakes: The essential guide to nutrient requirements.* Washington, D.C.: The National Academy Press. https://www.nap.edu/catalog/11537.html.

Jacob K, Periago MJ, Bohm V, Berruezo GR. 2008. "Influence of lycopene and vitamin C from tomato juice on biomarkers of oxidative stress and inflammation." *Br J Nutr* 99:137-146.

Jacob RA, Spinozzi GM, Simon VA, Kelley DS, Prior RL, Hess-Pierce B, Kader AA. 2003. "Consumption of cherries lowers plasma urate in healthy women." *J Nutr* 133:1826-1829.

Jakše B, Jakše B, Pajek M, Pajek J. 2019. "Uric acid and plant-based nutrition." *Nutrients* 11:1736.

Japanese Society of Nephrology. 2012. *Clinical practice guidebook for diagnosis and treatment of chronic kidney disease 2012.*Tokyo: Igakusha Co.Ltd.

Jenkins DJ, Kendall CW, Vidgen E, Augustin LS, van Erk M, Geelen A, Parker T, Faulkner D, Vuksan V, Josse RG, Leiter LA, Connelly PW. 2001. "High-protein diets in hyperlipidemia: effect of wheat gluten on serum lipids, uric acid, and renal function." *Am J Clin Nutr* 74:57-63.

Jhang J-J, Lin J-H, Yen G-C. 2018. "Beneficial properties of phytochemicals on NLRP3 inflammasome-mediated gout and complication." *J Agric Food Chem* 31, 765-772.

Joosten LAB, Crişan TO, Bjornstad P, Johnson RJ. 2020. "Asymptomatic hyperuricaemia: a silent activation of the innate immune system." *Nat Rev Rheumatol* 16:75-86.

Jordan KM, Cameron JS, Snaith M, Zhang W, Doherty M, Seckl J, Hingorani A, Jaques R, Nuki G, British Society for Rheumatology and British Health Professionals in Rheumatology Standards, Guidelines and Audit Working Group (SGAWG). 2007.

"British Society for Rheumatology and British health professionals in rheumatology guideline for the management of gout." *Rheumatology* 46:1372-1374.

Joseph SV, Edirisingle I, Burton-Freeman BM. 2016. "Fruit polyphenols: a review of anti-inflammatory effects in humans." *Crit Rev Food Sci Nutr* 56:419-444.

Juraschek SP, Gelber AC, Choi HK, Appel LJ, Miller ER 3rd. 2016. "Effects of the Dietary Approaches to Stop Hypertension (DASH) diet and sodium intake on serum uric acid." *Arthritis Rheumatol* 68:3002-3009.

Juraschek SP, White K, Tang O, Yeh H-C, Cooper LA, Miller ER 3rd. 2018. "Effects of a Dietary Approaches to Stop Hypertension (DASH) diet intervention on serum uric acid in African Americans with hypertension." *Arthritis Care Res* 70:1509-1516.

Kahleova H, Levin S, Barnard ND. 2018. "Vegetarian dietary patterns and cardiovascular disease." Prong Cardiovasc *Dis* 61:54-61.

Kanbara A, Seyama I. 2011. "Effect of urine pH on uric acid excretion by manipulating food materials." *Nucleosides Nucleotides Nucleic Acids* 30:1066-1071.

Kanbara A, Miura Y, Nyogo H, Chayama K, Seyama I. 2012. "Effect of urine pH changed by dietary intervention on uric acid clearance mechanism of pH-dependent excretion of urinary uric acid." *Nutr J* 11:39.

Kaneko K, Aoyagi Y, Fukuuchi T, Inazawa K, Yamaoka N. 2014. "Total purine and purine base content of common foodstuffs for facilitating nutritional therapy for gout and hyperuricemia." *Biol Pharm Bull* 37:709-721.

Karanja NM, Obarzanek E, Lin PH, McCullough ML, Phillips KM, Swain JF, Champagne CM, Hoben KP. 1999. "Descriptive characteristics of the dietary patterns used in the Dietary Approaches to Stop Hypertension Trial. DASH Collaborative Research Group." *J Am Diet Assoc* 99 (Suppl):519-527.

Kela U, Vijayvargiya R, Trivedi CP. 1980. "Inhibitory effects of methylxanthines on the activity of xanthine oxidase." *Life Sci* 27:2109-2119.

Kelly DS, Rasooly R, Jacob RA, Kader AA, Mackey BE. 2006. "Consumption of Bing sweet cherries lowers circulating concentrations of inflammation markers in healthy men and women." *J Nutr* 136:981-986.

Khanna D, Fitzgerald JD, Khanna PP, Bae S, Singh MK, Neogi T, Pillinger MH, Merill J, Lee S, Prakash S, Kaldas M, Gogia M, Perez-Ruiz F, Taylor W, Lioté F, Choi H, Singh JA, Dalbeth N, Kaplan S, Niyyar V, Jones D, Yarows SA, Roessler B, Kerr G, King C, Levy G, Furst DE, Edwards NL, Mandell B, Schumacher HR, Robbins M, Wenger N, Terkeltaub R. 2012. "2012 American College of Rheumatology guidelines for management of gout. Part 1: systematic nonpharmacologic and pharmacologic therapeutic approaches to hyperuricemia." *Arthritis Care Research* 64:1431-1446.

Kidney Disease Outcomes Quality Initiative (K/DOQI). 2004. "K/DOQI clinical practice guidelines on hypertension and antihypertensive agents in chronic kidney disease." *Am J Kidney Dis* 43: S1-S290.

Kiyohara C, Kono S, Honjo S, Todoroki I, Sakurai Y, Nishiwaki M, Hamada H, Nishikawa H, Koga H, Ogawa S, Nakagawa K. 1999. "Inverse association between coffee drinking and serum uric acid concentrations in middle-aged Japanese males." *Br J Nutr* 82:125-130.

Koguchi T. 2018. "Essentials of dietary habits for prevention and suppression of hyperuricemia." *Curr Top Pharmacol* 22:77-133.

Koguchi T. 2021. "Modification of dietary habits for prevention of gout in Japanese people: Gout and the Japanese diet." *Am J Health Res* 9:117-127.

Koguchi T. 2021. "Modification of dietary habits for prevention of gout in Japanese people; Gout and diet." *Am J Health Res* 9:176-189.

Koguchi T. 2022. "Modification of macronutrient intake for prevention of gout in Japanese people in 2019: 2022 update." *Am J Health Res* 10: 83-106.

Koguchi T. 2022. "Modification of micronutrient intake for prevention of gout in Japanese people in 2019: 2022 update." *Am J Health Res* 10:107-131.

Koguchi T. 2022. "Modification of animal product intake for prevention of gout in Japanese people in 2019: 2022 update." *Am J Health Res* 10:140-153.

Koguchi T. 2022. "Modification of plant-based food intake for prevention of gout in Japanese people in 2019: 2022 update." *Am J Health Res* 10:154-168.

Koguchi T, Koguchi H, Nakajima H, Takano S, Yamamoto Y, Innami S, Maekawa A, Tadokoro T. 2004. "Dietary fiber suppresses elevation of uric acid and urea nitrogen concentrations in serum of rats with renal dysfunction induced by dietary adenine." *Int J Vitam Nutr Res* 74:253-263.

Koguchi T, Nakajima H, Koguchi H, Wada M, Yamamoto Y, Innami S, Maekawa A. Tadokoro T. 2003. "Suppressive effect of viscous dietary fiber on elevations of uric acid in serum and urine induced by dietary RNA in rats is associated with strength of viscosity." *Int J Vitam Nutr Res* 73:369-376.

Koguchi T, Nakajima H, Wada M, Yamamoto Y, Innami S, Maekawa A, Tadokoro T. 2002. "Dietary fiber suppresses elevations of uric acid and allantoin in serum and urine induced by dietary RNA and increases its excretion to feces in rats." *J Nutr Sci Vitaminol* 48:184-193.

Koguchi T, Tadokoro T. 2019. "Beneficial effect of dietary fiber on hyperuricemia in rats and humans: A review." *Int J Vitam Nutr Res* 89:89-108.

Kontogianni MD, Chrysohoou C, Panagiotakos DB, Tsetsekou E, Zeimbekis A, Pitsavos C, Stefanadis C. 2012. "Adherence to the Mediterranean diet and serum uric acid: the ATTICA study." *Scand J Rheumatol* 41:442-449.

Kontogianni MD, Panagiotakos DB. 2014. "Dietary patterns and stroke: A systematic review and re-meta-analysis." *Maturitas* 79:41-47.

Kozarski M, Klaus A, Jakovljevic D, Todorovic N, Vunduk J, Petrović P, Niksic M, Vrvic MM, van Griensven L. 2016. "Antioxidants of edible mushrooms." *Molecules* 20:19489-19525.

Kramer H. 2017. "Kidney disease and the Westernization and industrialization of food." *Am J Kidney Dis* 70: 111-121.

Krishnan E, Pandya BJ, Chung L, Hariri A, Dabbous O. 2012. "Hyperuricemia in young adults and risk of insulin resistance, prediabetes, and diabetes: a 15-year follow-up study." *Am J Epidemiol* 176:108-116.

Krishnamurthy VMR, Wei G, Baird BC, Murtaugh M, Chonchol MB, Raphael KL, Greene T, Beddhu S. 2012. "High dietary fiber intake associated with decreased inflammation and all-cause mortality in patients with chronic kidney disease." *Kidney Int* 81:300-306.

Kuo CF, Grainge MJ, Zhang W, Doherty M. 2015. "Global epidemiology of gout: prevalence, incidence and risk factors." *Nat Rev Rheumatol* 11:649-662.

Lee C-YJ, Isaac HB, Huang SH, Long LH, Wang H, Gruber J, Ong CN, Kelly RP, Halliwell B. 2009. "Limited antioxidant effect after consumption of a single dose of tomato sauce by young males, despite a rise in plasma lycopene." *Free Radic Res* 43:622-628.

Li S, Li L, Yan H, Jiang X, Hu W, Han N, Wang D. 2019. "Anti-gouty arthritis and anti-hyperuricemia properties of celery seed extracts in rodent models." *Mol Med Rep* 20:4623-4633.

Li X, Song P, Li J, Wang P, Li G. 2015. "Relationship between hyperuricemia and dietary risk factors in Chinese adults: a cross-sectional study." *Rheumatol Int* 35:2079-1089.

Li M, Yang D, Mei L, Yuan L, Xie A, Yuan J. 2014. "Screening and characterization of purine nucleoside degrading lactic acid bacteria isolated from Chinese sauerkraut and evaluation of the serum uric acid lowering effect in hyperuricemic rats." *PLOS ONE* 9: e105577.

Li L, Zhang Y, Zeng C. 2020. "Update on the epidemiology, genetics, and therapeutic options of hyperuricemia." *Am J Transl Res* 12:3167-3181.

Li Q, Kang X, Shi C, Li Y, Majumder K, Ning Z, Ren J. 2018. "Moderation of hyperuricemia in rats via consuming walnut protein hydrolysate diet and identification of new antihyperuricemic peptides." *Food Funct* 24:107-116.

Li R, Yu K, Li C. 2018. "Dietary factors and risk of gout and hyperuricemia: a meta-analysis and systematic review." *Asia Pac J Clin Nutr* 27:1344-1356.

Liese AD, Nichols M, Sun X, D'Agostino RB Jr, Haffner SM. 2009. "Adherence to the DASH diet is inversely associated with incidence of type 2 diabetes: the insulin resistance atherosclerosis study." *Diabetes Care* 32:1434-1436.

Lin CM, Chen CS, Chen CT, Liang YC, Lin JK. 2002. "Molecular modeling of flavonoids that inhibits xanthine oxidase." *Biochem Biophys Res Commun* 294:167-172.

Liu ZM, Ho CS, Chen YM, Woo J. 2015. "Can soy intake affect serum uric acid level? Pooled analysis from two 6-month randomized controlled trials among Chinese postmenopausal women with prediabetes or prehypertension." *Eur J Nutr* 54:51-58.

Liu N, Meng B, Zeng L, Yin S, Hu Y, Li S, Fu Y, Zhang X, Xie C, Shu L, Yang M, Wang Y, Yang X. 2020. "Discovery of a novel rice-derived peptide with significant anti-gout potency." *Food Funct* 11:10542-10553.

Liu J, Sun LL, He LP, Ling WH, Liu ZM, Chen M. 2014. "Soy food consumption, cardiometabolic alterations and carotid intima-media thickness in Chinese adults." *Nutr Metab Cardiovasc Dis* 24:1097-1104.

Loenen HMJA, Eshuis H, Löwik MRH, Schouten EG, Hulshof KFAM, Odink J, Kok FJ. 1990. "Serum uric acid correlates in elderly men and women with special reference to body composition and dietary intake (Dutch Nutrition Surveillance System)." *J Clin Epidemiol* 43:1297-1303.

Lu N, Shai I, Zhang Y, Curhan G, Choi HK. 2014. "High-protein diet (Atkins diet) and uric acid response." *Am Coll Rheumatol*Meeting abstract 171.

Lyu LC, Hsu CY, Yeh CY, Lee MS, Huang SH, Chen CL. 2003. "A case-control study of the association of diet and obesity with gout in Taiwan." *Am J Clin Nutr* 78:690-701.

Major TJ, Topless RK, Dalbeth N, Merriman TR. 2018. "Evaluation of the diet wide contribution to serum urate levels: meta-analysis of population based cohorts." *BMJ* 363: k3951.

Marriott BP, Cole N, Lee E. 2009. "National estimates of dietary fructose intake increased from 1977 to 2004 in the United States." *J Nutr* 139 (Suppl):1228S-1235S.

Martin KR, Bopp J, Burrell I, Hook G. 2011. "The effect of 100% tart cherry juice on serum uric acid levels, biomarkers of inflammation and cardiovascular disease risk factors." *FASEB J* 25 (Meeting Abstract Supplement):339.2.

Mena-Sánchez G, Babio N, Becerra-Tomás N, Martinez-González MÁ, Díaz-López A, Corella D, Zomeño MD, Eomaguera D, Vioque J, Alonso-Gómez ÁM, Wärnberg J, Martínez JA, Serra-Majem L, Estruch R, Bernal R, Lapetra J, Pintó X, Tur JA, Lopez-Miranda J, Cano-Ibáñez N, Gaforio JJ, Matía-Martin P, Daimiel L, Caro JLL, Vidal J, Vázquez C, Ros E, Arellano AG, Palau A, Fernández-Carrión R, Pérez-Vega K, Morey M, Garícia de la Hera M, Vaquero-Luna J, Carmona-González FJ, Abete I, Álvarez-Pérez J, Casas R, Fernández-Garícia JC, Santos-Lozano JM, Corbella E, Sureda A, Ruiz-Canela M, Barragán R, Goday A, Martin M, Altozano Rodado MC, Toledo E, Fitó M, Salas-Salvadó J, & PREDIMED-PLUS investigators. 2020. "Association between dairy product consumption and hyperuricemia in an elderly population with metabolic syndrome." *Nutr Metab Cardiovasc Dis* 30:214-222.

Merriman TR, Dalbeth N, Johnson RJ. 2014. "Sugar-sweetened beverages, urate, gout and genetic interaction." *Pac Health Dialog* 20:31-38.

Messina M, Messina VL, Chan P. 2011. "Soyfoods, hyperuricemia and gout: a review of the epidemiologic and clinical data." *Asia Pac J Clin Nutr* 20:347-358.

Miao Z, Li C, Chen Y, Zhao S, Wang Y, Wang Z, Chen X, Xu F, Wang F, Sun R, Hu J, Song W, Yan S, Wang C-Y. 2008. "Dietary and lifestyle changes associated with high prevalence of hyperuricemia and gout in the Shandong coastal cities of Eastern China." *J Rheumatol* 35:1859.

Mitrou PN, Kipnis V, Thiebaut AC, Reedy J, Subar AF, Wirfält E, Flood A, Mouw T, Hollenbeck AR, Leitzmann MF, Schatzkin A. 2007. "Mediterranean dietary pattern and prediction of all-cause mortality in a US population: results from the NIH-AARP Diet and Health Study." *Arch Intern Med* 167:2461-2468.

Moi JH, Sriranganathan MK, Falzon I, Edwards CJ, van der Heijde DM, Buchbinder R. 2014. "Lifestyle interventions for the treatment of gout: a summary of 2 Cochrane systematic reviews." *J Rheumatol Suppl* 92: 26-32.

Mozaffarian D, Appel LJ, Van Horn L. 2011. "Components of a cardioprotective diet: new insights." *Circulation* 123:2870-2892.

Muscelli E, Natali A, Bianchi S, Bigazzi R, Galvan AQ, Sironi AM, Frascerra S, Ciociaro D, Ferrannini E. 1996. "Effect of insulin on renal sodium and uric acid handling in essential hypertension." *Am J Hypertens* 9:746-752.

Muszyńska B, Grzywacz-Kisielewska A, Kała K, Gduła-Argasińska J. 2018. "Anti-inflammatory properties of edible mushrooms: A review." *Food Chem* 243:373-381.

National Health and Medical Research Council (NHMRC), Australian Government. Australian Guide to Healthy Eating, Eat for Health, Australian Dietary Guidelines, 2013. 2023. Accessed April 27. https://www.eatforhealth.gov.au/sites/default/files/files/the_guidelines/n55_australian_dietary_guidelines.pdf.

Nguyen S, Choi HK, Lustig RH, Hsu CY. 2009. "Sugar-sweetened beverages, serum uric acid, and blood pressure in adolescents." *J Pediatr* 154:807-813.

Nicholls A, Scott JT. 1972. "Effect of weight-loss on plasma and urinary levels of uric acid." *Lancet* 2:1223-1224.

Nickolai B, Kiss C. 2016. "Nutritional therapy of gout." *Ther Umsch* 73:153-158.

Ogura T, Matsuura K, Matsumoto Y, Mimura Y, Kishida M, Otsuka F, Tobe, K. 2004. "Recent trends of hyperuricemia and obesity in Japanese male adolescents, 1991 through 2002." *Metabolism* 53:448-453.

Okura T, Higaki J, Kurata M, Irita J, Miyoshi K, Yamazaki T, Hayashi D, Kohro T, Nagai R, Japanese Coronary Artery Disease Study Investigators. 2009. "Elevated serum uric acid is an independent predictor for cardiovascular events in patients with severe coronary artery stenosis: subanalysis of the Japanese Coronary Artery Disease (JCAD) Study." *Circ J* 73:885-891.

Olfsson C, Anderstam B, Bragfors-Helin A-C, Eriksson M, Qureshi AR, Lindholm B, Hilding A, Wiczkowski W, Orsini N, Stenvinkel P, Ekberg NR. 2019. "Effects of acute fructose loading on levels of serum uric acid- a pilot study." *Eur J Clin Nutr* 49: e13040.

Orlich MJ, Jaceldo-Siegl K, Sabate J, Fan J, Singh PN, Fraser GE. 2014. "Patterns of food consumption among vegetarians and non-vegetarians." *Br J Nutr* 112: 1644-1653.

Pan WH, Wu HJ, Yeh CJ, Chuang SY, Chuang HY, Yeh NH, Hsieh YT. 2011. "Diet and health trends in Taiwan: comparison of two nutrition and health surveys from 1993-1996 and 2005-2008." *Asia Pac J Clin Nutr* 20:238-250.

Panza VS, Wazlawik E, Ricardo Schütz G, Comin L, Hecht KC, da Silva EL. 2008. "Consumption of green tea favorably affects oxidative stress markers in weight-trained men." *Nutrition* 24:433-442.

Pérez-Jiménez J. 2010. "Identification of the 100 richest dietary sources of polyphenols an application of the Phenol-Explorer database." *Eur J Clin Nutr* 64 Suppl 3: S112-120.

Pham NM, Yoshida D, Morita M, Yin G, Toyomura K, Ohnaka K, Takayanagi R, Kono S. 2010. "The relation of coffee consumption to serum uric acid in Japanese men and women aged 49-76 years." *J Nutr Metab* 2010: 930757.

Poole R, Kennedy OJ, Roderick P, Fallowfield JA, Hayes PC, Parkes J. 2017. "Coffee consumption and health: umbrella review of meta-analyses of multiple health outcomes." *BMJ* 359: j5024.

Price CA, Medici V, Nunez MV, Lee V, Sigala DM, Benyam Y, Keim NL, Mason AE, Chen S-Y, Parenti M, Slupsky C, Epel ES, Havel PJ, Stanhope KL. 2021. "A pilot study comparing the effects of consuming 100%.

orange juice or sucrose-sweetened beverage on risk factors for cardiometabolic disease in women." *Nutrients* 13:760.

Psaltopoulou T, Sergentanis TN, Panagiotakos DB, Sergentanis IN, Kosti R, Scameas N. 2013. "Mediterranean diet, stroke, cognitive impairment, and depression: A meta-analysis." *Ann. Neurol* 74:580-591.

Rai SK, Fung TT, Lu N, Keller SF, Curhan GC, Choi HK. 2017. "The dietary approaches to Stop Hypertension (DASH) diet, Western diet, and risk of gout in men: prospective cohort study." *BMJ* 357: j1794.

Reagan-Shaw S, Nihal M, Ahmad N. 2008. "Dose translation from animal to human studies revisited." *FASEB J* 22:659-661.

Rebholz CM, Crews DC, Grams ME, Steffen LM, Levey AS, Miller ER 3 rd, Appel LJ, Coresh J. 2016. "DASH (Dietary Approaches to Stop Hypertension) diet and risk of subsequent kidney disease." *Am J kidney Dis* 68:853-861.

Reedy J, Krebs-Smith SM, Miller PE, Liese AD, Kahle LL, Park Y, Subar AF. 2014. "Higher diet quality is associated with decreased risk of all-cause, cardiovascular disease, and cancer mortality among older adults." *J Nutr* 144:881-889.

Ren Z, Huang C, Momma H, Cui Y, Sugiyama S, Niu K, Nagatomi R. 2016. "The consumption of fish cooked by different methods was related to the risk of hyperuricemia in Japanese adults: A 3-year follow-up study." *Nutr Metab Cardiovasc Dis* 26:778-785.

Richette P, Bardin T. 2010. "Gout." *Lancet* 375:318-328.

Richette P, Doherty M, Pascual E, Barskova V, Becce F, Castaneda-Sanabria J, Coyfish M, Guillo S, Jansen TL, Jansens H, Lioté F, Mallen C, Nuki G, Perez-Ruiz F, Pimentao J, Punzi L, Pywell T, So A, Tausche AK, Uhlig T, Zavada J, Zhang W, Tubach F, Bardin T. 2017. "2016 updated EULAR evidence-based recommendations for the management of gout." *Ann Rheum Dis* 76:29-42.

Ríos-Hoyo A, Cortés MJ, Ríos-Ontiveros H, Meaney E, Ceballos G, Gutiérrez-Salmeán G. 2014. "Obesity, metabolic syndrome, and dietary therapeutical approaches with a special focus on nutraceuticals (polyphenols): a mini-review." *Int J Vitam Nutr Res* 84:113-123.

Rodriguez A, Curhan GC, Gambaro G, Taylor EN, Ferraro PM. 2020. "Mediterranean diet adherence and risk of incident kidney stones." *Am J Clin Nutr* 111:1100-1106.

Romaguera D, Norat T, Vergnaud AC, Mouw T, May AM, Agudo A, Buckland G, Slimani N, Rinaldi S, Couto E, Clavel-Chapelon F, Boutron-Ruault MC, Cottet V, Rohrmann S, Teucher B, Bergmann M, Boeing H, Tjønneland A, Halkjaer J, Jakobsen MU, Dahm CC, Travier N, Rodriguez L, Sanchez MJ, Amiano P, Barricarte A, Huerta JM, Luan J, Wareham N, Key TJ, Spencer EA, Orfanos P, Naska A, Trichopoulou A, Palli D, Agnoli C, Mattiello A, Tumino R, Vineis P, Boeno-de-Mesquita HB, Büchner FL, Manjer J, Wirfält E, Johansson I, Hellstrom V, Lund E, Braaten T, Engeset D, Odysseos A, Riboli E, Peeters PH. 2010. "Mediterranean dietary patterns and prospective weight change in participants of the EPIC-PANACEA study." *Am J Clin Nutr* 92:912-921.

Ros E. 2009. "Nuts and novel biomarkers of cardiovascular disease." *Am J Clin. Nutr* 89:1649S-1656S.

Ruggiero C, Cherubini A, Ble A, Bos AJ, Maggio M, Dixit VD, Lauretani F, Bandinelli S, Senin U, Ferrucci L. 2006. "Uric acid and inflammatory markers." *Eur Heart J* 27:1174-1181.

Saag KG, Choi HK. 2006. "Epidemiology, risk factors, and lifestyle modifications for gout." *Arthritis Res Ther* 8 (suppl 1): S2.

Sánchez-Moreno C, Cano MP, de Ancos B, Plaza L, Olmedilla B, Granado F, Martín A. 2004. "Consumption of high-pressurized vegetable soup increases plasma vitamin C and decreases oxidative stress and inflammatory biomarkers in healthy humans." *J Nutr* 134:3021-3025.

Santos HO, Genario R, Gomes GK, Schoenfeld BJ. 2021. "Cherry intake as a dietary strategy in sport and diseases: a review of clinical applicability and mechanisms of action." *Crit Rev Food Sci Nutr* 61:417-430.

Sattui SE, Singh JA, Gaffo AL. 2014. "Comorbidities in patients with crystal diseases and hyperuricemia." *Rheum Dis Clin North Am* 40:251-278.

Saura-Calixto F, Goñi I. 2009. "Definition of the Mediterranean diet based on bioactive compounds." *Crit Rev Food Sci Nutr* 49:145-152.

Schlesinger N. 2005. "Dietary factors and hyperuricemia." *Curr Pharm Des* 11:4133-4138.

Schmidt JA, Crowe FL, Appleby PN, Key TJ, Travis RC. 2013. "Serum uric acid concentrations in meat eaters, fish eaters, vegetarians and vegans: a cross-sectional analysis in the EPIC-Oxford cohort." *PLoS One* 8: e56339.

Seegmiller JE, Grayzel AI, Laster L, Liddle L. 1961. "Uric acid production in gout." *J Clin Invest* 40: 1304-1314.

Shao SS, Lin CZ, Zhu YF, Chen C, Wu QJ, Chen RR. 2022. "Higher dietary acid load is associated with hyperuricemia in Chinese adults: A case-control study." *BMC Endocr Disord* 22:286.

Sigie T, Imatou T, Miyazaki M, Une H. 2005. "The effect of alcoholic beverage type on hyperuricemia in Japanese male office workers." *J Epidemiol* 15:41-47.

Siqueira J, Pereira TSS, Veiasquez-Melendez G, Barreto SM, Benseñor IM, Mill JG, Molina MCB. 2021. "Sugar-sweetened soft drinks consumption and risk of hyperuricemia: Results of the ELSA-Brasil study." *Nutr Metab Cardiovasc Dis* 31:2004-2013.

Skerret PJ, Willett WC. 2010. "Essentials of healthy eating: A guide." *J Midwifery Womens Health* 55:492-501.

Smyth A, Griffin M, Yusuf S, Mann JF, Reddan D, Canavan M, Newell J, O'Donnell M. 2016. "Diet and major renal outcomes: A prospective cohort study. The NIH-AARP Diet and Health Study." *J Ren Nutr* 26: 288-298.

Sofi F, Cesari F, Abbate R, Gensini GF, Casini A. 2008. "Adherence to Mediterranean diet and health status: meta-analysis." *BMJ* 337: a1344.

Solfrizzi V, Custodero C, Lozupone M, Imbimbo BP, Valiani V, Agosti P, Schilardi A, D'Introno A, La Montagna M, Calvani M, Guerra V, Sardone R, Abbrescia D, Bellomo A, Greco A, Paniele A, Seripa D, Logroscino G, Sabbá C, Panza F. 2017. "Relationships of dietary patterns, foods, and micro-and macronutrients with Alzheimer's disease and late-life cognitive disorders: A systematic review." *J Alzheimers Dis* 59:815-849.

Soltani S, Arablou T, Jayedi A, Salehi-Abargouei A. 2020. "Adherence to the dietary approaches to stop hypertension (DASH) diet in relation to all-cause and cause-specific mortality: a systematic review and dose-response meta-analysis of prospective cohort studies." *Nutr J* 19:37.

Soltani S, Chitsazi MJ, Salehi-Abargouei A. 2018. "The effect of Dietary Approaches to Stop Hypertension (DASH) on serum inflammatory markers: A systematic review and meta-analysis of randomized trials." *Clin Nutr* 37:542-550.

Stamostergiou J, Theodoridis X, Ganochoriti V, Bogdanos DP, Sakkas LI. 2018. "The role of the Mediterranean diet in hyperuricemia and gout." *Mediterr J Pheumatol* 29:21-25.

Sun L, Ni C, Zhao J, Wang G, Chen W. 2022. "Probiotics, bioactive compounds and dietary patterns for the effective management of hyperuricemia: a review." *Crit Rev Food Sci Nutr* 8:1-16.

Sun SZ, Flickinger BD, Williamson-Hughes PS, Empie MW. 2010. "Lack of association between dietary fructose and hyperuricemia risk in adults." *Nutr Metab* 7:16.

Szeto YT, Kwok TCY, Benzie IFF. 2004. "Effects of a long-term vegetarian diet on biomarkers of antioxidant status and cardiovascular disease risk." *Nutrition* 20:863-866.

Tang O, Miller ER 3rd, Gelber AC, Choi HK, Appel LJ, Juraschek SP. 2017. "DASH diet and change in serum uric acid over time." *Clin Rheumatol* 36:1413-1417.

Tappy L, Morio B, Azzout-Mamiche D, Champ M, Gerber M, Houdart S, Mas E, Rizkalia S, Slama G, Mariotti F, Margaritis I. 2018. "French recommendations for sugar intake in adults: a novel approach chosen by ANSES." *Nutrients* 10:989.

Taylor EN, Fung TT, Curhan GC. 2009. "DASH-Style diet associates with reduced risk for kidney stones." *J Am Soc Nephrol* 20:2253-2259.

Tektonidis TG, Akesson A, Gigante B, Wolk A, Larsson SC. 2015. "A Mediterranean diet and risk of myocardial infarction, heart failure and stroke; A population-based cohort study." *Atherosclerosis* 243:93-98.

Teng GG, Tan CS, Santosa A, Saag KG, Yuan JM, Koh WP. 2013. "Serum urate levels and consumption of common beverages and alcohol among Chinese in Singapore." *Arthritis Care Res* 65:1432-1440.

Ter Maaten JC, Voorburg A, Heine RJ, Ter Wee PM, Donker AJ, Gans RO. 1997. "Renal handling of urate and sodium during acute physiological hyperinsulinaemia in healthy subjects." *Clin. Sci* 92. 51-58.

Terkeltaub R, Edwards NL. 2013. *Gout; Diagnosis and management of gouty arthritis and hyperuricemia.* (Terkeltaub R, Edwards NL., eds.) vol.3. NY: Professional Communications, Inc.

The Council for Science and Technology, Ministry of Education, Culture, Sports, Science and Technology in Japan. 2023. "Standard tables of food composition in Japan -2020- (Eighth Revised Edition), Report of the Subdivision Resources." Accessed April 28. https://www.mext.go.jp/content/20201225-mxt_kagsei-mext_01110_011.pdf.

The Ministry of Health, Labour and Welfare, Japan. 2023. "Dietary Reference Intakes for Japanese, 2020." Accessed April 28. https://www.mhlw.go.jp/file/06-Seisakujouhou-10900000-Kenkoukyoku/Overview.pdf.

The Ministry of Health, Labour and Welfare and Ministry of Agriculture, Forestry and Fisheries. 2023. "2010, Japanese Food Guide Spinning Top, Tokyo." Accessed April 28. http://www.maff.go.jp/j/balance_guide/b_sizai/attach/pdf/index-56.pdf.

Tonstad S, Stewart K, Oda K, Batech M, Herring RP, Fraser GE. 2013. "Vegetarian diets and incidence of diabetes in the adventist health study-2." *Nutr Metab Cardiovasc Dis* 23:292-299.

Tozser J, Benko S. 2016. "Natural compounds as regulators of NLRP3 inflammasome-mediated IL-1beta production." *Mediat Inflamm* 2016:5460302.

Tsai YT, Liu JP, Tu YK, Lee MS, Chen PR, Hsu HC, Chen MF, Chien LL. 2012. "Relationship between dietary patterns and serum uric acid concentrations among ethnic Chinese adults in Taiwan." *Asia Pac J Clin Nutr* 21:263-270.

Tyrovolas S, Bountziouka V, Papairakleous N, Zeimbekis A, Anastassiou F, Gotsis E, Metallinos G, Polychronopoulos E, Lionis C, Panagiotakos D. 2009. "Adherence to the Mediterranean diet is associated with lower prevalence of obesity among elderly people living in Mediterranean islands: the MEDIS study." *Int J Food Sci Nutr* 60 Suppl 6:137-150.

Underwood M. 2006. "Diagnosis and management of gout." *BMJ* 332:1315-1319.

Unger T, Borghi C, Charchar F, Khan NA, Poulter NR, Prabhakaran D, Ramirez A, Schlaich M, Stergiou GS, Tomaszewski M, Wainford RD, Williams B, Schutte AE. 2020. "2020 International Society of Hypertension global hypertension practice guidelines." *Hypertension* 75:1334-1357.

U.S. Department of Agriculture. 2005. *Dietary guidelines for Americans. Center for Nutrition Policy and Promotion*. Washington, DC: USDA.

U.S. Department of Agriculture. 2023. "Dietary Guidelines for Americans 2015-2020, eighth edition." Accessed April 28. https://health.gov/sites/default/files/2019-09/2015-2020_Dietary_Guidelines.pdf.

U.S. Department of Health & Human Services. National Institutes of Health. 2023. "Office of Dietary Supplements. Dietary Supplement Fact Sheets." Accessed April 28. https://ods.od.nih.gov/factsheets/list-all/.

Usharani P, Nutalapati C, Pokuri VK, Kumar CU, Taduri G. 2016. "A randomized, double-blind, placebo-, and positive-controlled clinical pilot study to evaluate the efficacy and tolerability of standardized aqueous extracts of *Terminalia chebula* and *Terminalia bellerica* in subjects with hyperuricemia." *Clinical Pharmacology: Advances and Applicvations* 8:51-59.

van Dam RM, Rimm EB, Willett WC, Stampfer MJ, Hu FB. 2002. "Dietary patterns and risk for type 2 diabetes mellitus in U.S. men." *Ann Intern Med* 136:201-209.

van der Gaag MS, van den Berg R, van den Berg H, Schaafsma G, Hendriks HF. 2000. "Moderate consumption of beer, red wine and spirits has counteracting effects on plasma antioxidants in middle-aged men." *Eur J Clin Nutr* 54:586-591.

Vedder D, Walrabenstein W, Heslinga M, de Vries R, Nurmohamed M, van Schaardenburg D, Gerritsen M. 2019. "Dietary interventions for gout and effect on cardiovascular risk factors: A systematic review." *Nutrients* 11: 2955.

Villegas R, Xiang Y-B, Elasy T, Xu WH, Cai H, Cai Q, Linton MF, Fazio S, Zheng W, Shu X-O. 2012. "Purine-rich foods, protein intake, and the prevalence of hyperuricemia: the Shanghai Men's Health Study." *Nutr Metab Cardiovasc Dis* 22:409-416.

Vinha AF, Barreira SV, Costa AS, Alves RC, Oliveira MBP. 2014. "Pre-meal tomato (Lycopersicon esculentum) intake can have anti-obesity effects in young women?" *Int J Food Sci Nutr* 65:1019-1026.

Vuorinen-Markkola H, Yki-Järvinen H. 1994. "Hyperuricemia and insulin resistance." *J Clin Endocrinol Metab* 78:25-29.

Wang C, Guo X-F, Yang T, Zhao T, Li D. 2021. "Nut intake and hyperuricemia risk in young adults." *Public Health Nutr* 15:1-19.

Willett WC, Stampfer MJ. 2003. "Rebuilding the food pyramid." *Sci Am* 288:64-71.

Williams PT. 2008. "Effects of diet, physical activity and performance, and body weight on incident gout in ostensibly healthy, vigorously active men." *Am J Clin Nutr* 87:1480-1487.

World Health Organization. 2007. *Prevention of cardiovascular disease. Guidelines for assessment and management of cardiovascular risk.* Geneva, Switzerland: WHO Press.

World Health Organization 2023. "Healthy diet." Accessed April 28. https://www.who.int/news-room/fact-sheets/detail/healthy-diet.

Wu Y, Ye Z, Feng P, Li R, Chen X, Tian X, Han R, Kakade A, Liu P, Li X. 2021. "*Limosilactobacillus fermentum* JL-3 isolated from 'Jiangshui' ameliorates hyperuricemia by degrading uric acid." *Gut Microbes* 13:1-1.

Xia Y, Wu Q, Wang H, Zhang S, Jiang Y, Gong T, Xu X, Chang Q, Niu K, Zhao Y. 2020. "Global, regional and national burden of gout, 1990-2017: a systematic analysis of the Global Burden of Disease Study." *Rheumatology* 59:1529-1538.

Xia Y, Xiang Q, Gu Y, Jia S, Zhang Q, Liu L, Meng G, Wu H, Bao X, Yu B, Sun S, Wang X, Zhou M, Jia Q, Wu Y, Song K, Niu K. 2018. "A dietary pattern rich in animal organ, seafood and processed meat products is associated with newly diagnosed hyperuricaemia in Chinese adults: a propensity score-matched case-control study." *Br J Nutr* 119:1177-1184.

Xiong Z, Zhu C, Qian X, Zhu J, Wi Z, Chen L. 2013. "Serum uric acid is associated with dietary and lifestyle factors in elderly women in suburban Guangzhou in Guangdong province of south China." *J Nutr Health Aging* 17:30-34.

Xu K, Cui X, Wang B, Tang Q, Cai J, Shen X. 2020. "Healthy adult vegetarians have better renal function than matched omnivores: a cross-sectional study in China." *BMC Nephrol* 21:268.

Yahfoufi N, Alsadi N, Jambi M, Matar C. 2018. "The immunomodulatory and anti-inflammatory role of polyphenols." *Nutrients* 10:1618.

Yamamoto T, Moriwaki Y, Ka T, Inokuchi T, Takahashi S, Tsutsumi Z, Fukuchi M, Hada T. 2004. "Effect of purine-free low-malt liquor (happo-shu) on the plasma concentrations and urinary excretion of purine bases and uridine—comparison between purine-free and regular happo-shu." *Horm Metab Res* 36:231-237.

Yamamoto T, Moriwaki Y, Takahashi S. 2005. "Effect of ethanol on metabolism of purine bases (hypoxanthine, xanthine, and uric acid)." *Clin Chim Acta* 356:35-57.

Yang S-Y, Zhang H-J, Sun S-Y, Wang L-Y, Yan B, Liu C-Q, Zhang W, Li X-J. 2011. "Relationship of carotid intima-media thickness and duration of vegetarian diet in Chinese male vegetarians." *Nutr Metab* 8:63.

Yi K, Cui S, Tang M, Wu Y, Xiang Y, Yu Y, Tong X, Jiang Y, Zhao Q, Zhao G. 2022. "Adherence to DASH dietary pattern and its association with incident hyperuricemia risk: a prospective study in Chinese community residents." *Nutrients* 14:4853.

Yokose C, McCormick N, Choi HK. 2021. "Dietary and lifestyle-centered approach in gout care and prevention." *Curr Rheumatol Rep* 23:51.

Yokose C, McCormick N, Rai SK, Lu N, Curhan G, Schwarzfuchs D, Shai I, Choi HK. 2020. "Effects of low-fat, Mediterranean, or low-carbohydrate weight loss diets on serum urate and cardiometabolic risk factors: A secondary analysis of the Dietary Intervention Randomized Controlled Trial (DIRECT)." *Diabetes Care* 43:2812-2820.

Yokoyama Y, Nishimura K, Barnard ND, Takegami M, Watanabe M, Sekikawa A, Okamura T, Miyamoto Y. 2014. "Vegetarian diets and blood pressure: a meta-analysis." *JAMA Intern Med* 174:577-587.

Yoo TW, Sung KC, Shin HS, Kim BJ, Kim BS, Kang JH, Lee MH, Park JR, Kim H, Rhee EJ, Lee WY, Kim SW, Ryu SH, Keum DG. 2005. "Relationship between serum uric acid concentration and insulin resistance and metabolic syndrome." *Circ J* 69:928-933.

Yu K-H, See L-C, Huang Y-C, Yang C-H, Sun J-H. 2008. "Dietary factors associated with hyperuricemia in adults." *Semin Arthritis Rheum* 37:243-250.

Yu JW, Yang TG, Diao WH, Cai XQ, Li T, Zhong H, Hu DL, Chen CQ, Chen ZX. 2010. "Epidemiological study on hyperuricemia and gout in Foshan areas, Guangdong province." *Chin J Epidemiol* 31:860-862.

Zgaga L, Theodoratou E, Kyle J, Farrington SM, Agakov F, Tenesa A, Walker M, McNeill G, Wright AF, Rudan I, Dunlop MG, Campbell H. 2012. "The association of dietary intake of purine-rich vegetables, sugar-sweetened beverages and dairy with plasma urate, in a cross-sectional study." *PLoS One* 7: e38123.

Zhang M, Chang H, Gao Y, Wang X, Xu W, Liu D, Li G, Huang G. 2012. "Major dietary patterns and risk of asymptomatic hyperuricemia in Chinese adults." *J Nutr Sci Vitaminol* 58:339-345.

Zhang M, Gao Y, Wang X, Liu W, Zhang Y, Huang G. 2016. "Comparison of the effect of high fruit and soybean products diet and standard diet interventions on serum uric acid in asymptomatic hyperuricemia adults: an open randomized controlled trial." *Int J Food Sci Nutr* 67:335-343.

Zhang T, Rayamajhi S, Meng G, Zhang Q, Liu L, Wu H, Gu Y, Wang Y, Zhang S, Wang X, Zhang J, Li H, Thapa A, Sun S, Wang X, Zhou M, Jia Q, Song K, Niu K. 2021. "Edible mushroom consumption and incident hyperuricemia: results from the TCLSIH cohort study." *Food Funct* 12:9178.

Zhang Y, Cui Y, Li X-A, Li L-J, Xie X, Huang Y-Z, Deng Y-H, Zeng C, Lei G-H. 2017. "Is tea consumption associated with the serum uric acid level, hyperuricemia, or the risk of gout? A systematic review and meta-analysis." *BMC Musculoskelet Disord* 18:95.

Zhou M, Huang X, Li R, Zhang Z, Zhang L, Gao X, Yang H, Ma Y. 2022. "Association of dietary patterns with blood uric acid concentration and hyperuricemia in northern Chinese adults." *Nutr J* 21: 42.

Zhu JN, Qi XY, Tan Y, Lyu XH. 2016. "Dietary factors associated with hyperuricemia and glycolipid metabolism disorder in middle-aged and elderly people." *Sichuan Da Xue Xue Bao Yi Xue Ban* 47:68-72.

Zhu Q, Yu L, Li Y, Man Q, Jia S, Liu B, Zong W, Zhou Y, Zuo H, Zhang J. 2023. "Association between Dietary Approaches to Stop Hypertension (DASH) diet and hyperuricemia among Chinese adults: findings from a nationwide representative study." *Nutr J* 22:21.

Zhu Y, Pandya BJ, Choi HK. 2011. "Prevalence of gout and hyperuricemia in the US general population: the National Health and Nutrition Examination Survey 2007-2008." *Arthritis Rheum* 63:3136-3141.

Zhu Y, Pandya BJ, Choi HK. 2012. "Comorbidities of gout and hyperuricemia in the US general population: NHANES 2007-2008." *Am J Med* 125:679-687.

Zou F, Zhao X, Wang F. 2021. "A review on the fruit components affecting uric acid level and their underlying mechanisms." *J Food Biochem* 45: e13911.

Zykova SN, Storhaug HM, Toft I, Chadban SJ, Jenssen TG, White SL. 2015. "Cross-sectional analysis of nutrition and serum uric acid in two Caucasian cohorts: the AusDiab Study and the Tromsø study." *Nutr J* 14:49.

Chapter 3

Dietary Nutrients for the Prevention and Management of Hyperuricemia

Takashi Koguchi*, **PhD**
Department of Human Education, Kokugakuin Tochigi Junior College, Tochigi-shi, Tochigi, Japan

Abstract

Hyperuricemia is the status of high serum uric acid (SUA) concentration and is recognized as a lifestyle-related disease. The prevalence of hyperuricemia has increased in various regions over the last 30 years and was different among various populations or regions. Taking into account the Acceptable Macronutrient Distribution Ranges (AMDRs), the Adequate Intakes (AIs), the Recommended Dietary Allowances (RDAs), and the Tolerable Upper Intake Levels (UL) of dietary reference intakes for nutrients set by the Institute of Medicine of the National Academy of Sciences in the U.S., dietary nutrient intake for the prevention and management of hyperuricemia in the general population (especially adults) is suggested as follows: the percentage of carbohydrate, protein, fat, and n-3 polyunsaturated fatty acids and n-6 polyunsaturated fatty acids in total energy intake should be within the range of the Acceptable Macronutrient Distribution Ranges (AMDRs) set by the Institute of Medicine of the National Academy of Sciences in the U.S.; pay attention to intake of total sugars intake; limiting or decreasing intake of fructose, animal fats, saturated fatty acids, cholesterol, and salt; replacement of saturated fatty acids (e.g., dairy fats, meat fat) with mono- and polyunsaturated fatty acids (particularly n-3 polyunsaturated fatty acids) (e.g., macadamia nuts, almonds, peanuts and peanut butter, olive oil,

* Corresponding Author's Email: echo130@nifty.com.

In: Hyperuricemia
Editor: Warren Y. Salinas
ISBN: 979-8-89113-239-9

canola oil, avocados); maintenance of good hydration; limiting or decreasing alcohol consumption; limiting intake of purine; pay attention to intake of vitamin A, vitamin B5 (pantothenic acid), and folate to avoid high serum vitamin A, vitamin B5 (pantothenic acid), and vitamin B9 levels, respectively; pay attention to vitamin D intake to avoid vitamin D deficiency; and recognizing encouraged intake of fiber, animal sources of protein (e.g., casein, lactalbumin), vegetable sources of protein (e.g., wheat gluten, rice endosperm protein), polyphenol, vitamin E, vitamin B1, vitamin B2, folate, vitamin B12, vitamin C, calcium, magnesium, iron, and zinc. This article describes the importance of nutrient intake for the prevention and management of hyperuricemia in the general population (especially adults), referencing the results of clinical research reported.

Keywords: alcohol, fiber, food, fructose, hyperuricemia, mineral, nutrient, polyphenol, purine, uric acid, vitamin

Introduction

Hyperuricemia is recognized as a lifestyle-related disease. The prevalence of hyperuricemia is influenced by multiple factors, such as genetics, gender, age, lifestyle, food, eating habits, and economic development (Liu et al. 2013). The prevalence of hyperuricemia has increased in various regions over the last 30 years and was different among various populations or regions (Roman 2019). For example, the total hyperuricemia prevalence in China was 11.1% in 2015-2016 and 14.0% in 2018-2019 (Zhang et al. 2022). The overall prevalence of hyperuricemia, defined as a serum uric acid (SUA) level > 7.0 mg/dL (416.4 μmol/L) in men and > 5.7 mg/dL (339.0 μmol/L) in women, in the US National Health and Nutrition Examination Survey (NHANES) 2007-2008 are higher than those in the NHANES-III (1988-1994) database, representing an increase of 3.2% in the prevalence of hyperuricemia (Zhu et al. 2011). According to the data from the US National Health and Nutrition Examination Survey (NHANES) 2007-2008 and 2015-2016, the overall prevalence of hyperuricemia, defined as a serum uric acid (SUA) level > 7.0 mg/dL (416.4 μmol/L) in men and > 5.7 mg/dL (339.0 μmol/L) in women, among US adults was 21.4% (43.3 million in total; men, 20.7 million; women, 22.6 million) in 2007-2008 and 20.1% (47.1 million in total; men, 22.8 million; women, 24.4 million) in 2015-2016, respectively (Zhu et al. 2011; Chen-Xu et al. 2019). The prevalence of hyperuricemia in the NHANES 2015-2016 is similar to that in 2007-2008 (Zhu et al. 2011; Chen-Xu et al. 2019). This result indicates that the prevalence of hyperuricemia in the U.S. remained substantial.

Hyperuricemia is classified into three types: "overproduction," or an excessive production of uric acid (UA); "underexcretion," an impairment of urinary uric acid (UUA) excretion; and "mixed," which is caused by both factors (Hisatome et al. 2018). The disease type classification is determined by results of the amount of UUA excretion, UA clearance, and creatinine clearance (Hisatome et al. 2018). Regardless of the disease type classification, renal underexcretion of UA is considered to be the most frequent mechanism for the genesis and development of hyperuricemia (Perez-Ruiz et al. 2002). In the U.S., hyperuricemia results from the overproduction of UA (10%), underexcretion of UA (90%), or often a combination of the two (Choi, Mount and Reginato 2005). Asymptomatic hyperuricemia can be detected in some cases and is caused by reduced renal UA excretion combined with increased UA synthesis from endogenous sources (breakdown of purines during cell turnover) or exogenous sources (food with high purine content) (Wolfram 1992).

Epidemiological studies have shown that dietary factors affect SUA levels parallel to the direction of the risk of hyperuricemia (Choi 2010). A decrease in high SUA concentrations lead to the prevention of hyperuricemia. Therefore, management of SUA concentrations is important for the prevention and suppression of hyperuricemia. This article summarizes the results of clinical research (clinical trials and epidemiological studies) of the association between SUA concentrations or hyperuricemia risk and dietary nutrients.

Physiology of Uric Acid

Uric acid (UA) is the end product of purine metabolism, largely derived from endogenous synthesis, but a minor part also arises from exogenous sources such as foods with purine content, alcohol, and fructose drinks (Jakše et al. 2019). Endogenous production of UA from degradation of purines usually contributes about two-thirds of the body urate pool, the remainder being dietary in origin (Doherty 2009). UA is synthesized mainly in the liver and intestines, but it is also synthesized in other tissues, such as muscles, kidneys, and the vascular endothelium (Zychowcz 2011; MacFariane 2014; El Ridi and Tallima 2017).

UA is a weak acid with a pKa of 5.75 and, at the physiological pH of 7.40 it exists mainly in the ionized form as urate (Doherty 2009). UA is the primary antioxidant in human plasma and accounts for more than 60% of the capacity to scavenge free oxidative radicals in the serum (Fabbrini et al. 2014). The antioxidant activity of UA is also overcome by the pro-oxidant and proinflammatory effects of reactive oxygen species accumulation under ischemic conditions (Lippi et al. 2008).

The antioxidant properties of UA can also protect against free radical damage to vessels, the heart, and neurons (Stocker and Keaney 2004; Tana et al. 2018; De Becker et al. 2019) and prevent bone loss and osteoporosis (Lin et al. 2019). The association of UA with health risks is biphasic, since low levels of UA are detrimental to neurons, due to impaired antioxidant capacity in the cell (Fang et al. 2013). High SUA levels are associated with neuroprotection against Parkinson's disease and Alzheimer's disease (Schlesinger and Schlesinger 2008; Du et al. 2016). These phenomena show immune activation as a potential mechanism for UA-induced neuroprotection (Cipriani et al. 2012). The mechanism of neuroprotection by UA remains largely unknown.

Serum uric acid (SUA) concentration reflects the interactions of four major processes: (1) dietary purine intake; (2) endogenous purine metabolism; (3) urinary UA excretion; (4) intestinal uricolysis (Wortmann and Kelley 2001). The serum uric acid (SUA) concentration is determined by the amount of production of UA and the efficiency of urinary UA excretion (Taniguchi and Kamatani 2008; Itakura 2009). Uric acid synthesis averages ~750 mg/day in adult males, but increased dietary purine intake stimulates higher production of UA (Terkeltaub. and Edwards 2013, 23-37). Renal uric acid excretion in normal adult men on a low-purine diet is ~400 mg/day, but the normal amount cleared renally is up to ~750 mg/day on a typical Western diet (Terkeltaub and Edwards 2013, 23-37). The maintenance of SUA levels within the normal physiological range (2-7 mg/dL for men and 2-6.5 mg/dL for women) depends on dietary purine intake, urate biosynthesis, and the rate of urate excretion (Ekpenyong and Daniel 2015). Physiologic limits to renal uric acid excretion promote hyperuricemia.

Urate transporter 1 (URAT1/SLC22A12) and Glucose transporter 9 (GLUT9/SLC2A9), which are key renal urate anion transporters promoting reabsorption by the proximal renal tubule epithelial cell, and ATP-binding cassette transporter G2 (ABCG2), which is the proximal tubule renal urate anion secretory transporter in the human kidney (Terkeltaub 2010). Urate transporter 1(URAT1/SLC22A12) is an organic anion exchanger localized at the apical (tubule lumen-facing) membrane of renal proximal tubule epithelial cells (Terkeltaub 2010; Terkeltaub and Edwards 2013, 23-37). URAT1-transduced urate anion reabsorption is stimulated by intracellular organic anions, including lactic acid and monocarboxylates (Terkeltaub 2010). Lactic acid can exchange with UA in the kidneys *via* sodium-dependent monocarboxylate transporters SLC5A8 and SLC5A12, which provide the main source of anions needed for urate transporter 1 (URAT 1) function (Le et al. 2008). Increased lactic acid and ketone acids in the filtrate enhances UA reabsorption *via* an anion-exchange transport system at the proximal tubule, resulting in a decrease in UUA excretion. A balance between proximal tubular secretion and reabsorption of filtered urate (mediated partly by GLUT9/SLC2A9 and ABCG2, respectively) ultimately determines net renal uric acid excretion (Terkeltaub and Edwards 2013, 23-37).

Inflammatory Response in Hyperuricemia

The serum uric acid (SUA) concentrations have been associated with several inflammatory markers [neutrophil count, C-reactive protein, interleukin-1 receptor antagonist (IL-1ra), interleukin-6 (IL-6), interleukin-18 (IL-18), tumor necrosis factor-alpha (TNF-α)] in individuals with or without hyperuricemia [SUA concentration > 7.5 mg/dL (450 μmol/L) in men and > 6.2 mg/dL (372 μmol/L) in women] (Ruggiero et al. 2006).

Uric acid (UA) can exert, along with its extracellular antioxidant activity, an intracellular prooxidant effect (Lin et al. 2019). Soluble UA has many proinflammatory and prooxidative effects in the intracellular environment. Intracellular pathways are oxidative stress, inflammatory signaling, autophagy and inflammasome, and intracellular immunometabolic sensors (Joosten et al. 2020). An increase in SUA concentration accompanied with the excess production of reactive oxygen species (ROS) promoted the activation of inflammasomes (Cui et al. 2020). These effects are the result of the accumulation of oxygen free radicals after xanthine dehydrogenase (EC1.17.1.4) converts to xanthine oxidase (EC1.17.3.2) in parallel with UA production as an effect of adenosine triphosphate degradation (Glantzounis et al. 2005). Abnormal activation of the NLRP inflammasome is related to cellular oxidative stress. Inflammasome components include nucleotide-binding and oligomerization domain-like receptor, leucine-rich repeat and pyrin domain-containing 3 (NLRP3), apoptosis-associated speck-like protein containing a caspase recruitment domain (ASC), Pro-caspase-1, which activate cysteine-containing aspartate-specific protease-1 (caspase-1), and

Pro-interleukin-1β (Pro-IL-1β)] (Tan et al. 2019). The NLRP3 inflammasome is a component of innate immunity and is responsible for producing mature IL-1β and IL-18 (Lim et al. 2018). The NLRP3 inflammasome is also a multiprotein complex to control caspase-1 activation step that is a prerequisite for the maturation of IL-1β and IL-18. Caspase-1 promotes the production of active inflammatory cytokine interleukin-1β (IL-1β), release it outside the cell, promotes the occurrence of inflammation, and accelerates the process of kidney disease (Tan et al. 2019). Therefore, UA induces immune system activation and alters the characteristics of resident kidney cells, such as tubular epithelial cells, endothelial cells, and vascular smooth muscle cells, toward a proinflammatory and profibrotic state (Jung et al. 2020). UA can oxidize low-density lipoprotein (LDL) in the presence of copper ions and lipid hydroperoxides, increasing the inflammatory status (Bagnati et al. 1999). Therefore, UA has pro-inflammatory, pro-oxidant and vasoconstrictive effects and may contribute to the development of cardiometabolic disorders (Shostak et al. 2022).

Hyperuricemia causes increased oxidative stress, endothelial dysfunction, inflammation, platelet adhesion and aggregation, and vasoconstriction (Feig 2014; So and Martinon 2017). The SUA can affect endothelial function, and hyperuricemia-induced endothelial dysfunction is involved in the pathogenesis of cardiovascular diseases (CVD) (Wang et al. 2022). High-sensitivity C-reactive protein (CRP) levels were positively associated with hyperuricemia risk (Ryu et al. 2011; Yang et al. 2016; Dai et al. 2020). One potential mechanism by which asymptomatic hyperuricemia contribute to disease is by stimulating inflammation (Joosten et al. 2020). Keenan (2020) has stated that hyperuricemia can result in the formation of monosodium urate (MSU) crystals that may be recognized as danger signals by the immune system; that is to say, this immune response results in the activation of the NLRP3 inflammasome and ultimately in the production and release of IL-1β and IL-18, that mediate both inflammation, pyroptotic cell death, and necroinflammation. Mechanism of soluble UA- and monosodium urate (MSU) crystal-induced inflammation were reviewed in detail by Cabău et al. (2020) and Joosten et al. (2020).

Gut Microbiota in Patients with Hyperuricemia

Faecalibacterium prausnitzii, *Clostridium* butyrate-producing bacterium and *Bifidobacterium pseudocatenulatum* were enriched in healthy individuals

(Guo et al. 2016). Gut microbiota imbalances exist in patients with hyperuricemia and gout (Chu et al. 2021; Yin et al. 2022). Gut microbiota can be altered after UA reduction (Yu et al. 2018). Gut microbiota dysbiosis (e.g., richness, diversity, composition of microbiota, and relative abundance of microbiota taxa) was associated with SUA concentrations (Wei et al. 2022).

Hyperuricemia decreased gut microbiota richness and diversity, altered composition of microbiota, and lowered relative abundances of genus *Coprococcus* compared to those with normouricemia (Wei et al. 2022). The relative abundances of *Faecalibacterium*, *Gemmiger*, *Bacteroides*, and *Roseburia* were significantly increased in asymptomatic hyperuricemia patients compared to the control group (healthy subjects) (Yang et al. 2021). On the other hand, the relative abundances of *Bifidobacterium* and *Akkermansia* were significantly decreased in asymptomatic hyperuricemia patients compared to the control group (healthy subjects) (Yang et al. 2021).

The microbial composition differs between asymptomatic hyperuricemia and gout patients; that is to say, an asymptomatic hyperuricemia group showed a higher *Firmicutes*-to-*Bacteroidetes* ratio and lower *Prevotella*-to-*Bacteroides* ratio than the gout group (Kim et al. 2022). Kim et al. (2022) have stated that the phenomena that higher *Firmicutes*-to-*Bacteroidetes* ratio and lower *Prevotella*-to-*Bacteroides* ratio in asymptomatic hyperuricemia patients than in gout patients indicate that the microbiome of asymptomatic hyperuricemia is associated with metabolic diseases, whereas that of gout patients is associated with an inflammatory immune-related disease. The differences of the gut microbiota may exist in purine metabolism, UA metabolism, and amino acid metabolism between hyperuricemia and gout patients, resulting in the transformation of gut microbiota (Wang et al. 2022).

Association between Dietary Nutrients and Plasma or Serum Uric Acid Concentrations or Hyperuricemia Risk

The Institute of Medicine of the National Academy of Sciences in the U.S. (2021) has set Dietary Reference Intakes values: the Estimated Average Requirement (EAR), the Recommended Dietary Allowance (RDA), the Adequate Intake (AI), the Tolerable Upper Intake Level (UL), the Acceptable Macronutrient Distribution Ranges (AMDRs) for vitamins, minerals, macronutrients, and energy in life stage and gender groups.

It is important to recognize dietary recommendations for prevention and management of hyperuricemia. Based on the results of clinical research (clinical trials and epidemiological studies), association between dietary nutrients, foods or dietary patterns and hyperuricemia were reviewed in detail by Koguchi (2018; 2021; 2022).

Energy

The Institute of Medicine of the National Academy of Sciences in the U.S. (2021) has determined that the Acceptable Macronutrient Distribution Ranges (AMDRs) for carbohydrates is 45-65 percent of total calories for adults (aged ≥ 1 year) and total protein is 10-35 percent of total calories for adults (aged ≥ 19 years) and at 20-35 percent of total calories for adults (aged ≥ 19 years), respectively. The World Health Organization recommendations for a healthy diet (World Health Organization 2023) has stated that energy intake should balance energy expenditure (and keep total fat intake to less than 30% of total energy intake, with a shift in fat consumption away from saturated fats to unsaturated fats, and towards the elimination of industrial trans fats).

Zhu et al. (2016) reported that excessive intake of energy was risk factors of hyperuricemia in middle-aged and elderly people in China.

Considering the viewpoint for the prevention and management of hyperuricemia, it seems that it is necessary to be aware of the intake of casein, lactalbumin, wheat gluten, rice endosperm protein in a diet maintaining the Acceptable Macronutrient Distribution Ranges (AMDRs) for fat, carbohydrate, and protein.

Carbohydrate

Total Carbohydrate

The Institute of Medicine of the National Academy of Sciences in the U.S. (2021) has determined that the Acceptable Macronutrient Distribution Ranges (AMDRs), which is defined as a range of intakes for a particular energy source that is associated with reduced risk of chronic disease while providing adequate intakes of essential nutrients, for carbohydrates in both adults aged ≥ 19 years and children aged 1-18 years is 45-65 percent of total calories.

A cross-sectional study from China showed that every 10g increase in energy-adjusted carbohydrate intakes caused a 5% decrease in hyperuricemia risk (Zhang et al. 2023).

Sugars

The World Health Organization (WHO) has stated that the term "sugars" includes intrinsic sugars, which are those incorporated within the structure of intact fruit and vegetables; sugars from milk (lactose and galactose); and free sugars, which are monosaccharides and disaccharides added to foods and beverages by the manufacturer, cook or consumer, and sugars naturally present in honey, syrups, fruit juices and fruit juice concentrates (World Health Organization 2015). On the other hand, the 2015-2020 Edition of the Dietary Guidelines for Americans (U.S. Department of Agriculture 2023) recommends consuming less than 10% calories per day from added sugar and does not include sugars from fruit juices.

Increased intake of sugars was associated with increased hyperuricemia risk (Tappy et al. 2018). Tappy et al. (2018) have proposed to set a maximum limit to the intake of total sugars containing fructose (sucrose, glucose fructose syrups, honey or other syrups, and natural concentrates, etc.) of 100g/day. The recommendation for added sugars naturally present that was established by the Institute of Medicine of the National Academy of Sciences in the U.S. suggests the limit to a maximal intake of no more than 25 percent total energy (Institute of Medicine of the National Academy of Sciences 2021). The WHO recommends reducing the intake of free sugars to less than 10% of total energy intake in both adults and children and suggests a further reduction of the intake of free sugars to below 5% of total energy intake (World Health Organization 2015; World Health Organization 2023).

Glucose, Fructose, and Sucrose

From an analysis of the NHANES (1999-2004), Sun et al. (2010) estimated that the mean intake of total sugars, total sucrose, and total fructose in the U.S. for adults ages 20-80 were 135.91g/day, 36.06g/day, and 43.1g/day, respectively.

Sucrose is commonly known as table sugar and is naturally contained in fruit and vegetables. When sucrose is consumed, the enzyme beta-fructosidase separates sucrose into its individual sugar units of glucose and fructose. Oral administration of sucrose at 1.5g/kg of body weight in healthy male volunteers increased plasma UA (PUA) concentrations and oxypurines (hypoxanthine and xanthine), suggesting that increased PUA concentration is attributed to enhanced purine degradation (Kobayashi et al. 2007). Increased intake of sucrose was associated with increased hyperuricemia risk (Stanhope 2016).

The metabolism of glucose and fructose in humans was reviewed in detail by Sun and Empie (2012) and Fang et al. (2022). Intake of fructose (250-290 g/day) increased SUA concentration by 8-41% compared to glucose in three healthy men (Emmerson 1974). This result suggests that an increasing effect of fructose on SUA concentration is greater than that of glucose. A meta-analysis reported by Schwingshackl et al. have indicated that replacing fructose with an equivalent energy amount of glucose reduced insulin resistance (HOMA-IR) and plasma or serum UA concentrations (Schwingshackl et al. 2020). This result suggests that substitution of fructose with glucose has a beneficial effect for prevention and suppression of hyperuricemia.

In epidemiological studies, increased fructose intake was associated with increased SUA concentrations (Choi et al. 2008; Zhang et al. 2018) and hyperuricemia risk (Choi et al. 2008; Zhang et al. 2018; Li, Yu and Li 2018; Zhang et al. 2020).

Fructose intake has been shown to increase SUA level via both decreased UA excretion and increased UA production (Le et al. 2008). In a systematic review and meta-analysis of controlled feeding trials, high fructose intake (213-219 g/day) under hypercaloric feeding conditions (+35% excess energy) raised SUA concentrations in people with and without diabetes mellitus (Wang et al. 2012). Fructose metabolism activates adenosine monophosphate deaminase, promoting purine degradation and inosine production and resulting in elevated SUA concentrations (Thottam et al. 2017). A large amount of fructose can activate nicotinamide adenine dinucleotide phosphate oxidase, which further prevents the excretion of UA through the ileum in rats, resulting in an increase in the SUA concentrations (Kaneko et al. 2017).

In subjects receiving a low-fructose diet after ingestion of high-fructose diet, fasting plasma UA concentration was increased and urinary UA clearance and fractional UA excretion were lowered, suggesting that decreased urinary UA excretion may contribute to fructose-induced hyperuricemia (Lecoultre et al. 2013). It has been reported that a higher-than-normal daily intake of fructose may lead to hyperuricemia in humans (Livesey 2009; Perez-Pozo et al. 2010). It is assumed that a high fructose intake (213-219g/d) under hypercaloric feeding conditions (+35% excess energy) leads to increase hyperuricemia risk.

Effects of sucrose, glucose and fructose on serum uric acid (SUA) levels and hyperuricemia risk are reviewed in detail by Sun and Empie (2012), Dornas et al. (2015), Caliceti et al. (2017), and Koguchi (2018; 2022).

Fructose-Rich Foods

Higher intake of foods high in fructose was associated with increased SUA concentrations (Choi et al. 2008; Nguyen et al. 2009; Chuang et al. 2011; Kontogianni et al. 2012; Zgaga et al. 2012; Merriman et al. 2014; Xia et al. 2020; Ebrahimpour-Koujan et al. 2021; Siqueira et al. 2021) and hyperuricemia risk (Stanhope 2016; Ebrahimpour-Koujan et al. 2020; Siqueira et al. 2021). Increased intake of high fructose corn syrup was associated with increased hyperuricemia risk (Stanhope 2016). These results suggest that excessive intake of fructose and fructose-rich foods (e.g., high-fructose corn syrup and sugar-sweetened beverages, soft drinks) may lead to hyperuricemia.

Foods high in fructose are as follows: raisins, date palms, dried figs, dried mangos, dried tomatoes, dried kanpyo, dried apricots, dried prunes, ginger powders, grapes, apples, dried bananas, lychees, cherimoyas, pears, cherries, kiwifruit, quinces, gooseberries, persimmons, figs, mangos, blueberries (The Council for Science and Technology, Ministry of Education, Culture, Sports, Science and Technology in Japan 2023).

Fiber

The U.S. Department of Agriculture (USDA) has recommended that daily dietary fiber intake is 14g/1000kcal, for an average age adult, this means a daily intake of 25g (female) or 38g (male) in the U.S. (U.S. Department of Agriculture 2023). The recommended Adequate Intakes (AIs) for total fiber (the sum of dietary fiber and functional fiber) in the U.S. population aged ≥ 1 year established by the Institute of Medicine of the National Academy of Sciences in the U.S. is 14g/1,000 kcal [men aged 14-50 years, 38g/day; men aged ≥ 51 years, 30g/day; women aged 9-18 years, 26g/day; women aged 19-50 years, 25g/day; women aged ≥ 51 years, 21g/day; pregnancy aged ≤ 18 years and 19-50 years, 28g/day; lactation aged ≤ 18 years and 19-50 years, 29g/day] (Institute of Medicine of the National Academy of Sciences in the U.S. 2021).

In clinical trials, dietary fiber decreased serum uric acid (SUA) concentrations (Yamaguchi et al. 2007; Carabin et al. 2009). In epidemiological studies, increased dietary fiber intake was associated with decreased serum uric acid (SUA) concentrations (Sun et al. 2010; Shatat et al. 2012; Zykova et al. 2015; So et al. 2020; Zhu et al. 2022) and hyperuricemia risk (Yu et al. 2008; Sun et al. 2010; Zykova et al. 2015; Sun et al. 2019; So et al. 2020; Zhu et al. 2022). A cross-sectional study from China showed that every 10g increase in energy-adjusted dietary fiber intakes caused a 13% decrease in hyperuricemia risk (Zhang et al. 2023).

The underlying mechanism for suppression of elevation of SUA concentrations and decrease in hyperuricemia risk by fiber intake is not fully elucidated. At the present time, a possible mechanism for the suppression of elevation of SUA concentrations of fiber ingested in experimental hyperuricemia model animals are presumed to be due to the following six reasons: (1) dietary fiber suppresses digestion and/or absorption of dietary purines in the digestive system (Koguchi et al. 2002; Koguchi et al. 2003; Koguchi et al. 2004; Koguchi et al. 2016; Koguchi and Tadokoro 2019); (2) inulin (Lin et al. 2014; Guo et al. 2021) and konjac glucomannan (Zhang et al. 2016; Zhang et al. 2018) suppresses uric acid (UA) production through inhibition of xanthine oxidase activity; (3) agarose increases the renal excretion efficiency of UA (Koguchi et al. 2016); (4) inulin (Guo et al. 2021) and mannuronate oligosaccharides (Wei et al. 2023) promote intestinal UA excretion; (5) inulin alleviates the inflammatory state because of increased short chain fatty acids (SCFAs) concentrations (acetate, propionate, and butyrate concentrations) and SCFAs-producing bacteria (e.g., *Akkermansia*, *Ruminococcus*, *Bifidobacterium*, *Parasutterella*) in the feces and modulation of gut microbiota, resulting in reduced SUA levels (Guo et al. 2021); (6) mannuronate oligosaccharides suppresses the inflammatory response in the kidney inflammation and increases SCFAs concentrations (acetic acid, propionic acid, and isovaleric acid concentrations) and modulate the gut microbiota (Wei et al. 2023). The mechanism may be related to SCFAs, especially propionate and butyrate, providing ATP to the cells of the intestinal wall to show beneficial effects on UA excretion (Hosomi et al. 2012; Nieuwdorp et al. 2014), and butyrate improves metabolism of UA through lowering UA concentrations in the colonic mucosa (Hamer et al. 2009). Dietary fiber increases production of SCFAs, which are acetate, propionate, and butyrate, by increasing bacteria that are beneficial to health (Schariau et al. 2009; Lattimer and Haub 2010). Butyrate can play a role in inhibiting the pathways that lead to the production of pro-inflammatory cytokines (Bander et al. 2020). The mechanism responsible for the anti-inflammatory effect of dietary fiber has not been fully elucidated but might involve the production of SCFAs by colonic fermentation in rodents (Ando, Bamba and Sasaki 1999; Hijova et al. 2013; Guo et al. 2021). Future investigations are needed to clarify how dietary fiber suppresses elevation of SUA concentrations and lowers hyperuricemia risk, other than the above-mentioned mechanisms.

Foods high in dietary fiber are as follows: seeds and nuts (pumpkin seeds, chia seeds, almonds, pistachio nuts, hazelnuts, peanuts), whole grains (high fiber-bran ready-to-eat cereals, shredded wheat ready-to-eat cereals, whole grain bread, oats, barley, rye), legumes (navy beans, small white beans, yellow beans, cranberry beans, adzuki beans, French beans, split peas, chickpeas, lentils, pinto beans), seaweed, mushrooms (wood ear, shitake mushrooms, maitake mushrooms), potatoes (konjac, potato with skin), fruit (avocados, apples, raspberries, blackberries, prunes, oranges, bananas, guavas), and vegetables (artichokes, pumpkins, tomatoes, broccoli, carrots, sweet corn, pears) (The Council for Science and Technology, Ministry of Education, Culture, Sports, Science and Technology in Japan 2023; U.S. Department of Health & Human Services. National Institutes of Health. Office of Dietary Supplements 2023).

Protein

Total Protein

The Institute of Medicine of the National Academy of Sciences in the U.S. (2021) has determined that the Acceptable Macronutrient Distribution Ranges (AMDRs) for total protein at 10-35 percent of total calories for adults aged ≥ 19 years and at 10-30 percent of total calories for children aged 4-18 years and 5-20 percent of total calories for children aged 1-3 years. In healthy adult men and women, protein intake should not exceed the World Health Organization (WHO) recommendation (0.83 g/kg body weight/day for adults) (World Health Organization, Food and Agriculture Organization, and United Nations University 2007).

Epidemiological studies showed that the total protein intake was not associated with the SUA level (Loenen et al. 1990; Choi, Liu and Curhan 2005; Zykova et al. 2015) and hyperuricemia risk (Yu et al. 2008; Sun et al. 2010; Villegas et al. 2012). A cross-sectional study from China showed that every 10g increase in energy-adjusted protein intakes caused a 17% increase in hyperuricemia risk (Zhang et al. 2023).

Animal Protein

The gastrointestinal hydrolysate of α-lactalbumin reduced serum UA, creatinine, and urea nitrogen concentrations in potassium oxonate- and hypoxanthine- induced hyperuricemic mice (Xie et al. 2023). Xie et al. (2023) have stated that the anti-hyperuricemia and nephroprotective functions of the gastrointestinal hydrolysate of α-lactalbumin are mediated by inhibiting xanthine oxidase activity in the liver, ameliorating oxidative stress and inflammation, regulating renal urate transporters, and modulating the gut microbiota in hyperuricemic mice.

Ingestion of milk protein (casein and lactalbumin) has been shown to decrease SUA levels in healthy subjects via the uricosuric effect of these proteins (Garrel et al. 1991). The intake of milk and cheese seems to be important for the prevention of hyperuricemia.

A cross-sectional study from China showed that every 10g increase in energy-adjusted animal protein intakes caused an 18% increase in hyperuricemia risk (Zhang et al. 2023).

Vegetable Protein

Jenkins et al. (2001) found that a high intake of gluten-derived protein (especially wheat gluten) reduced SUA concentrations. Ingestion of 10g/day of rice endosperm protein for 4 weeks significantly decreased SUA concentration compared with the casein group or the baseline in adult male subjects with risk factors for metabolic syndrome (Hosojima et al. 2016).

Greater consumption of soy protein (6.1 vs. 0.5g/day) was associated with a lower presence of hyperuricemia in women (Liu et al. 2014). A cross-sectional study from China showed that every 10g increase in energy-adjusted plant-derived protein intakes caused a 10% decrease in hyperuricemia risk (Zhang et al. 2023).

Protein-Rich Foods

The effect of protein on SUA concentration or hyperuricemia risk varies depending on the protein derived from food. For example, administration of 80 grams of casein and lactalbumin significantly reduced SUA concentration after a 3-hour period, while that of soy protein increased SUA concentration (Garrel et al. 1991). A positive association between protein intake from animal sources and the prevalence of hyperuricemia, as well as an inverse association with protein from plant sources has been revealed (Choi, Liu and Curhan 2005; Villegas et al. 2012). In a cross-sectional study, there was an inverse association between intake of protein-rich foods (egg and egg products, dairy products, soybean, and soybean products) and prevalence of hyperuricemia (Yu et al. 2008). These reports indicate that intake of protein from vegetable sources and milk proteins (casein and lactalbumin) may have a protective effect for hyperuricemia. Further clinical trials and prospective studies are needed to clarify the relationship between protein and SUA concentration or hyperuricemia risk.

Fat

Total Fat

The Institute of Medicine of the National Academy of Sciences in the U.S. (2021) has determined that the Acceptable Macronutrient Distribution Ranges (AMDRs) for total fat at 20-35 percent of total calories for adults aged ≥ 19 years and at 25-35 percent of total calories for children aged 4-18 years and 30-40 percent of total calories for children aged 1-3 years. The World Health Organization's recommendations for a healthy diet (World Health Organization 2023) has stated that we should keep total fat intake to less than 30% of total energy intake, with a shift in fat consumption away from saturated fats to unsaturated fats, and towards the elimination of industrial trans fats.

In an epidemiological study, increased intake of fat was associated with increased SUA concentrations (Zykova et al. 2015). Zhu et al. (2016) reported that excessive intake of fat was a risk factor of hyperuricemia in middle-aged and elderly people in China. A cross-sectional study from China showed that every 10g increase in energy-adjusted fat intakes caused a 10% increase in hyperuricemia risk (Zhang et al. 2023).

n-3 Polyunsaturated Fatty Acids

The Institute of Medicine of the National Academy of Sciences in the U.S. (2021) has established that the Adequate Intakes (AIs) for α-linolenic acid is 1.2-1.6g/day for males aged ≥ 9 years and 1.0-1.1g/day for females aged ≥ 9 years. Respectively, for males aged 9-13 years, 1.2 g/day; males aged ≥ 14 years, 1.6 g/day; females aged 9-13 years, 1.0 g/day; females aged ≥ 14 years, 1.1 g/day. The Institute of Medicine of the National Academy of Sciences in the U.S. (2021) has determined that the Acceptable Macronutrient Distribution Ranges (AMDRs) for n-3 polyunsaturated fatty acids (α-linolenic acid) both adults aged ≥ 19 years and children aged 4-18 years is 0.6-1.2 percent of total calories.

Plant-based source (e.g., flax, canola, soybean, and walnuts) contains α-linolenic acid (ALA) and fatty fish (e.g., tuna, mackerel, and salmon) are rich in eicosapentaenoic acid (EPA) and docosahexaenoic acid (DHA) (The Council for Science and Technology, Ministry of Education, Culture, Sports,

Science and Technology in Japan 2023; U.S. Department of Health & Human Services. National Institutes of Health. Office of Dietary Supplements 2023).

Eicosapentaenoic acid (EPA), α-linolenic acid (ALA), and docosahexaenoic acid (DHA) strongly inhibited URAT 1 activities and n-3 polyunsaturated fatty acids inhibited the function of URAT 1 more effectively than n-6 polyunsaturated fatty acids (Saito et al. 2020). Saito et al. (2020) have stated that n-3 polyunsaturated fatty acids will be preferable to n-6 polyunsaturated fatty acids for the prevention of hyperuricemia/gout as uricosuric agents.

One should consume at least 250 mg/day of long-chain n-3 polyunsaturated fatty acids or at least 2 servings/week of oily fish (Mozaffarian and Wu 2011).

n-6 Polyunsaturated Fatty Acids

The Institute of Medicine of the National Academy of Sciences in the U.S. (2021) has established that the Adequate Intakes (AIs) for linoleic acid is 12-17 g/day for males aged ≥ 9 years and 10-12 g/day for females aged ≥ 9 years. Respectively, for males aged 9-13 years,: 12.0 g/day; males aged 14-18 years, 16.0 g/day; males aged 19-50 years, 17.0 g/day; males aged ≥ 51 years, 14.0 g/day; females aged 9-13 years, 10.0 g/day; females aged 14-18 years, 11.0 g/day; females aged 19-50 years, 12.0 g/day; females aged ≥ 51 years, 11.0 g/day. The Institute of Medicine of the National Academy of Sciences in the U.S. (2021) has determined that the Acceptable Macronutrient Distribution Ranges (AMDRs) for n-6 polyunsaturated fatty acids (linoleic acid) both adults aged ≥ 19 years and children aged 4-18 years is 5-10 percent of total calories.

Conjugated Linoleic Acid

The Institute of Medicine of The National Academy in the U.S. (2021) has not set the Estimated Average Requirement (EAR) and the Recommended Dietary Allowances (RDAs) for conjugated linoleic acid.

Conjugated linoleic acid ameliorates high fructose-induced hyperuricemia and renal inflammation in rats via inhibition of NLRP3 inflammasome and TLR4/MyD88 signaling pathway (Tan et al. 2019).

Cholesterol

The Estimated Average Requirement (EAR), the Recommended Dietary Allowances (RDAs), the Adequate Intakes (AIs), and the Tolerable Upper Intake Levels (ULs) for cholesterol in the U.S. population established by the

Institutes of Medicine has not been set (The Institute of Medicine of The National Academy in the U.S., 2021). The Institute of Medicine of the National Academy of Sciences in the U.S. (2021) has stated that recommendation for dietary cholesterol is as low possible while consuming a nutritionally adequate diet.

Foods high in cholesterol are as follows: liver, egg yolk, dried herring roe, dried squid, anchovy, sardines, shrimp, abalone, salmon, mackerel, sea urchin, carp, sweet fish, lobster, and full-fat dairy products (The Institute of Medicine of the National Academy of Sciences in the U.S. 2021; The Council for Science and Technology, Ministry of Education, Culture, Sports, Science and Technology in Japan 2023).

Alcohol

In epidemiological studies, increased intake of alcohol was associated with increased serum uric acid (SUA) concentrations (Loenen et al. 1990; Shadick et al. 2000; Choi and Curhan 2004; Williams 2008; Sun et al. 2010; Villegas et al. 2012; Zykova et al. 2015; Beydoun et al. 2018: So et al. 2020; Xia et al. 2020) amd hyperuricemia risk (Campion, Glynn and DeLabry 1987; Shadick et al. 2000; Sigie et al. 2005; Sun et al. 2010: Villegas et al. 2012; Xiong et al. 2013; Liu et al. 2014; Li, Yu and Li 2018; So et al. 2020).

Heavy alcohol (ethanol) consumption increased the production of uric acid (UA), which resulted in an increase in SUA concentration and a decrease in urinary UA excretion, which led to hyperuricemia (Yamamoto et al. 2005). Proposed mechanisms of higher alcohol consumption associated with increased SUA levels and hyperuricemia risk are presumed to be due to the following reasons reviewed in detail by Yamamoto et al. (2005): (1) alcohol consumption increases UA liver production through ATP degradation, leading to an accumulation of ADP and AMP (Roman 2019), and it increases lactic acid production, which has a competitive inhibitory effect on UA excretion and ethanol can increase the rate of sputum synthesis in humans and increase UA production (Eastmond et al. 1995); (2) alcohol consumption leads to dehydration and metabolic acidosis, resulting in decreased UA excretion (Yamamoto et al. 2004).

Water Intake

The Recommended Adequate Intakes (AIs) for water intake in the U.S. population aged ≥ 0 month established by the Institute of Medicine of the National Academy of Sciences in the U.S. (2021) are based on the median water intake U.S. survey data (total water intake includes drinking water, water in beverages and formula, and water that is contained in food). Total water intake: males aged 14-18 years, 3.3 L g/day (approximately 2.6 L as total beverages, including drinking water); males aged ≥ 19 years, 3.7 L/day (approximately 3.0 L as total beverages, including drinking water); females aged 14-18 years, 2.3 L/day (approximately 1.8 L as total beverages, including drinking water); females aged ≥ 19 years, 2.7 L/day (approximately 2.2 L as total beverages, including drinking water). Terkeltaub and Edwards (Terkeltaub. and Edwards 2013, 152) have stated that maintenance of good hydration (five to eight 8-oz servings of water daily: 1183-1893g) is essential.

Purine

Purine, such as ribonucleic acid (RNA), adenosine-5'-monophosphate (5'-AMP), guanosine-5'-monophosphate (5'-GMP), inosine-5'-monophosphate (5'-IMP), hypoxanthine, and adenine, increased plasma uric acid (PUA) or serum uric acid (SUA) concentrations (Yü, Berger and Gutman 1962; Bowering et al. 1970; Edozien et al. 1970; Clifford et al. 1976; Liu et al. 2018; Zhang et al. 2018).

Bowering et al. (1970) found that daily administration of 4g of RNA to healthy subjects doubled the uric acid (UA) pool, increasing serum uric acid (SUA) concentration, and increasing urinary uric acid (UUA) excretion, which cause overproduction-type hyperuricemia. Brulé et al. (1988), Yokozawa et al. (1982), and Koguchi et al. (2004) reported that dietary adenine caused experimental underexcretion-type hyperuricemia through renal dysfunction in rats, which seems to be due to the 2.8-dihydroxyadenine nephrolithiasis. Considering the maximum recommended amount of nucleic acid from the daily diet, long-term excessive intake of adenine-rich foods which is containing 50 mg or more adenine in 100 g of food [e.g., animal liver, legumes (soybeans, peas, lentils, white beans, green beans, red beans, etc.) (Kaneko et al. 2014; Hisatome et al. 2018)] can cause elevated SUA levels due to decreased kidney function. It is necessary to limit the amount to one serving of purine-rich foods, especially adenine.

Purine-rich foods are animal meat (i.e., beef, pork, lamb, organ meats, and meat extracts), seafood (i.e., fish fillets, tuna, shrimp, lobster, clams, etc.), plants (i.e., yeast extracts, peas, beans, lentils, asparaguses, cauliflowers, spinach, mushrooms, bamboo shoots), seaweed (e.g., nori, wakame), seasonings (i.e., soup stock, oyster sauce, consommé, Chinese soup, etc.) (Kaneko et al. 2014; Hisatome et al. 2018). By contrast, dairy products (i.e., milk, cheese, yogurt, ice cream), grains and their products (i.e., bread, pasta, cereals), nuts, fruit, vegetables, sugars and sweets, sugar-sweetened beverages, and alcoholic beverages are low in purine (Kaneko et al. 2014; Hisatome et al. 2018). Eggs and milk contained no purine (Kaneko et al. 2014; Hisatome et al. 2018). The amounts of purines in distilled liquor (i.e., whiskey, brandy, shochu, awamori) and plum wine do not almost contain (0-0.4 mg/100mL) and those in beer and wine were 3.3-9.8 mg/100mL and 0.4-1.6 mg/100mL, respectively (Kaneko et al. 2014; Hisatome et al. 2018).

Intake of meat and fish, which are purine-rich foods, increased PUA or SUA concentrations in normal human subjects, respectively (Brulé et al., 1992). As management policy in patients with hyperuricemia, Neogi (2011) has stated that individuals with hyperuricemia should reduce the uptake of exogenous purine to reduce UA content contributing for the total UA pool of the body. Hisatome et al. (2018) have recommended that a daily intake of purines should keep less than 400mg.

Polyphenol

Plant foods contain polyphenols (Mehmood et al. 2019). The consumption of isoflavones was inversely associated with the presence of hyperuricemia in women (Liu et al. 2014).

In an *in vitro* study, apigenin (Adachi et al. 2021), caffeic acid (Mehmood et al. 2022), chlorogenic acid (Chan, Wen and Chiang 1995; Mehmood et al. 2022), chrysin (Nagao, Seki and Kobayashi 1999), curcumin (Shen and Ji 2009), gallic acid (Wu et al. 2022), isorhamnetin (Nagao, Seki and Kobayashi 1999), kaempferol (Nagao, Seki and Kobayashi, 1999), luteolin (Nagao, Seki and Kobayashi 1999; Adachi et al. 2021), myricetin (Nagao, Seki and Kobayashi, 1999), quercetin (Mehmood et al. 2022), tea catechins [e.g., catechin, epicatechin, (-)-epigallocatechin, (-)-epicatechin-3-gallate, (-)-epigallocatechin-3-gallate] (Wu et al. 2022), tea polyphenols (Wu et al. 2022), theaflavin (Wu et al. 2022) inhibit xanthine oxidase activity, thus suppressing uric acid (UA) production.

In experimental hyperuricemia with or without renal dysfunction (urate nephropathy) in mice or rats, anthocyanin extracts from purple sweet potato (Hwa et al. 2011; Zhang et al. 2015), astilbin (Chen et al. 2011; Wang et al. 2016), chrysin (Chang et al. 2021), curcumin (Chen et al. 2019; Xu et al. 2021), epigallocatechin gallate (Li et al. 2020), ferulic acid (Zhang et al. 2023), green tea polyphenols (Chen et al. 2015), kaempferol (Haidari et al. 2011), procyanidins from grape seeds (Wang et al. 2004), quercetin (Zhu et al. 2004; Hu et al. 2009; Haidari et al. 2011; Hu et al. 2012; Hu et al. 2012; Adachi, Yoshizawa and Yagasaki 2017), resveratrol (Shi et al. 2012; Xiao et al. 2021; Zhang et al. 2021), rutin (Zhu et al. 2004; Hu et al. 2009; Hu et al. 2012; Chen et al. 2013; Adachi et al. 2021), and sinapic acid (Ishaq et al. 2020) suppressed the elevation of SUA concentrations. Although the underlying mechanism for the suppression of elevation of SUA concentrations by polyphenol ingested in hyperuricemia is not fully elucidated, a possible mechanism for the suppression of elevation of SUA concentrations of polyphenol ingested in experimental hyperuricemia with or without renal dysfunction (urate nephropathy) in mice or rats are presumed to be due to the following three reasons: (1) certain polyphenol [anthocyanin extracts from purple sweet potato (Hwa et al. 2011; Zhang et al. 2015), curcumin (Chen et al. 2019), epigallocatechin gallate (Li et al. 2020), green tea polyphenols (Chen et al. 2015), kaempferol (Haidari et al. 2011), procyanidins from grape seeds (Wang et al. 2004), quercetin (Zhu et al. 2004; Haidari et al. 2011), resveratrol (Xiao et al. 2021), rutin (Zhu et al. 2004), sinapic acid (Ishaq et al. 2020)] can effectively inhibit xanthine oxidase activity in the liver, thereby reducing the production of UA; (2) certain polyphenol [chrysin (Chang et al. 2021), epigallocatechin gallate (Li et al. 2020), ferulic acid (Zhang et al. 2023), green tea polyphenols (Chen et al. 2015), resveratrol (Zhang et al. 2021), rutin (Chen et al. 2013)] reduces the reabsorption of UA by regulating UA-related transporters [urate transporter 1 (URAT1) and/or glucose transporter 9 (GLUT9)] and promotes the excretion of UA by regulating UA-related transporters [organic anion transporter 1 (OAT1) and/or ATP-binding cassette subfamily G, member 2 (ABCG2)], thus improving hyperuricemia; (3) certain polyphenol [chrysin (Chang et al. 2021), curcumin (Chen et al. 2019), quercetin (Hu et al. 2012), resveratrol (Xiao et al. 2021; Zhang et al. 2021), rutin (Hu et al. 2012)] can reduce the interleukin-1β (IL-1β) levels in serum and kidney by the reduction of oxidative stress and inflammation through suppressing NLRP3 inflammasome activation in the kidney. Mechanism of anti-hyperuricemic effects of polyphenols were reviewed in detail by Sun et al. (2022).

Table 1. Foods rich in polyphenols*

Polyphenol	Food items
	polyphenols (> 3.0 mg/100 g FW or > 3.0 mg/100mL)
Apigenin	Italian oregano, marjoram
Caffeic acid	common sage, common thyme, cumin, ginger, Italian oregano, nutmeg, oregano, rosemary, Spearmint, caraway, Ceylan cinnamon, sunflower seed, black chokeberry, lingonberry, plum prune juice (concentrate)
(+)-Catechin	red wine, chocolate dark, chocolate milk, cocoa powder, apple, grape, strawberry, nectarine, peach, plum, apple pure juice, chocolate milk beverage, plum pure juice, pecan nut, pistachio nut, common bean, broad bean seed, broad bean pod
Chlorogenic acid	rose wine, apricot, blackberry, blackcurrant, loquat, nectarine, peach, plum, quince, sour cherry, sweet cherry, coffee beverage, rowanberry pure juice, broccoli
Curcumin	turmeric, curry
(-)-Epicatechin	red wine, chocolate dark, chocolate milk, cocoa powder, apple, apricot, black elderberry, custard apple, European cranberry, grape (black), peach, pear, red raspberry, sweet cherry, apple pure juice, chocolate milk beverage, pear pure juice, black tea infusion, green tea infusion, broad bean seed, broad bean pod
(-)-Epicatechin-3-gallate	black tea infusion, green tea infusion, oolong tea infusion, peppermint tea infusion
(-)-Epigallocatechin	black tea infusion, green tea infusion, oolong tea infusion, pecan nut, broad bean seed, broad bean pod
(-)-Epigallocatechin-3-gallate	black tea infusion, green tea infusion, oolong tea infusion
Ferulic acid	barley whole grain flour, common wheat (refined flour), hard wheat (refined flour), hard wheat whole grain flour, common sage, common thyme, marjoram, oregano, olive (green), chocolate dark
Gallic acid	red wine, walnut liquor, blackberry, cloudberry, black tea infusion, common sage, oregano, clove, chestnut, chicory (green, red)
Genistein	soy paste, soy bacon, soy flour, soy meat, soy tempe, soy tofu, soybean roasted
Isorhamnetin	onion yellow
Kaempferol	caper, caraway, clove, cumin
Luteolin	common sage, common thyme, lemon verbena, Mexican oregano, rosemary, black olive, globe artichoke
Procyanidins (dimer B1-B5, trimer C1, T2, EEC)	red wine, chocolate dark, cocoa powder, apple, fox grape, nectarine, peach, plum, custard apple, quince jam, quince jelly, apple pure juice, black tea infusion, broad bean pod, barley whole grain flour
Quercetin	chocolate dark, black elderberry, Mexican oregano, caper, clove
Theaflavin	black tea infusion
Theaflavin-3,3'-digallate	black tea infusion

* INRA (2023).

The amount of Chrysin, Myricetin, Procyanidins (trimer C2, C-GC-C, GC-C-C, GC-GC-C), Puerarin, Pyrogallol, Theaflavin 3-gallate in food is below 3.0 mg/100 g FW or 3.0 mg/100mL.

Foods rich in polyphenols (> 3.0 mg/100 g FW or > 3.0 mg/100mL) are as follows (Table 1): beverages and infusion (apple pure juice, chocolate milk beverage, coffee beverage, pear pure juice, plum pure juice, rowanberry pure juice, black tea infusion, green tea infusion, oolong tea infusion, peppermint tea infusion), alcoholic beverages (red wine, rose wine, walnut liquor), cereals (barley whole grain flour, common wheat, hard wheat, hard wheat whole grain flour), legumes (common bean, broad bean seed), soy and soy products (soybean roasted, soy paste, soy bacon, soy flour, soy meat, soy tempe, soy tofu), seeds and nuts (sunflower seed, pecan nut, pistachio nut, broad bean seed, chestnut), fruit and fruit products (apple, apricot, blackberry, black chokeberry, black currant, black elderberry, cloudberry, custard apple, European cranberry, fox grape, grape, lingonberry, loquat, nectarine, peach, pear, plum, quince, red raspberry, sour cherry, strawberry, sweet cherry, quince jam, quince jelly), vegetables (black olive, green olive, broad bean pod, broccoli, chicory, globe artichoke, onion yellow), spices (caper, caraway, clove, cumin, Ceylan cinnamon, ginger, nutmeg, star anise, turmeric, curry), herbs (common sage, common thyme, lemon verbena, Italian oregano, marjoram, Mexican oregano, oregano, rosemary, spearmint), cocoa (chocolate dark, chocolate milk, cocoa powder) (INRA 2023). Dietary polyphenol intake in the US was ~1 g/day (Kuhnau 1976). Since it has reported that excessive intake of some polyphenols resulted in growth depression in animals (Yoon and Baek 2005), it must take care of excessive intake of polyphenols.

Vitamins

Vitamin A and β-Carotene

The Recommended Dietary Allowances (RDAs) for vitamin A in the U.S. men aged ≥ 14 years and women aged ≥ 14 years established by the Institute of Medicine of the National Academy of Sciences in the U.S. (2021) are 900 μgRAE/day and 700 μgRAE/day, respectively. The Tolerable Upper Intake levels (ULs) for vitamin A in men and women aged 14-18 years, men and women (aged ≥ 19 years), pregnancy and lactation aged ≤ 18 years, and pregnancy and lactation aged 19-50 years are 2,800μgRAE/day, 3,000 μgRAE/day, 2,800μgRAE/day, and 3,000 μgRAE/day, respectively (The Institute of Medicine of the National Academy of Sciences in the U.S. 2021).

Serum vitamin A (retinol) levels were positively associated with SUA concentrations (Ford and Choi 2013; Kim et al. 2020; Liu et al. 2021) and hyperuricemia risk (Kim et al. 2020). In contrast, β-carotene supplementation lowered SUA levels in healthy adult subjects (Elmadfa et al. 2004). A cross-sectional survey using Australian Diabetes, Obesity and Lifestyle Study (AusDiab) data (1999/00) collected for 9,734 subjects [4,295 males and 5,439 females aged ≥ 25 years] showed that increased intake of retinol showed a tendency to increase SUA levels, and increased intake of β-carotene did not lower SUA levels (Zykova et al. 2015).

Looking at results from the NHANES-Ⅲ (1988-1994) data, Choi et al. (2012) found that vitamin A supplementation and food fortification may contribute to the high frequency of hyperuricemia and β-carotene which is a precursor to vitamin A, intake may be beneficial against hyperuricemia. It must pay attention to vitamin A intake to avoid high serum vitamin A levels in general population and not to exceed the Tolerable Upper Intake levels (ULs) for vitamin A.

Foods high in vitamin A are as follows: organ meats (beef liver, pork liver, chicken liver, monkfish liver), seafood (herring, firefly squid, eel), potatoes (sweet potato), fruit (mangos, cantaloupes), vegetables (spinach, carrots, peppers), dairy products (milk, ricotta cheese), confectioneries (pumpkin pie, French vanilla ice cream) (The Council for Science and Technology, Ministry of Education, Culture, Sports, Science and Technology in Japan 2023; U.S. Department of Health & Human Services. National Institutes of Health. Office of Dietary Supplements 2023).

Vitamin D

The Adequate Intakes (AIs) for vitamin D in the U.S. men and women aged 0-50 years, men and women aged 51-70 years, and men and women aged ≥ 71 years established by the Institute of Medicine of the National Academy of Sciences in the U.S. (2021) are 5 μg/day, 10 μg/day, and 15 μg/day, respectively. The Tolerable Upper Intake levels (ULs) for vitamin D in men aged ≥ 1 year, women aged ≥ 1 year, pregnancy aged ≤ 18 years and 19-50 years, and lactation aged ≤ 18 years and 19-50 years are 50 μg/day, respectively (The Institute of Medicine of the National Academy of Sciences in the U.S. 2021).

Vitamin D deficiency can activate the parathyroid to induce the release of parathyroid hormone (Emilion and Emilion 2011), which was thought to increase SUA levels (Dalbeth et al. 2009; Hui et al. 2012). Vitamin D deficiency was associated with hyperuricemia (Isnuwardana et al. 2020). A review reported by Charoenngam (2021) suggests that correcting vitamin D deficiency (serum 25-hydroxyvitamin D concentration < 20 ng/mL) and insufficiency (serum 25-hydroxyvitamin D concentration 20- < 30 ng/mL) has a mild uric acid (UA)-lowering effect (~0.3-0.6 mg/dL), which is thought to be mediated by the suppression of parathyroid hormone, which is known to downregulate the ATP-binding cassette transporter G2 (ABCG2) in the kidneys, leading to a reduction in the renal clearance of UA (Ponvilawan and Charoenngam 2021).

Foods high in vitamin D are as follows: organ meats (beef liver, monkfish liver, chicken breast), fish (salmon, salmon roe, trout, herring, cuttlefish, tuna, sardines), fish oil (cod liver oil), mushrooms (wood ear), milks (whole milk, whole chocolate milk, soy milk, almond milk), dairy products (cheese), cereals (ready-to-eat cereal, fortified with 10% of the daily value for vitamin D), eggs (The Council for Science and Technology, Ministry of Education, Culture, Sports, Science and Technology in Japan 2023; U.S. Department of Health & Human Services. National Institutes of Health. Office of Dietary Supplements 2023). An overdose of vitamin D-rich foods and/or supplementation should be avoided so as not to exceed the Tolerable Upper Intake Levels (ULs).

Vitamin E

The Recommended Dietary Allowances (RDAs) for vitamin E in the U.S. men and women aged ≥ 14 years, pregnancy aged ≤ 18 years and 19-50 years, and lactation aged ≤ 18 years and 19-50 years established by the Institute of Medicine of the National Academy of Sciences in the U.S. (2021) are 15 mg/day, 15 mg/day, and 19 mg/day, respectively. The Tolerable Upper Intake levels (ULs) for vitamin E intake in men and women aged 14-18 years, men and women aged ≥ 19 years, pregnancy and lactation aged ≤ 18 years, and pregnancy and lactation aged 19-50 years are 800 mg/day, 1,000 mg/day, 800 mg/day, and 1,000 mg/day, respectively (The Institute of Medicine of the National Academy of Sciences in the U.S. 2021).

In the National Health and Nutrition Examination Survey (NHANES) 2009-2014, dietary vitamin E intake was inversely associated with hyperuricemia risk in the U.S. adult population aged ≥ 20 years, especially among males and participants aged ≥ 60 years (Zhang et al. 2020).

A possible mechanism of higher vitamin E intake associated with lower hyperuricemia risk could be that vitamin E inhibits the activity of xanthine oxidase (Mohd Fahami et al. 2012) and has uricosuric effect (increasing or promoting the excretion of UA in urine) (Seifi et al. 2011).

Foods high in vitamin E are as follows: fish (sweetfish), grains (wheat germ), oil (wheat germ oil, sunflower oil, safflower oil, corn oil, soybean oil), seeds and nuts (sunflower seeds, almonds, hazelnuts, peanuts), vegetables (spinach, broccoli, tomatoes, red pepper), fruit (kiwifruit, mangos), beverages (green tea), seasonings and condiments (peanut butter) (The Council for Science and Technology, Ministry of Education, Culture, Sports, Science and Technology in Japan 2023; U.S. Department of Health & Human Services. National Institutes of Health. Office of Dietary Supplements 2023). An overdose of vitamin E-rich foods and/or supplementation should be avoided so as not to exceed the Tolerable Upper Intake Levels (ULs).

Thiamin (Vitamin B_1)

The Recommended dietary allowances (RDAs) for thiamin in the U.S. men aged $\geq$ 14 years, women aged 14-18 years, women aged $\geq$ 19 years, and pregnancy and lactation aged $\leq$ 18 years and 19-50 years established by the Institute of Medicine of the National Academy of Sciences in the U.S. (2021) are 1.2 mg/day, 1.0 mg/day, 1.1 mg/day, and 1.4 mg/day, respectively. The Institute of Medicine of the National Academy of Sciences in the U.S. (2021) has not set the Tolerable Upper Intake Levels (ULs) for thiamin (vitamin B_1).

In Australian Diabetes, Obesity and Lifestyle Study (AusDiab) cohort, higher consumption of thiamin (vitamin B_1) was associated with lower SUA levels (Zykova et al. 2015).

Foods high in vitamin B_1 are as follows: meats (beef steak, pork), processed meats (pork chop), seafood (mussels, trout, tuna), mushrooms (maitake mushrooms), grains (white rice, egg noodles, bread, barley, wheat germ, macaroni), whole grains (brown rice, oatmeal, breakfast cereals), seeds (sunflower seeds, sesame seeds, chia seeds), legumes (black beans), vegetables (acorn squash), dairy products (milk, yogurt), beverages (orange juice), confectioneries (English muffin), seasonings and condiments (baker's yeast) (The Council for Science and Technology, Ministry of Education, Culture, Sports, Science and Technology in Japan 2023; U.S. Department of Health & Human Services. National Institutes of Health. Office of Dietary Supplements 2023).

Riboflavin (Vitamin B_2)

The Recommended dietary allowances (RDAs) for riboflavin in the U.S. men aged $\geq$ 14 years, women aged 14-18 years, women aged $\geq$ 19 years, pregnancy aged $\leq$ 18 years and 19-50 years, and lactation(aged $\leq$ 18 years and 19-50 years established by the Institute of Medicine of the National Academy of

Sciences in the U.S. (2021) are 1.3 mg/day, 1.0 mg/day, and 1.1 mg/day, 1.4 mg/day, and 1.6 mg/day, respectively. The Institute of Medicine of the National Academy of Sciences in the U.S. (2021) has not set the Tolerable Upper Intake Levels (ULs) for riboflavin (vitamin B_2).

In both the the AusDiab Study and the Tromsø study cohorts, higher consumption of riboflavin (vitamin B_2) was associated with lower SUA levels in most subject groups (Zykova et al. 2015). Results from these studies showed that the average reduction of SUA level was significant when riboflavin (vitamin B_2) intakes were above 2 mg per day (Zykova et al. 2015).

Foods high in vitamin B_2 are as follows: meats (beef steak, rotisserie chicken), organ meats (beef liver, pork liver, chicken liver), seafood (clams, salmon), mushrooms (maitake mushrooms), grains (quinoa), whole grains (oats, breakfast cereals), seeds and nuts (almonds), seaweed, vegetables (parsley), dairy products (milk, cheese, yogurt), eggs, confectioneries (bagel), seasonings and condiments (baker's yeast) (The Council for Science and Technology, Ministry of Education, Culture, Sports, Science and Technology in Japan 2023; U.S. Department of Health & Human Services. National Institutes of Health. Office of Dietary Supplements 2023).

Pantothenic Acid (Vitamin B_5)

The Adequate Intakes (AIs) for pantothenic acid (Vitamin B_5) in the U.S. men and women aged $\geq$ 14 years, pregnancy aged $\leq$ 18 years and 19-50 years, and lactation aged $\leq$ 18 years and 19-50 years established by the Institute of Medicine of the National Academy of Sciences in the U.S. (2021) are 5.0 mg/day and 5.0 mg/day, 6.0 mg/day, and 7.0 mg/day, respectively. The Institute of Medicine of the National Academy of Sciences in the U.S. (2021) has not set the Tolerable Upper Intake Levels (ULs) for pantothenic acid.

Serum vitamin B_5 (pantothenic acid) was positively associated with SUA concentrations (Liu et al. 2021). It must pay attention to vitamin B_5 (pantothenic acid) intake to avoid high serum vitamin B_5 (pantothenic acid) levels in general population.

Foods high in pantothenic acid are as follows: organ meats (beef liver, pork liver, chicken liver, chicken breast, beef kidney, pork kidney), seafood (tuna, anchovy), mushrooms (shitake mushrooms, mushrooms), potatoes, whole grains (breakfast cereals), seeds (sunflower seeds), soy products (natto), fruit (avocados), dairy products (milk, Greek yogurt), eggs, beverages (green tea), seasonings and condiments (baker's yeast) (The Council for Science and Technology, Ministry of Education, Culture, Sports, Science and Technology in Japan 2023; U.S. Department of Health & Human Services. National Institutes of Health. Office of Dietary Supplements 2023).

Vitamin B_6

The Recommended dietary allowances (RDAs) for vitamin B_6 in the U.S. men aged 14-50 years, men aged ≥ 51 years, women aged 14-18 years, women aged 19-50 years, women aged ≥ 51 years, pregnancy aged ≤ 18 years and 19-50 years, and lactation aged ≤ 18 years and 19-50 years established by the Institute of Medicine of the National Academy of Sciences in the U.S. (2021) are 1.3 mg/day, 1.7 mg/day, 1.2 mg/day, 1.3 mg/day, 1.5 mg/day, 1.9 mg/day, and 2.0 mg/day, respectively. The Tolerable Upper Intake levels (ULs) for vitamin B_6 in men and women aged 14-18 years, men and women aged ≥ 19 years, pregnancy and lactation aged ≤ 18 years, and pregnancy and lactation aged 19-50 years are 80 mg/day, 100 mg/day, 80 mg/day, and 100 mg/day, respectively (The Institute of Medicine of the National Academy of Sciences in the U.S. 2021).

In the National Health and Nutrition Examination Survey (NHANES) 2001-2014, there is no association between vitamin B_6 intake and hyperuricemia risk in both U.S. adult males and females aged 20-85 years (Zhang and Qiu 2018).

Foods high in vitamin B_6 are as follows: meats (turkey), organ meats (chicken breast, beef liver), seafood (tuna, salmon), grains (wheat germ), whole grains (breakfast cereals), potatoes (potatoes, konjac), seeds and nuts (sunflower seeds, pistachio nuts), legumes (chickpeas), vegetables (garlic, red pepper, ginger, parsley), fruit (bananas), beverages (green tea), seasonings and condiments (baker's yeast) (The Council for Science and Technology, Ministry of Education, Culture, Sports, Science and Technology in Japan 2023; U.S. Department of Health & Human Services. National Institutes of Health. Office of Dietary Supplements 2023). An overdose of vitamin B_6-rich foods and/or supplementation should be avoided so as not to exceed the Tolerable Upper Intake Levels (ULs).

Folate (Vitamin B_9)

The Recommended dietary allowances (RDAs) for folate in the U.S. males and females aged ≥ 14 years, pregnancy aged ≤ 18 years and 19-50 years, and lactation aged ≤ 18 years and 19-50 years) established by the Institute of Medicine of the National Academy of Sciences in the U.S. (2021) are 400 μg DFE (dietary folate equivalents: 1 DFE = 1μg food folate = 0.6 μg of folic acid from fortified food or as a supplement consumed with food = 0.5 μg of folic acid from a supplement taken on an empty stomach), 600μg DFE, and 500μg DFE, respectively. The Tolerable Upper Intake levels (ULs) of folate in males and females aged 14-18 years, males and females aged ≥ 19 years, pregnancy and lactation aged ≤ 18 years, and pregnancy and lactation aged 19-50 years are 800 μg DFE, 1.000 μg DFE, 800 μg DFE, and 1.000 μg DFE, respectively (The Institute of Medicine of the National Academy of Sciences in the U.S. 2021).

In the cross-sectional studies, increased folate intake was associated with decreased serum uric acid (SUA) concentrations (Zykova et al. 2015; Chae et al. 2022).

In the National Health and Nutrition Examination Survey (NHANES) 2001-2014, folate intake was inversely associated with hyperuricemia risk among U.S. adult males aged 20-85 years, but there is no association between folate intake and hyperuricemia risk among U.S. adult females aged 20-85 years (Zhang and Qiu 2018).

Folic acid (84 μg/kg) decreased SUA concentrations and serum adenosine deaminase and xanthine oxidase activities and enhanced the abundance of probiotics bacteria and reduced the abundance of pathogenic bacteria in high-purine diet-induced hyperuricemic rats (Sun et al. 2022).

Large amounts of supplemental folate (up to 80 mg/day) have reduced SUA levels, and the mechanism is presumed to be mediated through the inhibition of xanthine oxidase (Oster 1977). However, one intervention study showed that folate supplementation failed to lower blood UA concentrations in individuals with hyperuricemia (Boss et al. 1980). The reason for this discrepancy is not clear. Further randomized controlled trials will be required to evaluate the effect of folate on SUA concentrations.

Foods high in folate are as follows: meats (beef), organ meats (beef liver, chicken liver), grains (white rice, spaghetti, bread), whole grains (breakfast cereals), legumes (black-eyed peas), seaweed, fruit (avocados), vegetables (asparaguses, spinach, brussels sprouts, lettuces, broccoli, mustard greens, parsley), beverages (green tea) (The Council for Science and Technology, Ministry of Education, Culture, Sports, Science and Technology in Japan 2023; U.S. Department of Health & Human Services. National Institutes of Health. Office of Dietary Supplements 2023). Serum vitamin B_9 was positively associated with SUA concentrations (Liu et al. 2021). It must pay attention to folate intake to avoid high serum folate levels in general population and not to exceed the Tolerable Upper Intake levels (ULs) for folate in general population.

Vitamin B_{12}

The Recommended Dietary Allowances (RDAs) for vitamin B_{12} in the U.S. men and women aged ≥ 14 years, pregnancy aged ≤ 18 years and aged 19-50 years, and lactation aged ≤ 18 years and 19-50 years established by the Institute of Medicine of the National Academy in the U.S. (2021) are 2.4 μg/day, 2.6 μg/day, and 2.8 μg/day, respectively. The Institute of Medicine of the National Academy of Sciences in the U.S. (2021) has not set the Tolerable Upper Intake Levels (ULs) for vitamin B_{12}.

In the National Health and Nutrition Examination Survey (NHANES) 2001-2014, vitamin B_{12} intake was inversely associated with hyperuricemia risk among U.S. adult males aged 20-85 years, but no association between vitamin B_{12} intake and hyperuricemia risk among U.S. adult females aged 20-85 years (Zhang and Qiu 2018).

Foods high in vitamin B_{12} are as follows: meats (beef, turkey), organ meats (beef liver, chicken liver), seafood (clams, tuna, salmon, anchovy, sweetfish, lamprey), whole grains (breakfast cereals), legumes and soybean processed foods (tempeh), seaweed, dairy products (milk, yogurt, cheese), eggs, seasonings and condiments (nutritional yeast) (The Council for Science and Technology, Ministry of Education, Culture, Sports, Science and Technology in Japan 2023; U.S. Department of Health & Human Services. National Institutes of Health. Office of Dietary Supplements 2023).

Vitamin C

The Recommended dietary allowances (RDAs) for vitamin C in the U.S. men aged 14-18 years, men (≥ 19 years, women aged 14-18 years, women aged ≥ 19 years, pregnancy aged ≤ 18 years, pregnancy aged 19-50 years, lactation aged ≤ 18 years, and lactation aged 19-50 years established by the Institute of Medicine of the National Academy of Sciences in the U.S. (2021) are 75.0 mg/day, 90.0 mg/day, 65.0 mg/day, 75.0 mg/day, 80.0 mg/day, 85.0 mg/day, 115 mg/day, and 120 mg/day, respectively. The Institute of Medicine of the National Academy of Sciences in the U.S. (2021) has shown the Tolerable Upper Intake Levels (ULs) for healthy individuals [men and women aged 14-18 years, 1800 mg/day; men and women aged ≥ 19 years, 2000 mg/day; pregnancy and lactation aged ≤ 18 years, 1800 mg/day; and pregnancy and lactation aged 19-50 years, 2000 mg/day].

Vitamin C intake has been found to reduce SUA levels in clinical trials (Stein, Hasan and Fox 1976; Mitch et al. 1981; Sutton, Basu and Dickerson 1983; Huang et al. 2005; Juraschek et al. 2011). Huang et al. (2005) found that supplementation with 500 mg/day of vitamin C for 2 months reduced SUA concentration by 0.5 mg/dL compared to no change in the placebo group in a randomized controlled trial. Vitamin C lowers SUA concentration through a uricosuric effect by competing with SUA on the urate transporter 1 (also known as solute carrier family 22, member 12, or SLC22A12) for re-absorption in the kidney proximal tubule (Mitch et al. 1981; Enomoto et al. 2002; Huang et al. 2005; Juraschek et al. 2011). Vitamin C inhibits the pro-oxidant actions of uric acid (UA) during copper-mediated low density lipoprotein cholesterol (LDL-cholesterol) oxidation, and could reduce oxidative stress and inflammation, and may be related to lower UA production (Hayden and Tyagi 2004). Vitamin C, which exerts as an antioxidant, reduced uric acid-induced inflammation by inhibiting activation of responsible nucleotide-binding and oligomerization domain-like receptor, leucine-rich repeat and pyrin domain-containing 3 (NLRP3) inflammasome in monosodium urate (MSU)-induced inflammation (Kim et al. 2018). Brzezińska et al. (2021) have stated that a higher serum vitamin C level has a positive effect on purine metabolism and favors the reduction of UA level. It is speculated that UA-lowering effect of vitamin C is associated with uricosuric properties, antioxidant property, and lower UA production.

In epidemiological studies, increased intake of vitamin C was associated with decreased SUA concentrations (Gao et al. 2008; Beydoun et al. 2018; Zhang et al. 2018; So et al. 2020) and hyperuricemia risk (Yu et al. 2008; Sun et al. 2018; Zhang et al. 2018; So et al. 2020). Gao et al. (2008) found that total vitamin C intake of 500 mg/day or higher was associated with a ~0.6-0.7 mg/dL lower level of SUA and was over 42% less likely to be hyperuricemia relative to those with intake < 90 mg/day. However, a randomized trial of vitamin C 500 mg daily as an adjunct to allopurinol demonstrated no reduction in SUA levels with vitamin C (Stamp et al. 2013). It is unclear whether the ingestion of large amounts of vitamin C is what influences individuals with hyperuricemia. Terkeltaub and Edwards (2013, 148-149) have stated that it is not known if combined effects on urine pH, oxalate generation, and uricosuria of high vitamin C intake can promote urolithiasis. Overdose of vitamin C-rich foods and/or supplementation should be avoided so as not to exceed the Tolerable Upper Intake Levels (ULs).

Foods high in vitamin C are as follows: seaweed, fruit (acerolas, guavas, kiwifruit, strawberries, orange, grapefruit, cantaloupes, citron), vegetables (green pepper, parsley, broccoli, cauliflowers, brussels sprouts, cabbage, red pepper), beverages (orange juice, grapefruit juice, tomato juice, green tea) (The Council for Science and Technology, Ministry of Education, Culture, Sports, Science and Technology in Japan 2023; U.S. Department of Health &

Human Services. National Institutes of Health. Office of Dietary Supplements 2023).

Minerals

Sodium and Salt

The Adequate Intakes (AIs) for sodium in the U.S. men and women aged 4-8 years), men and women aged 9-50 years, men and women aged 51-70 year, men and women aged ≥ 71 years, and pregnancy and lactation aged ≤ 18 years and 19-50 years established by the Institute of Medicine of the National Academy of Sciences in the U.S. (2021) are 1.2 g/day, 1.5 mg/day, 1.3 g/day, 1.2 g/day, and 1.5 g/day, respectively. The Tolerable Upper Intake levels (ULs) of sodium in men and women aged 4-8 years, men and women aged 9-13 years, men and women aged ≥ 14 years, and pregnancy and lactation aged ≤ 18 years and 19-50 years are 1.9 g/day, 2.2 mg/day, 2.3 mg/day, and 2.3 g/day, respectively (The Institute of Medicine of the National Academy of Sciences in the U.S. 2021).

A study of 27 men showed that increasing sodium intake from 20 mmoles/day to 200 mmoles/day decreased UA levels by 1 mg/dL (Egan et al. 1991). In a crossover trial of 147 nonobese, normotensive adults, it was found that 7 days of low versus high sodium intake (20 mmoles/day versus 300 mmoles/day) significantly increased serum UA by ~1 mg/dL (Ruppert et al. 1991). A randomized trial analysis also found that high sodium intake lowerd serum UA concentration (Appel et al. 1997).

The World Health Organization recommendations for a healthy diet (World Health Organization 2023) has stated that salt intake should be less than 5 g/day.

Calcium

The Adequate Intakes (AIs) for calcium in the U.S. men and women aged 1-3 years, men and women aged 4-8 years, men and women aged 9-18 years, men and women aged 19-50 years, men and women aged ≥ 51 years, pregnancy and lactation aged ≤ 18 years, and pregnancy and lactation aged 19-50 years established by the Institute of Medicine of the National Academy of Sciences in the U.S. (2021) are 500 mg/day, 800 mg/day, 1,300 mg/day, 1,000 mg/day, 1,200 mg/day, 1,300 mg/day, and 1,000 mg/day, respectively. The Tolerable Upper Intake levels (ULs) of calcium in men aged ≥ 1 year), women aged ≥ 1 year, pregnancy aged 1-50 years, and lactation aged 1-50 years are 2,500 mg/day. (The Institute of Medicine of the National Academy of Sciences in the U.S. 2021).

In a randomized, placebo controlled clinical trial, 323 healthy men aged > 40 years ingested a dose level of 1200 mg per day of calcium for 24 months (Dalbeth et al. 2009). No significant differences were detected in serum uric acid (SUA) levels between placebo group and calcium group (Dalbeth et al. 2009). Regression analysis indicated that a difference of calcium intake of 1200 mg per day was associated with a difference in SUA levels of 0.022 mmol/L (Dalbeth et al. 2009). In epidemiological studies, increased intake of calcium was associated with decreased SUA concentrations (Zgaga et al. 2012; Zykova et al. 2015; Chae et al. 2022) and hyperuricemia risk (Yu et al. 2008). The minimal intake associated with SUA reduction was at a level of approximately 1000 mg of calcium per day for men and 650 mg per day for women (Zykova et al. 2015).

Foods high in calcium are as follows: seafood (sardines, salmon, dried shrimp), potatoes (konjac), whole grains (breakfast cereals), legumes (soybeans, peas), seeds (sesame seeds, chia seeds), vegetables (spinach, kales, turnip greens, parsley, Chinese cabbage), dairy products (milk, cottage cheese, yogurt, frozen yogurt, Mozzarella part skim), soy products (soy milk, tofu), beverages (orange juice), seasonings and condiments (baking powder, basil, thyme, cinnamon) (The Council for Science and Technology, Ministry of Education, Culture, Sports, Science and Technology in Japan 2023; U.S. Department of Health & Human Services. National Institutes of Health. Office of Dietary Supplements 2023). An overdose of calcium-rich foods and/or supplementation should be avoided so as not to exceed the Tolerable Upper Intake Levels (ULs).

Magnesium

The Recommended Dietary Allowances (RDAs) for magnesium in the U.S. men and women aged 9-13 years, men aged ≥ 14 years, women aged ≥ 14 years, pregnancy aged ≤ 18 years, pregnancy aged 19-50 years, lactation aged ≤ 18 years, and lactation aged 19-50 years established by the Institute of Medicine of the National Academy of Sciences in the U.S. (2021) are 240 mg/day, 400-420 mg/day, 310-360 mg/day, 400 mg/day, 350-360 mg/day, 360 mg/day, and 310-320 mg/day, respectively. The Institute of Medicine of the National Academy of Sciences in the U.S. (2021) has shown the Tolerable Upper Intake Levels (ULs) for magnesium in men and women aged ≥ 9 years, and pregnancy and lactation aged ≤ 18 years and 19-50 years are 350 mg/day, respectively.

In epidemiological studies, increased magnesium intake was associated with decreased serum uric acid (SUA) concentrations (Wang et al. 2015) and hyperuricemia risk (Wang et al. 2015; Zhang and Qiu 2018). A meta-analysis and systematic review reported that dietary magnesium intake was inversely associated with serum C-reactive protein levels as biomarker of inflammation (Dibaba, Xun and He 2014). The SUA level is positively associated with several inflammatory markers (e.g., white blood cell count, C-reactive protein, interleukin-6) (Ruggiero et al. 2006). It is speculated that UA-lowering effect of magnesium is associated with lower inflammation.

Foods high in magnesium are as follows: potatoes, seeds and nuts (pumpkin seeds, chia seeds, sunflower seeds, almonds, peanuts, cashew nuts, sesame seeds, chia seeds, Brazil nuts), whole grains (brown rice, breakfast cereals, oatmeal, cereal shredded wheat), legumes (black beans, kidney beans, edamame), seaweed, fruit (bananas), vegetables (spinach, pumpkin), dairy products (yogurt), soy products (soy milk), beverages (cocoa, coffee), seasonings and condiments (peanut butter) (The Council for Science and Technology, Ministry of Education, Culture, Sports, Science and Technology in Japan 2023; U.S. Department of Health & Human Services. National Institutes of Health. Office of Dietary Supplements 2023). An overdose of magnesium-rich foods and/or supplementation should be avoided so as not to exceed the Tolerable Upper Intake Levels (ULs).

Iron

The Recommended Dietary Allowances (RDAs) for iron in the U.S. men aged 14-18 years, men aged ≥ 15 years, women aged 14-18 years, women aged 19-50 years, women aged ≥ 51 years, pregnancy aged ≤ 18 years and 19-50 years, lactation aged ≤ 18 years, and lactation aged 19-50 years established by the Institute of Medicine of the National Academy of Sciences in the U.S. (2021) are 11 mg/day, 8 mg/day, 15 mg/day, 18 mg/day, 8 mg/day, 27 mg/day, 10 mg/day, and 9 mg/day, respectively. The Institute of Medicine of the National Academy of Sciences in the U.S. (2021) has shown the Tolerable Upper Intake Levels (ULs) for iron in men and women aged ≥ 14 years, and pregnancy and lactation aged ≤ 18 years and 19-50 years are 45 mg/day.

Consumption of iron above 11g per day was inversely associated with the SUA level (10-30 μmol/L) in the Australian cohort (Zykova et al. 2015).

Foods high in iron are as follows: lean meat and meats (beef), organ meats (beef liver), seafood (oysters, sardines, sweetfish, abalone, clams, lamprey), potatoes (potato, konjac), nuts (cashew nuts), whole grains (Iron-fortified ready-to-eat cereals and breads), mushrooms (wood ear), legumes (kidney beans, white beans, lentils, chickpeas), seaweed, vegetables (spinach, tomatoes), soy products (tofu), beverages (green tea), confectioneries (dark chocolate), seasonings and condiments (basil, thyme) (The Council for Science and Technology, Ministry of Education, Culture, Sports, Science and Technology in Japan 2023; U.S. Department of Health & Human Services. National Institutes of Health. Office of Dietary Supplements 2023). An overdose of iron-rich foods and/or supplementation should be avoided so as not to exceed the Tolerable Upper Intake Levels (ULs).

Zinc

The Recommended Dietary Allowances (RDAs) for zinc in the U.S. men aged ≥ 14 years, women aged 14-18 years, women (aged ≥ 19 years), pregnancy aged 14-50 years, and lactation aged 14-50 years established by the Institute of Medicine of the National Academy of Sciences in the U.S. (2021) are 11.0 mg/day, 9.0 mg/day, 8.0 mg/day, 11-12 mg/day, and 12-13 mg/day, respectively. The Institute of Medicine of the National Academy of Sciences in the U.S. (2021) has shown the Tolerable Upper Intake Levels (ULs) for zinc in men and women aged ≥ 14 years, pregnancy and lactation aged 14-18 years, and pregnancy and lactation aged 19-50 years are 34-40 mg/day, 34 mg/day, and 40 mg/day, respectively.

In an epidemiological study, increased zinc intake was associated with decreased hyperuricemia risk (Xie et al. 2015). Acting as an antioxidant and anti-inflammatory agent in humans, zinc may be associated with the the SUA level, which may function as a prooxidant and proinflammatory factor under certain circumstances (Sautin and Johnson 2008; Prasad 2014).

Foods high in zinc are as follows: meats (beef, pork), organ meats (turkey breast), seafood (oysters, blue crab, shrimp, sardines), seeds and nuts (pumpkin seeds, peanuts), whole grains (breakfast cereals, oats cereals, brown rice), grains (bread, wheat germ), legumes (lentils, kidney beans), vegetables (pumpkin), dairy products (milk, cheese, Greek yogurt, parmesan cheese), eggs, beverages (cocoa), seasonings and condiments (baker's yeast) (The Council for Science and Technology, Ministry of Education, Culture, Sports, Science and Technology in Japan 2023; U.S. Department of Health & Human Services. National Institutes of Health. Office of Dietary Supplements 2023). An overdose of zinc-rich foods and/or supplementation should be avoided so as not to exceed the Tolerable Upper Intake Levels (ULs).

Conclusion

Data from clinical research have revealed an association between dietary factors and SUA levels or hyperuricemia risk. Large-scale epidemiological studies have shown that dietary factors affect SUA levels parallel to the direction of risk of hyperuricemia (Choi 2010).

Table 2. Dietary nutrient intake for prevention and management of hyperuricemia in the general population (especially adults)

Nutrient	Behaviour
Energy	Carbohydrates is 45-65 percent of total calories, total protein is 10-35 percent of total calories, and at 20-35 percent of total calories, respectively (The Institute of Medicine of the National Academy of Sciences in the U.S. 2021).
Total sugars	Maximum limit to the intake of 100 g/day (Tappy et al. 2018). Pay attention to total sugars intake.
Fructose	Limiting or decreasing intake.
Fiber	Recognizing encouraged intake.
Protein	Recognizing encouraged intake of milk protein (casein and lactalbumin) and protein from vegetable sources.
Fat	Replacement of saturated fatty acids with mono- and polyunsaturated ones (especially n-3 polyunsaturated fatty acids).
Animal fats, Saturated fatty acids, Cholesterol	Limiting or decreasing intake.
Alcohol	Limiting or decreasing consumption.
Water intake	Maintenance of good hydration (five to eight 8-oz servings of water daily: 1183-1893 g) is essential (Terkeltaub. and Edwards 2013, 152). Total water intake: males (aged $\geq$ 19 years): 3.7 L/day (approximately 3.0 L as total beverages, including drinking water); females (aged $\geq$ 19 years): 2.7 L/day (approximately 2.2 L as total beverages, including drinking water) (Institute of Medicine of the National Academy of Sciences in the U.S. 2021).
Purine	Limiting intake. Daily purine intake should be approximately 400 mg (Hisatome et al. 2018).
Polyphenol	Recognizing encouraged intake. Dietary polyphenol intake in the US was ~1 g/day (Kuhnau 1976).
Vitamin A	Pay attention to vitamin A intake to avoid high serum vitamin A levels.
Vitamin D	Pay attention to vitamin D intake to avoid vitamin D deficiency.
Vitamin E	Recognizing encouraged intake.
Vitamin B_1	Recognizing encouraged intake.
Vitamin B_2	Recognizing encouraged intake.
Pantothenic acid	Pay attention to vitamin B_5 (pantothenic acid) intake to avoid high serum vitamin B_5 (pantothenic acid) levels.
Vitamin B_6	Pay attention to vitamin B_6 intake so as not to exceed the Tolerable Upper Intake Levels (ULs) for vitamin B_6.

Table 2. (Continued)

Nutrient	Behaviour
Folate	Recognizing encouraged intake. Pay attention to folate intake to avoid high serum vitamin B_9 levels.
Vitamin B_{12}	Recognizing encouraged intake.
Vitamin C	Recognizing encouraged intake
Salt	Limiting or decreasing intake. Keep less than 5 g/day (World Health Organization 2023).
Calcium	Recognizing encouraged intake.
Magnesium	Recognizing encouraged intake.
Iron	Recognizing encouraged intake.
Zinc	Recognizing encouraged intake.

The Institute of Medicine of the National Academy of Sciences in the U.S. has set Dietary Reference Intake values in life stage and gender groups (2021). Considering Dietary Reference Intake values for the nutrients of individuals, choosing and eating foods containing nutrients which decrease SUA concentration seems to be important for the prevention and management of hyperuricemia. Terkeltaub and Edwards (2013, 151) have stated the view that the expected maximal SUA concentration lowering with diet alone is typically 1 mg/dL (and up to ~18%, especially if coupled with effective weight loss).

It is necessary to recognize what food is important as a potential dietary habit to prevent hyperuricemia in the general population (especially adults). Dietary nutrient intake for the prevention and management of hyperuricemia described in this article is shown in Table 2.

Dietary nutrient intake for the prevention and management of hyperuricemia in the general population (especially adults) is suggested as follows: the percentage of carbohydrate, protein, fat, and n-3 polyunsaturated fatty acids and n-6 polyunsaturated fatty acids in total energy intake should be within the range of the Acceptable Macronutrient Distribution Ranges (AMDRs) set by the Institute of Medicine of the National Academy of Sciences in the U.S.: Pay attention to intake of total sugars intake [maximum limit to the intake of 100 g/day (Tappy et al. 2018)]; limiting or decreasing intake of fructose, animal fats, saturated fatty acids, cholesterol, and salt; replacement of saturated fatty acids (e.g., dairy fats, meat fat) with mono- and polyunsaturated fatty acids (particularly n-3 polyunsaturated fatty acids) (e.g., macadamia nuts, almonds, peanuts and peanut butter, olive oil, canola oil, avocados); maintenance of good hydration; limiting or decreasing alcohol consumption; limiting intake of purine; pay attention to intake of vitamin A, vitamin B_5 (pantothenic acid), and folate to avoid high serum vitamin A, vitamin B_5 (pantothenic acid), and vitamin B_9 levels, respectively; pay attention to vitamin D intake to avoid vitamin D deficiency; and recognizing encouraged intake of fiber, animal sources of protein (e.g., casein, lactalbumin), and vegetable sources of protein (e.g., wheat gluten, rice endosperm protein), polyphenol, vitamin E, vitamin B_1;, vitamin B_2, folate, vitamin B_{12}, vitamin C, calcium, magnesium, iron, and zinc. Further animal experiments, large-scale prospective cohort studies, and randomized controlled trials are required to evaluate the effect of dietary nutrients on SUA concentration.

Disclaimer

None.

References

Adachi S, Oyama M, Kondo S, Yagasaki K. 2021. "Comparative effects of quercetin, luteolin, apigenin and their related polyphenols on uric acid production in cultured hepatocytes and suppression of purine bodies-induced hyperuricemia by rutin in mice." *Cytotechnology* 73:343-351.

Adachi S, Yoshizawa F, Yagasaki K. 2017. "Assay systems for screening food and natural substances that have anti-hyperuricemic activity: uric acid production in cultured hepatocytes and purine bodies-induced hyperuricemic model mice." *Cytotechnology* 69:435-442.

Ando A, Bamba T, Sasaki M. 1999. "Physiological and anti-inflammatory roles of dietary fiber and butyrate in intestinal functions." *JPEN J Parenter Enteral Nutr* 23: S70-S73.

Appel LJ, Moore TJ, Obarzanek E, Vollmer WM, Svetkey LP, Sacks FM, Bray GA, Vogt TM, Cutler JA, Windhauser MM, Lin PH, Karanja N. 1997. "A clinical trial of the effects of dietary patterns on blood pressure. DASH Collaborative Research Group." *N Engl J Med* 336:1117-1124.

Bagnati M, Perugini C, Cau C, Bordone R, Albano E, Bellomo G. 1999. "When and why a water-soluble antioxidant becomes pro-oxidant during copper-induced low-density lipoprotein oxidation: a study using uric acid." *Biochem J* 340:143-152.

Bander ZA, Nitert MD, Mousa A, Naderpoor N. 2020. "The gut microbiota and inflammation: An overview." *Int J Environ Res Public Health* 17:7618.

Beydoun MA, Fanelli-Kuczmarski MT, Canas J-A, Beydoun HA, Evans MK, Zonderman AB. 2018. "Dietary factors are associated with serum uric acid trajectory differentially by race among urban adults." *Br J Nutr* 120:935-945.

Boss GR, Ragsdale RA, Zettner A, Seegmiller JE. 1980. "Failure of folic acid (pteroylglutamic acid) to affect hyperuricemia." *J Lab Clin Med* 96:783-789.

Bowering J, Calloway DH, Margen S, Kaufmann NA. 1970. "Dietary protein level and uric acid metabolism in normal man." *J Nutr* 100:249-261.

Brulé D, Sarwar G, Savoie L, Campbell J, Zeggelaar MV. 1988. "Differences in uricogenic effects of dietary purine bases, nucleosides and nucleotides in rats." *J Nutr* 118:780-786.

Brulé D, Sarwar G. Savoie L. 1992. "Changes in serum and urinary uric acid levels in normal human subjects fed purine-rich foods containing different amounts of adenine and hypoxanthine." *J Am Coll Nutr* 11: 353-358.

Brzezińska, O., Styrzyński, F., Makowska, J, Walczak, K. 2021. "The role of vitamin C in prophylaxis and treatment of gout- A literature review." *Nutrients* 13: 701.

Cabău G, Crişan TO, Klück V, PoppRA, Joosten LAB. 2020. "Urate-induced immune programming: Consequences for gouty arthritis and hyperuricemia." *Immunol Rev* 294:92-105.

Caliceti C, Calabria D, Roda A, Cicero A. 2017. "Fructose intake, serum uric acid, and cardiometabolic disorders: A critical review." *Nutrients* 9:395.

Campion EW, Glynn RJ, DeLabry LO. 1987. "Asymptomatic hyperuricemia: Risks and consequences in the Normative Aging Study." *Am J Med* 82:421-426.

Carabin IG, Lyon MR, Wood S, Pelletier X, Donazzolo Y, Burdock GA. 2009. "Supplementation of the diet with the functional fiber PolyGlycoplex is well tolerated by healthy subjects in a clinical trial." *Nutr J* 8:9.

Chae S-J, Lee G-S, Kim S-H, Ryu H-S, Yun M-E. 2022. "The association between serum uric acid levels and the nutrients adequacy ration among male adult Koreans -Based on the 2016-2019 Korea National Health and Nutrition Examination Survey." *J Korean Diet Assoc* 28:169-181.

Chan WS, Wen PC, Chiang HC. 1995. "Structure-activity relationship of caffeic acid analogues on xanthine inhibition." *Anticancer Res* 15:703-705.

Chang Y-H, Chiang Y-F, Chen H-Y, Huang Y-J, Wang K-L, Hong Y-H, Ali M, Shieh T-M, Hsia S-M. 2021. "Anti-inflammatory and anti-hyperuricemic effects of chrysin on a high fructose corn syrup-induced hyperuricemia rat model via the amelioration of urate transporters and inhibition of NLRP3 inflammasome signaling pathway." *Antioxidants* 10: 564.

Charoenngam N. 2021. "Vitamin D and rheumatic diseases: A review of clinical evidence." *Int J Mol Sci* 22: 10659.

Chen G, Tan M-L, Li K-K, Leung P-C, Ko C-H. 2015. "Green tea polyphenols decreases uric acid level through xanthine oxidase and renal urate transporters in hyperuricemic mice." *J Ethnopharmacol* 175:14-20.

Chen L, Lan Z, Zhou Y, Li F, Zhang X, Zhang C, Yang Z, Li P. 2011. "Astilbin attenuates hyperuricemia and ameliorates nephropathy in fructose-induced hyperuricemic rats." *Planta Med* 77:1769-1773.

Chen Y, Li C, Duan S, Yuan X, Liang J, Hou S. 2019. "Curcumin attenuates potassium oxonate-induced hyperuricemia and kidney inflammation in mice." *Biomed Pharmacother* 118:109195.

Chen Y-S, Hu Q-H, Zhang X, Zhu Q, Kong L-D. 2013. "Beneficial effect of rutin on oxonate-induced hyperuricemia and renal dysfunction in mice." *Pharmacology* 92:75-83.

Chen-Xu M, Yokose C, Rai SK, Pillinger MH, Choi HK. 2019. "Contemporary prevalence of gout and hyperuricemia in the United States and decadal trends: the National Health and Nutrition Examination Survey, 2007-2016." *Arthritis Rheumatol* 71:991-999.

Choi HK, Curhan G. 2004. "Beer, liquor, and wine consumption and serum uric acid level; The Third National Health and Nutrition Examination Survey." *Arthritis Rheum* 51:1023-1029.

Choi HK, Liu S, Curhan G. 2005. "Intake of purine-rich foods, protein, and dairy products and relationship to serum levels of uric acid: The Third National Health and Nutrition Examination Survey." *Arthritis Rheum* 52:283-289.

Choi HK, Mount DB, Reginato AM. 2005. "Pathogenesis of gout." *Ann Intern Med* 143:499-516.

Choi HK. 2010. "A prescription for lifestyle change in patients with hyperuricemia and gout." *Curr Opin Rheumatol* 22:165-172.

Choi JWJ, Ford ES, Gao X, Choi HK. 2008. "Sugar-sweetened soft drinks, diet soft drinks, and serum uric acid level: The third national health and nutrition examination survey." *Arthritis. Rheum* 59:109-116.

Choi WJ, Ford ES, Curhan G, Rankin JI, Choi HK. 2012. "Independent association of serum retinol and β-carotene levels with hyperuricemia: A national population study." *Arthritis Care Res* 64:389-398.

Chu Y, Sun S, Huang Y. 2021. "Metagenomic analysis revealed the potential role of gut microbiome in gout." *NPJ Biofilms Microbiomes* 7, 1,66.

Chuang SY, Lee SC, Hsieh YT, Pan WH. 2011. "Trends in hyperuricemia and gout prevalence: Nutrition and Health Survey in Taiwan from 1993-1996 to 2005-2008." *Asia Pac J Clin Nutr* 20:301-308.

Cipriani S, Desjardins CA, Burdett TC, Xu Y, Xu K, Schwarzschild MA. 2012. "Protection of dopaminergic cells by urate requires its accumulation in astrocytes." *J Neurochem* 123: 172-181.

Clifford AJ, Riumallo JA, Young VR, Scrimshaw NS. 1976. "Effect of oral purines on serum and urinary uric acid of normal, hyperuricemic and gouty humans." *J Nutr* 106:428-434.

Cui D, Liu S, Tang M, Lu Y, Zhao M, Mao R, Wang C, Yuan Y, Li L, Chen Y, Cheng J, Lu Y, Liu J. 2020. "Phloretin ameliorates hyperuricemia-induced chronic renal dysfunction through inhibiting NLRP3 inflammasome and uric acid reabsorption." *Phytomedicine* 66:153111.

Dai HX, Zhao ZY, Xia Y, Wu QJ, Zhao YH. 2020. "Higher levels of high-sensitivity C-reactive protein is positively associated with the incidence of hyperuricemia in Chinese population: a report from the China Health and Retirement Longitudinal Study." *Mediat Inflamm* 2020:3854982.

Dalbeth N, Horne A, Gamble GD, Ames R, Reid IR. 2009. "The effect of calcium supplementation on serum urate; analysis of a randomized controlled trial." *Rheumatology* 48:195-197.

De Becker B, Borghi C, Bumier M, van de Borne P. 2019. "Uric acid hypertension: a focused review and practical recommendations." *J Hypertens* 37:878-883.

Dibaba DT, Xun P, He K. 2014. "Dietary magnesium intake is inversely associated with serum C-reactive protein levels: Meta-analysis and systematic review." *Eur J Clin Nutr* 68:510-516.

Doherty M. 2009. "New insights into epidemiology of gout." *Rheumatology* 48 (suppl 2): ii2-ii8.

Dornas WC, de Lima WG, Pedrosa ML, Silva ME. 2015. "Health implications of high-fructose intake and current research." *Adv Nutr* 6:729-737.

Du N, Xu D, Hou X, Song X, Liu C, Chen Y, Wang Y, Li X. 2016. "Inverse association between serum uric acid levels and Alzheimer's disease risk." *Mol Neurobiol* 53:2594-2599.

Eastmond CJ, Garton M, Robins S, Riddoch S. 1995. "The effects of alcoholic beverages on urate metabolism in gout sufferers." *Br J Rheumatol* 34:756-759.

Ebrahimpour-Koujan S, Saneei P, Larijani B, Esmaillzadeh A. 2020. "Consumption of sugar sweetened beverages and dietary fructose in relation to risk of gout and hyperuricemia: a systematic review and meta-analysis." *Crit Rev Food Sci Nutr* 60:1-10.

Ebrahimpour-Koujan S, Saneei P, Larijani B, Esmaillzadeh A. 2021. "Consumption of sugar-sweetened beverages and serum uric acid concentrations: a systematic review and meta-analysis." *J Hum Nutr Diet* 34: 305-313.

Edozien JC, Udo UU, Young VR, Scrimshaw NS. 1970. "Effects of high levels of yeast feeding on uric acid metabolism of young men." *Nature* 228:180.

Egan BM, Weder AB, Petrin J, Hoffman RG. 1991. "Neurohumoral and metabolic effects of short-term dietary NaCl restriction in men: relationship to salt-sensitivity status." *Am J Hypertens* 4:416-421.

Ekpenyong CE, Daniel N. 2015. "Roles of diets and dietary factors in the pathogenesis, management and prevention of abnormal serum uric acid levels." *Pharma Nutrition* 3:29-45.

El Ridi R, Tallima H. 2017. "Physiological functions and pathogenic potential of uric acid: A review." *J Adv Res* 8:487-493.

Elmadfa I, Rust P, Majchrzak D, Wagner KH, Genser D, Lettner R, Pinter M. 2004. "Effects of beta-carotene supplementation on free radical mechanism in healthy adult subjects." *Int J Vitam Nutr Res* 74:147-152.

Emilion E, Emilion R. 2011. "Estimation of the 25(OH) Vitamin D threshold below which secondary hyperparathyroidism may occur among African Migrant Women in Paris." *Int J Vitam Nutr Res* 81: 218-224.

Emmerson BT. 1974. "Effect of oral fructose on urate production." *Ann Rheum Dis* 33:276-280.

Enomoto A, Kimura H, Chairoungdua A, Shigeta Y, Jutabha P, Cha SH, Hosoyamada M, Takeda M, Sekine T, Igarashi T. 2002. "Molecular identification of a renal urate anion exchanger that regulates blood urate levels." *Nature* 417:447-452.

Fabbrini E, Serafini, M, Colic Baric C, Hazen SL, Klein S. 2014. "Effect of plasma uric acid on antioxidant capacity, oxidative stress, and insulin sensitivity in obese subjects." *Diabetes* 63:976-981.

Fang P, Li X, Luo JJ, Wang H, Yang X-F. 2013. "A Double-edged sword: uric acid and neurological disorders." *Brain Disord Ther* 2:109.

Fang X-Y, Qi L-W, Chen H-F, Gao P, Zhang Q, Leng R-X, Fan Y-G, Li B-Z, Pan H-F, Ye D-Q. 2022. "The interaction between dietary fructose and gut microbiota in hyperuricemia and gout." *Front Nutr* 9:890730.

Feig DI. 2014. "Serum uric acid and the risk of hyperuricemia and chronic kidney disease." *Curr Opin Rheumatol* 26:176-185.

Ford ES, Choi HK. 2013. "Associations between concentrations of uric acid with concentrations of vitamin A and beta-carotene among adults in the United States." *Nutr Res* 33:995-1002.

Gao X, Curhan G, Forman JP, Ascherio A, Choi HK. 2008. "Vitamin C intake and serum uric acid concentration in men." *J Rheumatol* 35:1853-1858.

Garrel DR, Verdy M, PetitClerc C, Martin C, Brulé D, Hamet P. 1991. "Milk-and soy-protein ingestion; Acute effect on serum uric acid concentration." *Am J Clin Nutr* 53:665-669.

Glantzounis GK, Tsimoyiannis EC, Kappas AM, Galaris DA. 2005. "Uric acid and oxidative stress." *Curr Pharm Des* 11:4145-4151.

Guo Y, Yu Y, Li H, Ding X, Li X, Jing X, Chen J, Liu G, Lin Y, Jiang C, Liu Z, He Y, Li C, Tian Z. 2021. "Inulin supplementation ameliorates hyperuricemia and modulates gut microbiota in *Uox*-knockout mice." *Eur J Nutr* 60:2217-2230.

Guo Z, Zhang J, Wang Z, Ang KY, Huang S, Hou Q, Su X, Qiao J, Zheng Y, Wang L, Koh E, Danliang H, Xu J, Lee YK, Zhang H. 2016. "Intestinal microbiota distinguish gout patients from healthy humans." *Sci Rep* 6:20602.

Haidari F, Keshavarz SA, Shahi MM, Mahboob S-A, Rashidi M-R. 2011. "Effects of parsley (Petroselinum crispum) and its flavonol constituents, kaempferol and quercetin, on serum uric acid levels, biomarkers of oxidative stress and liver xanthine oxidoreductase activity in oxonate-induced hyperuricemic rats." *Iran J Pharm Res* 10:811-819.

Hamer HM, Jonkers DM, Bast A, Vanhoutvin SA, Fischer MA, Kodde A, Troost F, Venema K, Brummer R-JM. 2009. "Butyrate modulates oxidative stress in the colonic mucosa of healthy humans." *Clin Nutr* 28:88-93.

Hayden MR, Tyagi SC. 2004. "Uric acid: A new look at an old risk marker for cardiovascular disease, metabolic syndrome, and type 2 diabetes mellitus: The urate redox shuttle." *Nutr Metab* 1:10.

Hijova E, Szabadosova V, Štofilová J, Hrčková G. 2013. "Chemopreventive and metabolic effects of inulin on colon cancer development." *J Vet Sci* 14:387-393.

Hisatome I, Ichida K, Mineo I, Ohtahara A, Ogino K, Kuwabara M, Ishizaka N, Uchida S, Kurajoh M, Kohagura K, Sato Y, Taniguchi A, Tsuchihashi T, Terai C, Nakamura T, Hamaguchi T, Hamada T, Fujimori S, Masuda I, Moriwaki Y, Yamamoto T. on behalf of guideline development group. 2018. *Japanese Society of Gout and Uric & Nucleic Acids Guidelines for Management of Hyperuricemia and Gout: 3 rd edition.* Tokyo: SHINDAN TO CHIRYO SHA, Inc.

Hosojima M, Kaseda R, Kondo H, Fujii M, Kubota M, Watanabe R, Tanabe N, Kadowaki M, Suzuki Y, Saito A. 2016. "Beneficial effects of rice endosperm protein intake in Japanese men with risk factors for metabolic syndrome: a randomized, crossover clinical trial." *BMC Nutr* 2:25.

Hosomi A, Nakanishi T, Fujita T, Tamai I, Hosomi A. 2012. "Extra-renal elimination of uric acid via intestinal efflux transporter BCRP/ABCG2." *PLoS ONE* 7: e30456.

Hu Q-H, Wang C, Li J-M, Zhang D-M, Kong L-D. 2009. "Allopurinol, quercetin and rutin attenuate hyperuricemia and renal dysfunction in rats induced by fructose intake: renal organic ion transporter involvement." *Am J Physiol Renal Physiol* 297: F1080-F1091.

Hu Q-H, Zhang X, Pan Y, Li Y-C, Kong L-D. 2012. "Allopurinol, quercetin and rutin ameliorate renal NLRP3 inflammasome activation and lipid accumulation in fructose-fed rats." *Biochem Pharmacol* 84: 113-125.

Hu Q-H, Zhang X, Wang X, Jiao R-Q, Kong L-D. 2012. "Quercetin regulates organic ion transporter and uromodulin expression and improves renal function in hyperuricemic mice." *Eur J Nutr* 51:593-606.

Huang HY, Appel LJ, Choi MJ, Gelber AC, Charleston J, Norkus EP, Miller ER 3 rd. 2005. "The effects of vitamin C supplementation on serum concentrations of uric acid: results of a randomized controlled trial." *Arthritis Rheum* 52:1843-1847.

Hui JY, Choi JW, Mount DB, Zhu Y, Zhang Y, Choi HK. 2012. "The independent association between parathyroid hormone levels and hyperuricemia: a national population study." *Arthritis Res Ther* 14: R56.

Hwa KS, Chung D-M, Chung YC, Chun HK. 2011. "Hypouricemic effects of anthocyanin extracts of purple sweet potato on potassium oxonate-induced hyperuricemia in mice." *Phytother Res* 25:1415-1417.

INRA. 2023. "Phenol-Explorer database." Accessed April 27. http://phenol-explorer.eu/compounds.

Institute of Medicine of the National Academy of Sciences. 2021. *Food and Nutrition Board. Dietary Reference Intakes: The essential guide to nutrient requirements.* Washington, D.C.: The National Academy Press. https://www.nap.edu/catalog/11537.html.

Ishaq M, Mehmood A, Rehman AL, Zad OD, Li J, Zhao L, Wang C, Hossen I, Naveed M, Lian Y. 2020. "Antihyperuricemic effect of dietary polyphenol sinapic acid commonly present in various edible food plants." *J Food Biochem* 44: e13111.

Isnuwardana R, Bijukchhe S, Thadanipon K, Ingsathit A, Thakkinstian A. 2020. "Association between vitamin D and uric acid in adults: A systematic review and meta-analysis." *Horm Metab Res* 52:732-741.

Itakura M. 2009. "Metabolic pathway and regulation of uric acid production." *Hyperuricemia and Gout* 17:106-111.

Jakše B, Jakše B, Pajek M, Pajek J. 2019. "Uric acid and plant-based nutrition." *Nutrients* 11:1736.

Jenkins DJ, Kendall CW, Vidgen E, Augustin LS, van Erk M, Geelen A, Parker T, Faulkner D, Vuksan V, Josse RG, Leiter LA, Connelly PW. 2001. "High-protein diets in hyperlipidemia: effect of wheat gluten on serum lipids, uric acid, and renal function." *Am J Clin Nutr* 74:57-63.

Joosten LAB, Crişan TO, Bjornstad P, Johnson RJ. 2020. "Asymptomatic hyperuricaemia: a silent activation of the innate immune system." *Nat Rev Rheumatol* 16:75-86.

Jung SW, Kim S-M, Kim YG, Lee S-H, Moon J-Y. 2020. "Uric acid and inflammation in kidney disease." *Am J Physiol Renal Physiol* 318: F1327-F1340.

Juraschek SP, Miller ER 3rd, Gelber AC. 2011. "Effect of oral vitamin C supplementation on serum uric acid: a meta-analysis of randomized controlled trials." *Arthritis Rheum* 63:1295-1306.

Kaneko C, Ogura J, Sasaki S, Okamoto K, Kobayashi M, Kuwayama K, Narumi K, Iseki K. 2017. "Fructose suppresses uric acid excretion to the intestinal lumen as a result of the induction of oxidative stress by NADPH oxidase activation." *Biochim Biophys Acta Gen Subj* 1861:559-566.

Kaneko K, Aoyagi Y, Fukuuchi T, Inazawa K, Yamaoka N. 2014. "Total purine and purine base content of common foodstuffs for facilitating nutritional therapy for gout and hyperuricemia." *Biol Pharm Bull* 37:709-721.

Keenan R. 2020. "The biology of urate." *Semin Arthritis Rheum* 50: S2-S10.

Kim H. W, Yoon E-J, Jeong SH, Park M-C. 2022. "Distinct gut microbiota in patients with asymptomatic hyperuricemia: A potential protector against gout development." *Yonsei Med J* 63:241-251.

Kim S.-K, Choe J.-Y, Park K.-Y. 2018. "TXNIP-mediated nuclear factor-κB signaling pathway and intracellular shuttling of TXNIP in uric acid-induced NLRP3 inflammasome." *Biochem Biophys Res Commun* 511:725-731.

Kim Y, Choi JH, Kang J, Kim G-T, Lee S-G. 2020. "Associations serum retinol and α-tocopherol levels with uric acid concentrations: analysis of a population-based, nationally representative sample." *Nutrients* 12:1797.

Kobayashi T, Inokuchi T, Yamamoto A, Takahashi S, Ka T, Tsutsumi Z, Saito H, Moriwaki Y, Yamamoto T. 2007. "Effects of sucrose on plasma concentrations and urinary excretion of purine bases." *Metabolism* 56:439-443.

Koguchi T, Koguchi H, Nakajima H, Takano S, Yamamoto Y, Innami S, Maekawa A, Tadokoro T. 2004. "Dietary fiber suppresses elevation of uric acid and urea nitrogen concentrations in serum of rats with renal dysfunction induced by dietary adenine." *Int J Vitam Nutr Res* 74:253-263.

Koguchi T, Nakajima H, Koguchi H, Wada M, Yamamoto Y, Innami S, Maekawa A. Tadokoro T. 2003. "Suppressive effect of viscous dietary fiber on elevations of uric acid in serum and urine induced by dietary RNA in rats is associated with strength of viscosity." *Int J Vitam Nutr Res* 73:369-376.

Koguchi T, Nakajima H, Takano S, Ota T, Wada M, Innami S, Tadokoro T. 2016. "Suppressive effect of agarose and cellulose on hyperuricemia induced by dietary RNA in rats." *Curr Top Pharmacol* 20:57-66.

Koguchi T, Nakajima H, Wada M, Yamamoto Y, Innami S, Maekawa A, Tadokoro T. 2002. "Dietary fiber suppresses elevations of uric acid and allantoin in serum and urine induced by dietary RNA and increases its excretion to feces in rats." *J Nutr Sci Vitaminol* 48:184-193.

Koguchi T, Tadokoro T. 2019. "Beneficial effect of dietary fiber on hyperuricemia in rats and humans: A review." *Int J Vitam Nutr Res* 89:89-108.

Koguchi T. 2018. "Essentials of dietary habits for prevention and suppression of hyperuricemia." *Curr Top Pharmacol* 22:77-133.

Koguchi T. 2021. "Modification of dietary habits for prevention of gout in Japanese people: Gout and the Japanese diet." *Am J Health Res* 9:117-127.

Koguchi T. 2021. "Modification of dietary habits for prevention of gout in Japanese people; Gout and diet." *Am J Health Res* 9:176-189.

Koguchi T. 2022. "Modification of animal product intake for prevention of gout in Japanese people in 2019: 2022 update." *Am J Health Res* 10:140-153.

Koguchi T. 2022. "Modification of macronutrient intake for prevention of gout in Japanese people in 2019: 2022 update." *Am J Health Res* 10: 83-106.

Koguchi T. 2022. "Modification of micronutrient intake for prevention of gout in Japanese people in 2019: 2022 update." *Am J Health Res* 10:107-131.

Koguchi T. 2022. "Modification of plant-based food intake for prevention of gout in Japanese people in 2019: 2022 update." *Am J Health Res* 10:154-168.

Kontogianni MD, Chrysohoou C, Panagiotakos DB, Tsetsekou E, Zeimbekis A, Pitsavos C, Stefanadis C. 2012. "Adherence to the Mediterranean diet and serum uric acid: the ATTICA study." *Scand J Rheumatol* 41:442-449.

Kuhnau J. 1976. "The flavonoids. A class of semi-essential food components: their role in human nutrition." *World Rev Nutr Diet* 24:117-191.

Lattimer JM, Haub MD. 2010. "Effects of dietary fiber and its components on metabolic health." *Nutrients* 2: 1266-1289.

Le MT, Shafiu M, Mu W, Johnson RJ. 2008. "SLC2A9—a fructose transporter identified as a novel uric acid transporter." *Nephrol Dial Transplant* 23:2746-2749.

Lecoultre V, Egli I, Theytaz F, Despland C, Schneiter P, Tappy I. 2013. "Fructose-induced hyperuricemia is associated with a decreased renal uric acid excretion in humans." *Diabetes Care* 36: e149-e150.

Li F, Liu Y, Xie Y, Liu Z, Zou G. 2020. "Epigallocatechin gallate reduces uric acid levels by regulating xanthine oxidase activity and uric acid excretion in vitro and in vivo." *Ann Palliat Med* 9:331-338.

Li R, Yu K, Li C. 2018. "Dietary factors and risk of gout and hyperuricemia: a meta-analysis and systematic review." *Asia Pac J Clin Nutr* 27:1344-1356.

Lim H, Min DS, Park H, Kim HP. 2018. "Flavonoids interfere with NLRP3 inflammasome activation." *Toxicol Appl Pharmacol* 355:93-102.

Lin K-M, Lu C-L, Hung K-C, Wu P-C, Pan C-F, Wu C-J, Syu R-S, Chen J-S, Hsiao P-J, Lu, K-C. 2019. "The paradoxical role of uric acid in osteoporosis." *Nutrients* 11:2111.

Lin Z, Zhang B, Liu X, Jin R, Zhu W. 2014. "Effects of chicory inulin on serum metabolites of uric acid, lipids, glucose, and abdominal fat deposition in quails induced by purine-rich diets." *J Med Food* 17:1214-1221.

Lippi G, Montagnana M, Franchini M, Favaloro EJ, Targher G. 2008. "The paradoxical relationship between serum uric acid and cardiovascular disease." *Clin Chim Acta* 392:1-7.

Liu H, Zhang XM, Wang YL, Liu BC. 2014. "Prevalence of hyperuricemia among Chinese adults: a national cross-sectional survey using multistage, stratified sampling." *J Nephrol* 27:653-658.

Liu J, Sun LL, He LP, Ling WH, Liu ZM, Chen M. 2014. "Soy food consumption, cardiometabolic alterations and carotid intima-media thickness in Chinese adults." *Nutr Metab Cardiovasc Dis* 24:1097-1104.

Liu L, Lou S, Xu K, Meng Z, Zhang Q, Song K. 2013. "Relationship between lifestyle choice and hyperuricemia in Chinese men and women." *Clin Rheumatol* 32:233-239.

Liu Y, Xia Y, Wu Q, Chang Q, Zhao Y. 2021. "Associations between serum vitamins and serum uric acid in a population of Shenyang, China." *J Nutr Sci Vitaminol* 67:77-83.

Liu Z, Que S, Zhou L, Zheng S. 2018. "Dose-response relationship of serum uric acid with metabolic syndrome and non-alcoholic fatty liver disease incidence: a meta-analysis of prospective studies." *Sci Rep* 5: 14325.

Livesey G. 2009. "Fructose ingestion: dose-dependent responses in healthy research." *J. Nutr* 139: 1246S-1252S.

Loenen HMJA, Eshuis H, Löwik MRH, Schouten EG, Hulshof KFAM, Odink J, Kok FJ. 1990. "Serum uric acid correlates in elderly men and women with special reference to body composition and dietary intake (Dutch Nutrition Surveillance System)." *J Clin Epidemiol* 43:1297-1303.

MacFariane LA. 2014. "Gout: a review of nonmodifiable and modifiable risk factors." *Rheum Dis Clin N Am* 40:581-604.

Mehmood A, Li J, Rehman AU, Kobun R, Liah IU, Khan I, Althobaiti F, Albogami S, Usman M, Alharthi F, Soliman MM, Yaqoob S, Awan KA, Zhao L, Zhao L. 2022. "Xanthine oxidase inhibitory study of eight structurally diverse phenolic compounds." *Front Nutr* 9:966557.

Mehmood A, Zhao I, Wang C, Nadeem M, Raza A, Ali N, Shah AA. 2019. "Management of hyperuricemia through dietary polyphenols as a natural medicament: A comprehensive review." *Crit Rev Food Sci Nutr* 59:1433-1455.

Merriman TR, Dalbeth N, Johnson RJ. 2014. "Sugar-sweetened beverages, urate, gout and genetic interaction." *Pac Health Dialog* 20:31-38.

Mitch WE, Johnson MW, Kirshenbaum JM, Lopez RE. 1981. "Effect of large oral doses of ascorbic acid on uric acid excretion by normal subjects." *Clin Pharmacol Ther* 29:318-321.

Mohd Fahami NA, Ibrahim IA, Kamisah Y, Mohd Ismail N. 2012. "Palm vitamin E reduces catecholamines, xanthine oxidase activity and gastric lesions in rats exposed to water-immersion restraint stress." *BMC Gastroenterol* 12: 54.

Mozaffarian D, Wu JHY. 2011. "Omega-3 fatty acids and cardiovascular disease." *J Am Coll Cardiol* 58:2047-2067.

Nagao A, Seki M, Kobayashi H. 1999. "Inhibition of xanthine oxidase by flavonoids." *Biosci Biotehnol Biochem* 63:1787-1790.

Neogi T. 2011. "Gout." *N Engl J Med* 364:443-452.

Nguyen S, Choi HK, Lustig RH, Hsu CY. 2009. "Sugar-sweetened beverages, serum uric acid, and blood pressure in adolescents." *J Pediatr* 154:807-813.

Nieuwdorp M, Gilijamse PW, Pai N, Kaplan LM. 2014. "Role of the microbiome in energy regulation and metabolism." *Gastroenterology* 146:1525-1533.

Oster KA. 1977. "Xanthine oxidase and folic acid." *Ann Intern Med* 87:252-253.

Perez-Pozo SE, Schold J, Nakagawa T, Sánchez-Lozada LG, Johnson RJ, Lillo JI. 2010. "Excessive fructose intake induces the features of metabolic syndrome in healthy adult men: role of uric acid in the hypertensive response." *Int. J. Obes* 34:454-461.

Perez-Ruiz F, Calabozo M, Erauskin GG, Ruibal A, Herrero-Beites AM. 2002. "Renal underexcretion of uric acid is present in patients with apparent high urinary uric acid output." *Arthritis Rheum* 47:610-613.

Ponvilawan B, Charoenngam N. 2021. "Vitamin D and uric acid: Is parathyroid hormone the missing link?" *J Clin Transl Endocrinol* 25:100263.

Prasad AS. 2014. "Zinc: an antioxidant and anti-inflammatory agent: role of zinc in degenerative disorders of aging." *J Trace Elem Med Biol* 28:364-371.

Roman YM. 2019. "Perspectives on the epidemiology of gout and hyperuricemia." *Hawaii J Med Public Health* 78:71-76.

Ruggiero C, Cherubini A, Ble A, Bos AJ, Maggio M, Dixit VD, Lauretani F, Bandinelli S, Senin U, Ferrucci L. 2006. "Uric acid and inflammatory markers." *Eur Heart J* 27:1174-1181.

Ruppert M, Diehl J, Kolloch R, Overlack A, Kraft K, Göbel B, Hittel N, Stumpe KO. 1991. "Short-term dietary sodium restriction increases serum lipids and insulin in salt-sensitive and salt-resistant normotensive adults." *Klin Wochenschr* 69 (Suppl 25):51-57.

Ryu S, Chang Y, Zhang Y, Kim SG, Cho J, Son HJ, Shin H, Guallar E. 2011. "A cohort study of hyperuricemia in middle-aged South Korean men." *Am J Epidemiol* 175:133-143.

Saito H, Toyoda Y, Takada T, Hirata H, Ota-kontani A, Miyata H, Kobayashi N, Tsuchiya Y, Suzuki H. 2020. "n-3 polyunsaturated fatty acids inhibit the function of human URAT 1, a renal urate re-absorber." *Nutrients* 12:1601.

Sautin YY, Johnson RJ. 2008. "Uric acid: the oxidant-antioxidant paradox." *Nucleosides Nucleotides Nucleic Acids* 27:608-619.

Schariau D, Borowicki A, Habermann N, Hofmann T, Klenow S, Miene C, Munjal U, Stein K, Glei M. 2009. "Mechanisms of primary cancer prevention by butyrate and other products formed during gut flora-mediated fermentation of dietary fiber." *Mutat Res* 582:39-53.

Schlesinger I, Schlesinger N. 2008. "Uric acid in Parkinson's disease." *Mov Disord* 23:1653-1657.

Schwingshackl L, Neuenschwander M, Hoffmann G, Buyken A, Schlesinger S. 2020. "Dietary sugars and cardiometabolic risk factors: a network meta-analysis on isocaloric substitution interventions." *Am J Clin Nutr* 111:187-196.

Seifi B, Kadkhodace M, Zahmatkesh M. 2011. "Effect of vitamin E therapy on serum uric acid in DOCA-salt-treated rats." *Acta Physiol Hung* 98:214-220.

Shadick NA, Kim R, Weiss S, Liang MH, Sparrow D, Hu H. 2000. "Effect of low level lead exposure on hyperuricemia and gout among middle aged and elderly men: the normative aging study." *J Rheumatol* 27:1708-1712.

Shatat IF, Abdallah RT, Sas DJ, Hailpern SM. 2012. "Serum uric acid in US adolescents: distribution and relationship to demographic characteristics and cardiovascular risk factors." *Pediatric Research* 72:95-100.

Shen L, Ji H-F. 2009. "Insights into the inhibition of xanthine oxidase by curcumin." *Bioorg Med Chem Lett* 19:5990-5993.

Shi Y-W, Wang C-P, Liu L, Liu Y-L, Wang X, Hong Y, Li Z, Kong L-D. 2012. "Antihyperuricemic and nephroprotective effects of resveratrol and its analogues in hyperuricemic mice." *Mol Nutr Food Res* 56:1433-1444.

Shostak NA, Pravdyuk NG, Loginova TK, Lazarenko GN. 2022. "Hyperuricemia, gout and comorbidity." *Clinician* 16:58-64.

Sigie T, Imatou T, Miyazaki M, Une H. 2005. "The effect of alcoholic beverage type on hyperuricemia in Japanese male office workers." *J Epidemiol* 15:41-47.

Siqueira J, Pereira TSS, Veiasquez-Melendez G, Barreto SM, Benseñor IM, Mill JG, Molina MCB. 2021. "Sugar-sweetened soft drinks consumption and risk of hyperuricemia: Results of the ELSA-Brasil study." *Nutr Metab Cardiovasc Dis* 31:2004-2013.

So AK, Martinon F. 2017. "Inflammation in gout: mechanisms and therapeutic targets." *Nat Rev Rheumatol* 13:639-647.

So MW, Lim D-H, Kim S-H, Lee S. 2020. "Dietary and nutritional factors associated with hyperuricemia: The seventh Korean National Health and Nutrition Examination Survey." *Asia Pac J Clin Nutr* 29:609-617.

Stamp LK, O'Donnell JL, Frampton C, Drake JM, Zhang M, Chapman PT. 2013. "Clinically insignificant effect of supplemental vitamin C on serum urate in patients with gout." *Arthritis Rheum* 65:1636-1642.

Stanhope KL. 2016. "Sugar consumption, metabolic disease and obesity: The state of the controversy." *Crit Rev Clin Lab Sci* 53:52-67.

Stein HB, Hasan A, Fox IH. 1976. "Ascorbic acid-induced uricosuria. A consequency of megavitamin therapy." *Ann Intern Med* 84:385-388.

Stocker R, Keaney JF Jr. 2004. "Role of oxidative modifications in atherosclerosis." *Physiol Rev* 84:1381-1478.

Sun L, Ni C, Zhao J, Wang G, Chen W. 2022. "Probiotics, bioactive compounds and dietary patterns for the effective management of hyperuricemia: a review." *Crit Rev Food Sci Nutr* 8:1-16.

Sun SZ, Empie MW. 2012. "Fructose metabolism in humans-what isotopic tracer studies tell us." *Nutr Metab* 9:89.

Sun SZ, Flickinger BD, Williamson-Hughes PS, Empie MW. 2010. "Lack of association between dietary fructose and hyperuricemia risk in adults." *Nutr Metab* 7:16.

Sun X, Wen J, Guan B, Li J, Luo J, Li J, Wei M, Qiu H. 2022. "Folic acid and zinc improve hyperuricemia by altering the gut microbiota of rats with high-purine diet-induced hyperuricemia." *Front Microbiol* 13: 907952.

Sun Y, Sun J, Wang J, Gao T, Zhang H, Ma A. 2018. "Association between vitamin C intake and risk of hyperuricemia in US adults." *Asia Pac J Clin Nutr* 27:1271-1276.

Sun Y, Sun J, Zhang P, Zhong F, Cai J, Ma A. 2019. "Association of dietary fiber intake with hyperuricemia in U.S. adults." *Food Funct* 10:4932-4940.

Sutton JL, Basu TK, Dickerson JW. 1983. "Effect of large doses of ascorbic acid in man on some nitrogenous components of urine." *Hum Nutr Appl Nutr* 37:136-140.

Tan J, Wan L, Chen X, Li X, Hao X, Li X, Li J, Ding H. 2019. "Conjugated linoleic acid ameliorates high fructose-induced hyperuricemia and renal inflammation in rats via NLRP3 inflammasome and TLR4 signaling pathway." *Mol Nutr Food Res* 63: e1801402.

Tana C, Ticinesi A, Prati B, Nouvenne A, Meschi T. 2018. "Uric acid and cognitive function in older individuals." *Nutrients* 10:975.

Taniguchi A, Kamatani N. 2008. "Control of renal uric acid excretion and gout." *Curr Opin Rheumatol* 20:192-197.

Tappy L, Morio B, Azzout-Mamiche D, Champ M, Gerber M, Houdart S, Mas E, Rizkalia S, Slama G, Mariotti F, Margaritis I. 2018. "French recommendations for sugar intake in adults: a novel approach chosen by ANSES." *Nutrients* 10:989.

Terkeltaub R, Edwards NL. 2013. *Gout; Diagnosis and management of gouty arthritis and hyperuricemia*. (Terkeltaub R, Edwards NL., eds.) vol.3. NY: Professional Communications, Inc.

Terkeltaub R. 2010. "Update on gout.; new therapeutic strategies and options." *Nat Rev Rheumatol* 6:30-38.

The Council for Science and Technology, Ministry of Education, Culture, Sports, Science and Technology in Japan. 2023. "Standard tables of food composition in Japan -2020- (Eighth Revised Edition), Report of the Subdivision Resources." Accessed April 28. https://www.mext.go.jp/content/20201225-mxt_kagsei-mext_01110_011.pdf.

Thottam GE, Krasnokutsky S, Pillinger MH. 2017. "Gout and metabolic syndrome: a tangled web." *Curr Rheumatol Rep* 19:60.

U.S. Department of Agriculture. 2023. "Dietary Guidelines for Americans 2015-2020, eighth edition." Accessed April 28. https://health.gov/sites/default/files/2019-09/2015-2020_Dietary_Guidelines.pdf.

U.S. Department of Health & Human Services. National Institutes of Health. 2023. "Office of Dietary Supplements. Dietary Supplement Fact Sheets." Accessed April 28. https://ods.od.nih.gov/factsheets/list-all/.

Villegas R, Xiang Y-B, Elasy T, Xu WH, Cai H, Cai Q, Linton MF, Fazio S, Zheng W, Shu X-O. 2012. "Purine-rich foods, protein intake, and the prevalence of hyperuricemia: the Shanghai Men's Health Study." *Nutr Metab Cardiovasc Dis* 22:409-416.

Wang DD, Sievenpiper JL, de Souza RJ, Chiavaroli L, Ha V, Cozma AI, Mirrahimi A, Yu ME, Carleton AJ, Buono MD, Jenkins AL, Leiter LA, Wolever TMS, Beyene J, Kendall CWC, Jenkins DJA. 2012. "The effects of fructose intake on serum uric acid vary among controlled dietary trials." *J Nutr* 142:916-923.

Wang M, Zhao J, Zhang N, Chen J. 2016. "Astilbin improves potassium oxonate-induced hyperuricemia and kidney injury through regulating oxidative stress and inflammation response in mice." *Biomed Pharmacother* 83:975-988.

Wang W, Jing Z, Liu W, Zhu L, Ren H, Hou X. 2022. "Hyperuricemia is an important risk factor of the erectile dysfunction: A systematic review and meta-analysis." *Andrologia* 54: e14384.

Wang Y, Zhu JX, Kong LD, Yang C, Cheng CHK, Zhang X. 2004. "Administration of procyanidins from grape seeds reduces serum uric acid levels and decreases hepatic xanthine dehydrogenase/oxidase activities in oxonate-treated mice." *Basic Clin Pharmacol Toxicol* 94:232-237.

Wang YL, Zeng C, Wei J, Yang T, Li H, Deng ZH, Yang Y, Zhang Y, Ding X, Xie DX, Yang TB, Lei GH. 2015. "Association between dietary magnesium intake and hyperuricemia." *PLoS One* 10: e0141079.

Wang Z, Li Y, Liao W, Huang J, Liu Y, Li Z, Tang J. 2022. "Gut microbiota remodeling: A promising therapeutic strategy to confront hyperuricemia and gout." *Front Cell Infect Microbiol* 12: 935723.

Wei B, Ren P, Yang R, Gao Y, Tang Q, Xue C, Wang Y. 2023. "Ameliorative effect of mannuronate oligosaccharides on hyperuricemic mice via promoting uric acid excretion and modulating gut microbiota." *Nutrients* 15:417.

Wei J, Zhang Y, Dalbeth N, Terkeltaub R, Yang T, Wang Y, Yang Z, Li J, Wu Z, Zeng C, Lei G. 2022. "Association between gut microbiota and elevated serum urate in two independent cohorts." *Arthritis Rheumatol* 74:682-691.

Williams PT. 2008. "Effects of diet, physical activity and performance, and body weight on incident gout in ostensibly healthy, vigorously active men." *Am J Clin Nutr* 87:1480-1487.

Wolfram G. 1992. "Das moderne Konzept der Ernährung bei Gicht." *Akt Ernährungsmed* 17:24-32.

World Health Organization 2023. "Healthy diet." Accessed April 28. https://www.who.int/news-room/fact-sheets/detail/healthy-diet.

World Health Organization, Food and Agriculture Organization, and United Nations University. 2007. "Protein and amino acid requirements in human nutrition." *Tech Rep Ser* 935.

World Health Organization. 2015. *Guideline: Sugars intake for adults and children.* Geneva, Switzerland: WHO Press.

Wortmann RL, Kelley WN. 2001. "Gout and hyperuricemia, sixth edition" In: *Kelley's textbook of rheumatology*, edited by Ruddy S, Harris Jr ED, Sledge CB, 1339-1376. Philadelphia: P. W. B. Saunders.

Wu D, Chen R, Zhang W, Lai X, Sun L, Li Q, Zhang Z, Cao J, Wen S, Lai Z, Li Z, Cao F, Sun S. 2022. "Tea and its components reduce the production of uric acid by inhibiting xanthine oxidase." *Food Nutr Res* 66:8239.

Xia Y, Wu Q, Wang H, Zhang S, Jiang Y, Gong T, Xu X, Chang Q, Niu K, Zhao Y. 2020. "Global, regional and national burden of gout:, 1990-2017: a systematic analysis of the Global Burden of Disease Study." *Rheumatology* 59:1529-1538.

Xiao B, Ma W, Zheng Y, Li Z, Li D, Zhang Y, Li Y, Wang D. 2021. "Effects of resveratrol on the inflammatory response and renal injury in hyperuricemic rats." *Nutr Res Pract* 15:26-37.

Xie D, Shen Y, Su E, Du L, Xie J, Wei D. 2023. "Anti-hyperuricemic, nephroprotective, and gut microbiota regulative effects of separated hydrolysate of α-lactalbumin on potassium oxonate- and hypoxanthine-induced hyperuricemic mice." *Mol Nutr Food Res* 67: e2200162.

Xie D-X, Xiong Y-L, Zeng C, Wei J, Yang T, Li H, Wang Y-L, Gao S-G, Li Y-S, Lei G-H. 2015. "Association between low dietary zinc and hyperuricaemia in middle-aged and older males in China: a cross-sectional study." *BMJ Open* 5: e008637.

Xiong Z, Zhu C, Qian X, Zhu J, Wi Z, Chen L. 2013. "Serum uric acid is associated with dietary and lifestyle factors in elderly women in suburban Guangzhou in Guangdong province of south China." *J Nutr Health Aging* 17:30-34.

Xu X, Wang H, Guo D, Man X, Liu J, Li J, Luo C, Zhang M, Zhen L, Liu X. 2021. "Curcumin modulates gut microbiota and improves renal function in rats with uric acid nephropathy." *Ren Fail* 43:1063-1075.

Yamaguchi Y, Ando C, Tsukamoto S, Nagao J, Ueda T, Yamaguchi H, Akaoka I. 2007. "The effect on the serum uric acid level of long-term intake of chitosan-supplemented food and its safety in adults." *J Jpn Soc Clin Nutr* 29:104-113 (in Japanese).

Yamamoto T, Moriwaki Y, Ka T, Inokuchi T, Takahashi S, Tsutsumi Z, Fukuchi M, Hada T. 2004. "Effect of purine-free low-malt liquor (happo-shu) on the plasma concentrations and urinary excretion of purine bases and uridine comparison between purine-free and regular happo-shu." *Horm Metab Res* 36:231-237.

Yamamoto T, Moriwaki Y, Ka T, Takahashi S, Tsutsumi Z, Cheng J, Inokuchi T, Yamamoto A, Hada T. 2004. "Effect of sauna bathing and beer ingestion on plasma concentrations of purine bases." *Metabolism* 53: 772-776.

Yamamoto T, Moriwaki Y, Takahashi S. 2005. "Effect of ethanol on metabolism of purine bases (hypoxanthine, xanthine, and uric acid)." *Clin Chim Acta* 356:35-57.

Yang H-Y, Xiu W-J, Liu J-K, Yang Y, Hou X-G, Zheng Y-Y, Wu T-T, Xie X. 2021. "Gut microbiota characterization in patients with asymptomatic hyperuricemia: probiotics increased." Bioengineered 12:7363-7275.

Yang T, Ding X, Wang YL, Zeng C, Wei J, Li H, Xiong YL, Gao SG, Li YS, Lei GH. 2016. "Association between high-sensitivity C-reactive protein and hyperuricemia." *Rheumatol Int* 36:561-566.

Yin H, Liu N, Chen J. 2022. "The role of the intestine in the development of hyperuricemia." *NPJ Biofilms Microbiomes* 13:845684.

Yokozawa T, Oura H, Nakagawa H, Okada T. 1982. "Adenine-induced hyperuricemia and renal damage in rats." *J Jpn Soc Biosci Biotech Agrochem* 56:655-663 (in Japanese).

Yoon J-H, Baek SJ. 2005. "Molecular targets of dietary polyphenols with anti-inflammatory properties." *Yonsei Med J* 46:585-596.

Yu K-H, See L-C, Huang Y-C, Yang C-H, Sun J-H. 2008. "Dietary factors associated with hyperuricemia in adults." *Semin Arthritis Rheum* 37:243-250.

Yü TF, Berger L, Gutman AB. 1962. "Renal function in gout. II. Effect of uric acid loading on renal excretion of uric acid." *Am J Med* 33:829-844.

Yu Y, Liu Q, Li H, Wen C, He Z. 2018. "Alterations of the gut microbiome associated with the treatment of hyperuricemia in male rats." *Front Microbiol* 9:2233.

Zgaga L, Theodoratou E, Kyle J, Farrington SM, Agakov F, Tenesa A, Walker M, McNeill G, Wright AF, Rudan I, Dunlop MG, Campbell H. 2012. "The association of dietary intake of purine-rich vegetables, sugar-sweetened beverages and dairy with plasma urate, in a cross-sectional study." *PLoS One* 7: e38123.

Zhang C, Li L, Zhang Y, Zeng C. 2020. "Recent advances in fructose intake and risk of hyperuricemia." *Biomed Pharmacother* 131:110795.

Zhang L, Shi X, Yu J, Zhang P, Ma P, Sun Y. 2020. "Dietary vitamin E intake was inversely associated with hyperuricemia in U.S. adults: NHANES 2009-2014." *Ann Nutr Metab* 76:354-360.

Zhang M, Ye C, Wang R., Zhang Z, Huang X, Halimulati M, Sun M, Ma Y, Zhang Z. 2023. "Association between dietary acid load and hyperuricemia in Chinese adults: Analysis of the China Health and Nutrition Survey (2009)." *Nutrients* 15:1806.

Zhang M, Zhu X, Wu J, Huang Z, Zhao Z, Zhang X, Xue Y, Wan W, Li C, Zhang W, Wang L, Zhou M, Zou, H, Wang L. 2022. "Prevalence of hyperuricemia among Chinese adults; Findings from two nationally representative cross-sectional surveys in 2015-16 and 2018-19." *Front Immunol* 12:791983.

Zhang N, Zhou J, Zhao L, Zhao Z, Wang S, Zhang L, Zhou F. 2023. "Ferulic acid supplementation alleviates hyperuricemia in high-fructose/fat det-fed rats via promoting uric acid excretion and mediating the gut microbiota." *Food Funct* 14:1710-1725.

Zhang X, La Q, Zhang Z, Chen Y, Wang Y, Wang Y, Li Z, Jiang L. 2018. "Value of three-dimensional speckle tracking echocardiography to assess left ventricular function in hyperuricemia patients." *Clin Rheumatol* 37: 2539-2545.

Zhang X, Nie Q, Zhang Z, Zhao J, Zhang F, Wang C, Wang X, Song G. 2021. "Resveratrol affects the expression of uric acid transporter by improving inflammation." *Mol Med Rep* 24:564.

Zhang Y, Deng L, Wu CM, Zheng L, Zhong G. 2018. "Konjac glucomannan improves hyperuricemia through regulating xanthine oxidase, adenosine deaminase and urate transporters in rats." *Journal of Functional Foods* 48:566-575.

Zhang Y, Qiu H. 2018. "Dietary magnesium intake and hyperuricemia among US adults." *Nutrients* 10:296.

Zhang Y, Qiu H. 2018. "Folate, vitamin B6 and vitamin B12 intake in relation to hyperuricemia." *J Clin Med* 7: 210.

Zhang Y, Shuai TG, Wu CM, Shen JJ, Zhong G. 2016. "Effect of konjac glucomannan on hyperuricemic rats." *Journal of Food and Dairy Technology* 4:18-25.

Zhang Z, Harman JL, Coresh J, Köttgen A, McAdams-DeMarco MA, Correa A, Young BA, Katz R, Rebholz CM. 2018. "The dietary fructose: vitamin C intake ratio is associated with hyperuricemia in African American adults." *J Nutr* 148:419-426.

Zhang Z-C, Su G-H, Luo C-L, Pang Y-L, Wang L, Li X, Wen J-H, Zhang J-L. 2015. "Effects of anthocyanins from purple sweet potato (Ipomoea batatas L,. cultivar Eshu No. 8) on the serum uric acid level and xanthine oxidase activity in hyperuricemic mice." *Food Funct* 6:3045-3055.

Zhu JN, Qi XY, Tan Y, Lyu XH. 2016. "Dietary factors associated with hyperuricemia and glycolipid metabolism disorder in middle-aged and elderly people." *Sichuan Da Xue Xue Bao Yi Xue Ban* 47:68-72.

Zhu JX, Wang Y, Kong LD, Yang C, Zhang X. 2004. "Effects of Biota orientalis extract and its flavonoid constituents, quercetin and rutin on serum uric acid levels in oxonate-induced mice and xanthine dehydrogenase and xanthine oxidase activities in mouse liver." *J Ethnopharmacol* 93:133-140.

Zhu Q, Yu L, Li Y, Man Q, Jia S, Zhou Y, Zuo H, Zhang J. 2022. "Association between dietary fiber intake and hyperuricemia among Chinese adults: Analysis of the China Adult Chronic Disease and Nutrition Surveillance (2015)." *Nutrients* 14:1433.

Zhu Y, Pandya BJ, Choi HK. 2011. "Prevalence of gout and hyperuricemia in the US general population: the National Health and Nutrition Examination Survey 2007-2008." *Arthritis Rheum* 63:3136-3141.

Zychowcz ME. 2011. "Gout: No longer the disease of kings." *Orthop Nurs* 30:322-330.

Zykova SN, Storhaug HM, Toft I, Chadban SJ, Jenssen TG, White SL. 2015. "Cross-sectional analysis of nutrition and serum uric acid in two Caucasian cohorts: the AusDiab Study and the Tromsø study." *Nutr J* 14:49.

Biographical Sketch

Takashi Koguchi

Affiliation:
Department of Human Education, Kokugakuin Tochigi Junior College

Education:
Department of Agricultural Chemistry, Graduate School of Agriculture, Tokyo University of Agriculture- Tokyo, JAPAN 1990-1996
Bachelor of Agricultural Chemistry
Master of Agricultural Chemistry
Doctor of Agricultural Chemistry

Business Address: 608 Hirai-cho, Tochigi-shi, Tochigi 328-8588, Japan.
Phone: +81-282-22-5511/Email: echo130@nifty.com

Research and Professional Experience:

Research:
I reported the suppressive effect of dietary fiber (DF) on experimental hyperuricemia in rats. My findings are that DF was of much benefit to hyperuricemia of rats induced by dietary purines. Recently, clinical studies have revealed that intake of DF lowers serum uric acid (SUA) concentrations of healthy subjects and hyperuricemic subjects. Epidemiological studies have found that increased DF intake is associated with decreased SUA concentration and hyperuricemia risk. My hypothesis is supported as the possible mechanism by the reports of epidemiological and clinical studies. It seems that the basic research results of our series concerning the suppressive effect of DF on hyperuricemia stimulated subsequent clinical research into this matter. Nobody has ever shown the report on relationship between DF intake and SUA concentration or hyperuricemia. These contents were reported in a review article entitled "Beneficial effect of dietary fiber on hyperuricemia in rats and humans" in the International Journal of Vitamin and Nutrition Research in 2019. In the review article, I also reported the association of dietary factors with hyperuricemia (Essentials of dietary habits for prevention and suppression of hyperuricemia. Curr. Top. Pharmacol. 22, 77-133, 2018). I reported about the modification of dietary habits for prevention of gout in Japanese people in the American Journal of Health Research in 2021 and 2022.

Professional Experience:
2016-present
Kokugakuin Tochigi Junior College
Visiting Professor
Lectures of nutrition, food science, and my field of expertise

Professional Appointments:
(Editorial Activities)
Reviewer
2020-present
International Journal of Nutrition and Food Sciences
Science Publishing Group. NY, USA

Special Editorial Board
2020-2023 (August/7/2023)
International Journal of Food Science and Agriculture
Hill Publishing Group. NY, USA

Honors: None

Publications from the Last 3 Years:

1) Koguchi, T. (2021) Modification of dietary habits for prevention of gout in Japanese people; Gout and the Japanese diet. *Am. J. Health Res.* 9, 117-127.
2) Koguchi, T. (2021) Modification of dietary habits for prevention of gout in Japanese people; Gout and macronutrient intake. *Am. J. Health Res.* 9, 128-142.
3) Koguchi, T. (2021) Modification of dietary habits for prevention of gout in Japanese people; Gout and micronutrient intake or alcohol consumption. *Am. J. Health Res.* 9, 143-157.
4) Koguchi, T. (2021) Modification of dietary habits for prevention of gout in Japanese people; Gout and food intake. *Am. J. Health Res.* 9, 158-175.
5) Koguchi, T. (2021) Modification of dietary habits for prevention of gout in Japanese people; Gout and diet. *Am. J. Health Res.* 9, 176-189.
6) Koguchi, T. (2022) Modification of macronutrient intake for prevention of gout in Japanese people in 2019: 2022 update. *Am J Health Res,* 10, 83-106.
7) Koguchi, T. (2022) Modification of micronutrient intake for prevention of gout in Japanese people in 2019: 2022 update. *Am J Health Res,* 10, 107-131.
8) Koguchi, T. (2022) Modification of animal product intake for prevention of gout in Japanese people in 2019: 2022 update. *Am J Health Res,* 10, 140-153.
9) Koguchi, T. (2022) Modification of plant-based food intake for prevention of gout in Japanese people in 2019: 2022 update. *Am J Health Res,* 10, 154-168.

Chapter 4

Uric Acid and the Kidney – Causes and Consequences, and the Role of the Immune Response

Milena K. Nikolova[1,*]
Kaloyan M. Davidoff[2]
Julian R. Ananiev[3]
and Yordan D. Vlahov[4]

[1]Clinic of Nephrology, University Hospital St. Ivan Rilski, Medical University-Sofia, Bulgaria
[2]Clinic of Urology, Sofiamed University Hospital, Faculty of Medicine, Sofia University St. Kliment Ohridski, Sofia, Bulgaria
[3]Department of General and Clinical Pathology, Medical Faculty, Trakia University, Stara Zagora, Bulgaria
[4]Clinic of Endocrinology and Metabolic Diseases, Sofiamed University Hospital, Faculty of Medicine, Sofia University St. Kliment Ohridski, Sofia, Bulgaria

Abstract

Hyperuricemia is a well-known risk factor for the development of acute and chronic renal diseases and for the progression of chronic kidney disease. The relationship between hyperuricemia and renal diseases is complex and sometimes it is unclear who the victim is and who is the culprit, as both hyperuricemia can harm the kidney, and renal diseases can lead to an increase in uric acid levels.

Three major types of renal involvement have been described in patients with hyperuricemia:

* Corresponding Author: Dr. Milena Nikolova, MD, PhD, MBA, Assoc. Prof. Clinic of Nephrology, University Hospital St. Ivan Rilski Medical University-Sofia, Bulgaria, EU; e-mail: milena_i_dani@abv.bg.

In: Hyperuricemia
Editor: Warren Y. Salinas
ISBN: 979-8-89113-239-9

acute renal injury (due to tubular obstruction in terms of precipitation of monosodium urate crystals in the renal distal tubules and collecting ducts),

chronic kidney injury (due to urate crystal deposition within the tubule lumen and in the tubulointerstitial spaces with subsequent inflammatory changes and formation of fibrosis and nephrocalcinosis; development of granulomatous tubulointerstitial nephritis resembling the soft tissue tophi in gout; and rarely, glomerular changes),

formation of renal stones.

Moreover, hyperuricemia and gout are associated with significant co-morbidity in the spectrum of the metabolic syndrome, and with the development of renal changes secondary to arterial hypertension, diabetes, accelerated atherosclerosis, heart failure and their treatment. The use of non-steroid anti-inflammatory medications in patients with gout is also potentially harmful for both tubulointerstitial and glomerular structures.

Novel studies have shown that hyperuricemia can lead to both local and systemic activation of the innate immune system (including stimulation of the NLRP3 inflammasome and secretion of interleukin-1β and interleukin-18 via caspace-1 pathway with subsequent cytokine release and both local and systemic inflammatory response), and to pro-inflammatory changes in resident renal cells with fibrogenesis.

The authors discuss the current knowledge on the interactions between hyperuricemia and the kidney and the role of the immune response in this relationship.

Keywords: hyperuricemia, gout, kidney, immune response, acute and chronic kidney disease

Introduction

Uric acid (UA) in humans is the end product of adenine and guanine metabolism and is derived from three major pathways: cellular nucleic acids (cell turnover – from dead, dying or damaged cells), hepatic synthesis, food (rich in purines and/or fructose and sucrose) [1, 2]. Purines are metabolized to xantine which is further converted to uric acid via the xantine oxidase pathway. While in most other mammals UA is further metabolized to the soluble and non-toxic allantoin, humans lack the enzyme uricase (urate oxidase) and purine metabolism stops to the end product UA which can crystallize in the form of monosodium urate (MSU) in the tissues under certain conditions when the solubility threshold is exceeded and/or factors increasing precipitation are present, including plasma oversaturation (due to overproduction, dehydration and/or decreased renal excretion), acidosis, decreased local blood flow, low temperature, local inflammation and/or trauma, edema and stasis, changes in joint cartilage [3]. Therefore, the risk of crystallization increases in dehydration, acidosis, decreased blood flow/stasis, hypothermia and local tissue damage. MSU crystals can deposit in joints, periarticular structures and soft tissues (tophi), and kidneys, (Figure 1) and cause local inflammatory reaction, leading to the development of granuloma-like tissue reaction and perpetuation of low-grade inflammation that further increases cardiovascular risk [3, 4, 5]. Further unfavorable effect of hyperuricemia and hyperuricosuria is the increased risk for the formation of calcium oxalate containing stones due to formation of nidus for calcium oxalate nucleation and increased precipitation crystallization of calcium oxalate in medium with high levels of dissolved UA [1].

The endogenous production of UA is relatively constant – up to 400 mg a day, and accounts for approximately half of the total amount of uric acid in human body, with the other half originating from food sources (including purine-rich and fructose-containing food) [1]. On the other hand, the renal excretion is relatively stable and in the Western world is approximately 10 mg/kg/24 hours [1]. Therefore, the major determinant of UA blood and urine levels in humans is the dietary intake of UA-generating substances.

Hyperuricemia is a well-known risk factor for the development of acute and chronic renal diseases and for the progression of chronic kidney disease. The relationship between hyperuricemia and renal diseases is complex and sometimes it is unclear who is the victim and who is the culprit, as both hyperuricemia can harm the kidney, and renal diseases can lead to an increase in uric acid levels.

Three major types of renal involvement have been described in patients with hyperuricemia: acute renal injury, chronic kidney injury, formation of renal stones.

Moreover, hyperuricemia and gout are associated with significant co-morbidity in the spectrum of the metabolic syndrome, and with the development of renal changes secondary to arterial hypertension, diabetes, accelerated atherosclerosis, heart failure and their treatment. The use of non-steroid anti-inflammatory medications in patients with gout is also potentially harmful for both tubulointerstitial and glomerular structures.

Novel studies have shown that hyperuricemia can lead to both local and systemic activation of the innate immune system (including stimulation of the NLP3 inflammasome and secretion of interleukin-1β and interleukin-18 via caspace-1 pathway with subsequent cytokine release and an both local and systemic inflammatory response), and to pro-inflammatory changes in resident renal cells with fibrogenesis.

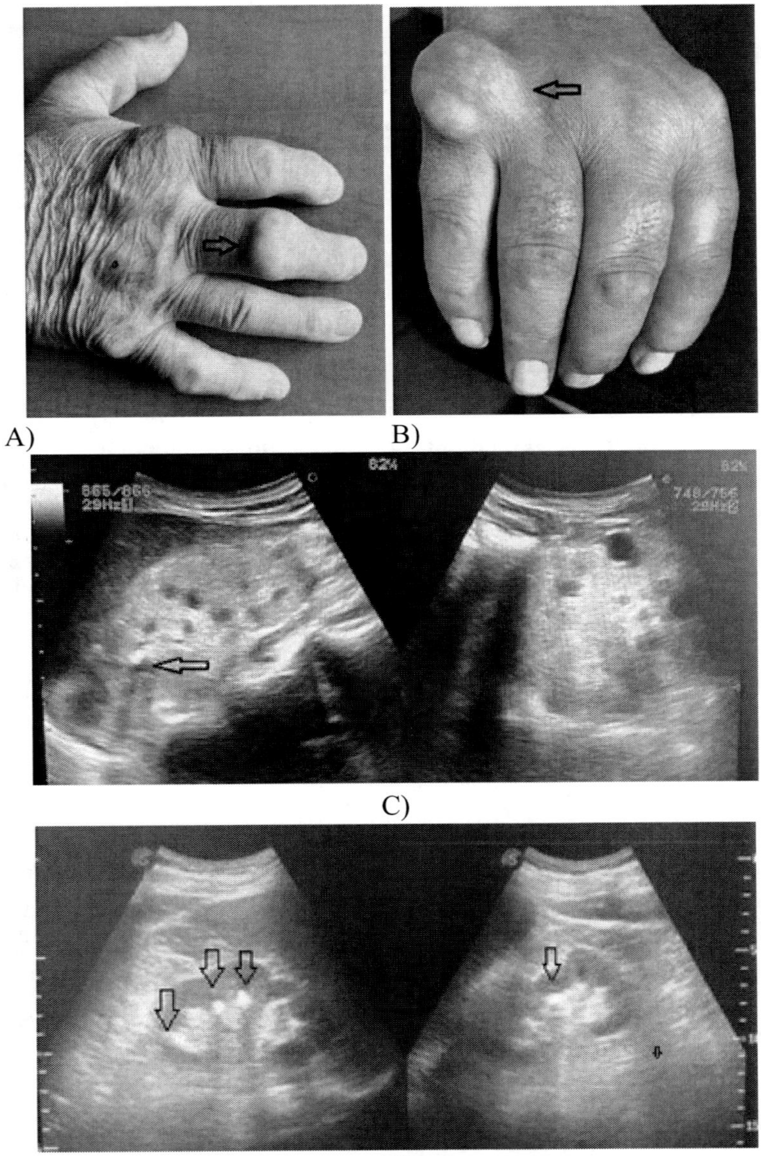

Figure 1. Sites of deposition of uric acid (UA). A) Acute gout arthritis of a finger (arrow). B) Tophi – deposition of UA in periarticular and soft tissues (arrow). C) Renal stone (arrow). D) Nephrocalcinosis (arrows).

The Kidney and UA – Causes and Consequences

Handling UA in Physiological Conditions

In the human body, UA is generated mainly the hepatic and intestinal structures and the vascular endothelium [6]. Approximately two thirds of the produced uric acid is excreted by the kidneys, and the remaining one third has intestinal clearance – excretion with feces with further intestinal urocolysis by the resident microbiota of the gut [7]. The urinary excretion of UA is performed via four-step process of glomerular filtration, pre-secretory reabsorption, secretion and post-secretary reabsorption [7]. Several defects in tubular transport proteins have been associated with hyperuricemia, including SLC2A9 gene encoding GLUT9, SLC22A12 gene encoding URAT1, SLC17A1 encoding NPT1, and ABCG2.

Estrogens are uricosuric and uric acid concentrations are higher in men and post-menopausal women.

And finally, not all patients with hyperuricemia progress to gout and the reason why the majority of individuals do not develop gout is unclear but certain genetic polymorphisms are thought to be responsible [8].

Thus, UA levels in human body are influenced mainly by diet, alcohol and diuretic consumption, levels of hydration, increased cell turnover, enzyme defects in purine metabolism, changes in renal function and estrogen levels. The complicated mechanism of renal handling of uric acid excretion in the kidney could lead to increased risk for deposition of uric acid crystals inside tubular structures and/or sedimentation within the renal tubules, interstitial spaces, calyces and renal pelvis, leading to the development of tubulointerstitial nephritis, acute tubular obstruction and development of renal stones.

The kidney can play the role of both culprit, causing an increase in UA levels in renal dysfunction, and the victim of hyperuricemia.

What Is the Physiological Role of UA in Humans?

UA has several physiological roles in humans [6, 7,8, 9, 10]:

- Antioxidant properties: UA is one of the major extracellular antioxidant molecules, especially in the spaces, where radical oxygen species are generated, including the liver, nasal secretions, and vascular endothelium. UA is also present in normal liver, intestinal and endothelial cells and can interfere with the activity of lipoxygenases and serve as a substrate for the cyclooxygenase, therefore serving as antioxidant. Yet, in high levels inside the cells UA can have pro-oxidant effect.

- Protection of endothelial function: UA has crucial role in tissue repair due to its antioxidant properties, its ability to scavenge oxygen free radicals and to stimulate progenitor endothelial cells [9]. S. Sugihara et al., [9] and T. Iso et al., [10] have shown that extremely low UA levels are related to severe endothelial dysfunction. Nonetheless, high UA levels are also associated with severe endothelial dysfunction, which is particularly visible in patients with multiple components of metabolic syndrome plus hyperuricemia [3] and in preeclampsia [11].
- Induction of type 2 immune response: it has been hypothesized that UA is important for the development of type 2 immune response to cysteine peptidases in the absence of adjuvant. This process is thought to be associated with the liberation of uric acid from damaged, dying and dead cells. Under such circumstances, UA acts as a signal for danger and stimulates the generation of inflammatory monocyte-derived dendritic cells [12, 13]. It has been shown that MSU crystals in combination with harmless inhalatory protein allergens can induce potent type 2 immune response via activating spleen tyrosine kinase (Syk) and the phosphoinositol 3 (PI3)-kinase, thus making UA a major initiator and amplifier of allergic inflammation [14]. It is well-known that many cysteine proteaseses and cysteine peptidases can stimulate barrier epithelial cells to produce type 2 cytokines (thymic stromal lymphopoietin (TSLP), interleukin (IL)-25, and IL-33) that can shift the immune environment towards type 2 response and hypersensitivity reactions. Since allergens and cysteine peptidases can induce barrier cell damage, they could lead to release of UA that can further increase the immune response functioning as alarming, danger signal for ongoing cellular damage and death and engage epithelial, innate lymphoid cells, eosinophils, basophils, and mast cells [13,14,15,16]. This has been proven in models of allergic and vaccine-induced response of the airways [13, 14, 15, 16].
- Resistance to parasites, including Schistosoma mansoni and Schictosoma haematobium and Fasciola hepatica: the non-specific immune defense mechanisms, including eosinophils, basophils and

mast cells, secrete toxic and pro-oxidant substances in response to the invasion of parasites and lead to endothelial injury in the adjacent vessels which causes release and accumulation of UA. UA increases in damaged cells and is released by all damaged, dying and dead cells, and can interfere with the synthesis of arachidonic acid, which in turn can mediate the damage of parasite cells. This has been proven in experimental studies [17,18]. Defense against autoimmune diseases: as mentioned above, UA acts as natural antioxidant [6, 7,8], and hypouricemia has been detected in patients with various autoimmune diseases, including multiple sclerosis, pemphigus vulgaris, and lichen planus, as well as in neurological diseases, such as Alzheimer's diseases and Parkinson's disease [19, 20, 21, 22]. The presumed mechanism of neuroprotective effect of UA is blockage of peroxynitrites and radical oxygen species that are responsible for the damage and destruction of myelin and other nervous system components, along with regulation of calcium homeostasis, mitochondrial function and counteracting glutamate toxicity on neuronal cells [8].

What Is the Pathological Role of Uric Acid in Humans?

Uric acid is a risk factor for adverse outcome in cardiovascular disease and in all components of the metabolic syndrome [4, 6, 8, 24, 25, 27]. High UA levels are associated with unfavorable outcome in patients with chronic kidney disease [4, 6, 24, 25, 27]. Despite its role as natural antioxidant and immune response modulator, when in high levels UA has potent pro-oxidative properties, including formation of free radicals and reacting with lipids, increasing lipid oxidation and protein nitrosylation, stimulation of NADH oxidase dependent ROS and generation of ROS via xantine oxidoreductase activation, activation of MAPK p38, ERK 1 / 2, decreased in nitric oxide (NO) synthesis and bioavailability [8]. As mentioned above, UA can modulate immune response and in both very low and very high levels can induce pro-oxidant and pro-inflammatory reactions. Thus, the pro-oxidant and pro-inflammatory effects of UA significantly prevail over its protective role in humans and define it as a pro-inflammatory and vascular risk factor.

High levels of uric acid are known to cause microvascular injury via stimulation of the rennin-angiotensin system (RAS), increased expression of rennin in glomerular cells and increased expression of (pro) rennin receptor in endothelial cells, inhibition of NO synthesis and decreased expression of NO-synthase-1 in renal macula, stimulation of smooth-muscle cell proliferation [8, 24].

UA can activate monocytes and macrophages and induce the generation of NRLP3 inflammasome with subsequent secretion of IL-1β and IL-18 via caspace-1 pathway with subsequent cytokine release and both local and systemic inflammatory response. The pro-inflammatory effects of UA on tubular cells are mediated by HMGM1 (high mobility group box chromosomal protein 1) and NF-kB (nuclear factor kappa-B). The pro-inflammatory state in chronic kidney disease (CKD) and hyperuricemia, especially with changes in gut microbiota that is known to participate in UA clearance has been confirmed by the high levels of acute-phase and pro-inflammatory cytokines in such patients [25].

The Kidney and Uric Acid

The kidney is a key regulator of uric acid levels via changes in UA excretion [8]. In terms of renal failure uric acid serum levels tend to increase due to decrease in both glomerular filtration and tubular transport. Marked increase in UA levels is observed in tubulointerstitial diseases. On the other hand, uric acid itself is toxic for the renal tubular cells, it can precipitate within the renal tubules (usually within the collecting ducts) and cause glomerular injury and fibrogenesis, and in terms of hyperuricemia and hyperuricosuria UA can cause several types of kidney damage [8, 23, 24]:

- acute kidney injury due to tubular toxicity or to precipitation/ crystallization within the tubular lumens (usually in the collecting ducts), frequently observed in patients with massive tissue damage and/or dehydration, chemotherapy. This type is potentially reversible with rehydration, urine alkalization and temporary dialysis.
- chronic kidney injury due to chronic tubular toxicity with tubular atrophy and fibrosis, development of granulomatous interstitial nephritis in response to UA crystals (resembling the changes in soft tissue depositions presenting as tophi), or glomerular involvement in the form of mesangioproliferative glomerulonephritis or glomerulosclerosis. In the presence of inflammatory changes the process is potentially reversible with UA lowering agents and short-

term corticosteroid treatment aimed at suppression of the lymphoid inflammatory infiltrate (Figure 2).

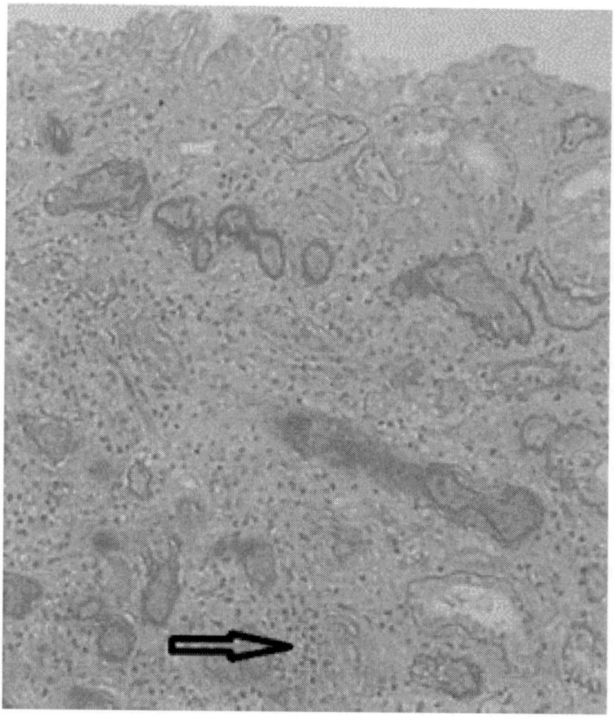

Figure 2. Advanced chronic tubulointerstitial nephritis in a patient with gout – clearly visible mononuclear lymphoid infiltration (arrow). PAS, x100.

- renal stones and nephrocalcinosis. The development of nephrolithiasis has been explained by oversaturation of urine with uric acid with subsequent sedimentation and crystallization and/or facilitation of calcium oxalate crystal formation by the UA. Nephrocalcinosis in hyperuricemia can develop as a result of tubular and interstitial damage or secondary to vascular occlusions in arteriolosclerosis. Uric acid stones are potentially soluble with urine alkalization, but sometimes may require surgical treatment, especially if severe complications are present, i.e., forniceal rupture or pyonephrosis. The development and treatment of uric acid stones is reviewed in a separate Chapter.

- Moreover, the levels of uric acid correlate with the degree of tubular atrophy and fibrosis [26], and hyperuricemia can worsen the prognosis and increase the rate of progression of IgA glomerulonephritis and CKD of other causes [26, 27, 28] and with a greater risk of CKD, especially in older patients [29]. An interesting finding is the higher prevalence of hyperuricemia in patients with IgA glomerulonephritis with negative impact on both disease course and progression [26], more severe histopathological findings on renal biopsy, especially in female patients [28], and higher prevalence of glomerular ischemic lesions [30]. The more sever pathological changes in hyperuricemic patients could be could be explained by the activation of immune response and fibrogeneris, the vascular and hemodynamic effects of UA, initiation of free-radical pathways and pro-inflammatory state [31, 32] and the presence of comorbidities in the spectrum of metabolic syndrome, associated with hyperuricemia.

The Role of the Immune System in Hyperuricemia-Induced Renal and Systemic Complications

Uric acid is a well-known nephrotoxic and cardio-vascular risk factor [2, 3, 4, 5, 6, 23-32]. Its effects on the kidney and on the vascular structures are due to renal afferent arteriosclerosis, precipitation within and obstruction of renal tubules, crystallization in the tubulointerstitial spaces and induction of focal inflammatory response, pro-oxidant state with changes in mitochondrial metabolism and disruption of cellular energetic balance, endothelial function and endothelial cell damage and death with subsequent decrease in NO levels, vascular smooth-muscle cell proliferation, platelet activation, pro-inflammatory action. Moreover, UA can worsen and induce the development of metabolic syndrome, hypertension and diabetes [32]. These effects lead to increased vascular risk and rate of progression of CKD. Nevertheless, the immune system plays central role in the development of both renal and vascular complications of hyperuricemia [31, 32]. The innate immune system plays crucial role in the protection against pathogens and stress factors released by damaged cells and tissues. Such stress-molecules derived from damaged or dead cells and tissues are a wide range of proteins and non-protein molecules, including ATP, uric acid, heparin sulfate and DNA. They are recognized by component of the immune system, including Toll-like receptors

(TLRs) on cell surface or in the endosoma and trigger immediate response from macrophages, fibroblasts, mast cells, and dendritic cells in the tissues, and circulating leukocytes. Therefore, UA can serve as stress-signal or alarming signal that in the past has had beneficial role in the fight against infections and cellular death. With the significant increase of UA serum levels on population level, due to the higher consumption of purine-rich and fructose-rich foods, this adaptive evolutionary mechanism has gradually turned into harmful pathway, leading to multiple immune, metabolic and vasculoendothelial complications. The NRLs (NOD-like receptors) are of particular interest in the recognition of both protein and non-protein stress-signals because they represent a second line of defense against pathogens that have entered the cells and against the residues of non-pathogenic, amicrobial injury. These intracellular receptors form inflammasomes aimed at fighting the residues of cellular damage and death and are named after the protein initiating the cascade signalling (e.g., NLRP1, NLRC4, NLRP3). Among the best studied is the NLRP3 inflammasome that has been detected in leukocytes (including monocytes and macrophages) and dendritic cells. It consists of three parts: a sensor protein (NRLP molecule recognizing the stress-signal), adapter protein (Apoptosis-associated Speck-like protein containing a CARD, ASC – linking NRLP to caspase-1) and caspace-1 (IL1-converting enzyme that cleaves precursor proteins and turns them into active forms of the inflammatory cytokine molecules, including IL1β and IL-18). The generated inflammatory molecules can act both locally and enter the circulation and trigger acute and chronic inflammatory cascades that can amplify the inflammatory response and induce systemic complications, such as arthritis or vascular damage in chronic inflammation in patients with gout [32]. Therefore, the chronic low-grade inflammation in patients with hyperuricemia due to high UA levels and deposition in the joints, renal tissue and soft tissues can lead to systemic vascular changes and increased cardio-vascular risk as a consequence of IL1 β (and subsequent NKFkb and leukocyte activation) and IL18 pathway initiation as a result of NRLP3 activation. Probably via this very mechanism, the prolonged activation of the intrarenal inflammasome due to the deposition of uric acid and/or calcium oxalate [32]. It has been speculated that in patients with acute and chronic nephropathies the liberation of alarm-signals (stress-signals, danger-signals), such as ROS, extracellular ATP, UA, nucleic acids and matrix components, from the parenchymal structures can trigger NLRP3 activation with subsequent liberation of IL1β and IL18, further amplification of the inflammatory signal, engaging macrtophages/monocytes, neutrophils, fibroblasts and dendritic cells and development of local and systemic vascular and fibrotic complications due to uncontrolled synthesis and release of cytokines and other pro-inflammatory signals [32]. These speculations require further verification and give suggestions for future research work aimed at finding novel treatment modalities and agent directed against inflammatory dysregulation.

The role of hyperuricemia in the development of renal and systemic and metabolic complications is summarized in Figure 3 [4, 8, 24, 25, 31, 32].

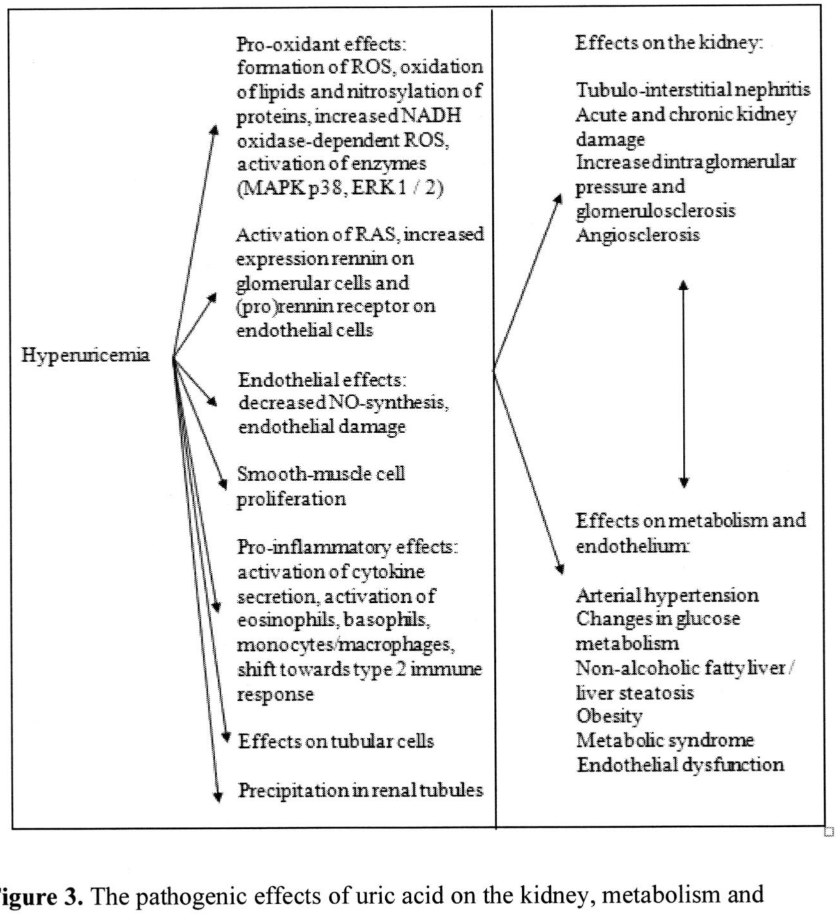

Figure 3. The pathogenic effects of uric acid on the kidney, metabolism and endothelium [4, 8, 24, 25, 31, 32].

Possible Interventions

Several strategies have been proposed for the treatment of hyperuricemia both as a cause and as a consequence of renal diseases, including inhibition of UA synthesis (xantine oxidase inhibitors], uricosuric medications, treatment of the underlying diseases and risk factors, and nephroprotective strategies.

Inhibition of Uric Acid Synthesis

Several agents blocking uric acid synthesis have been introduced in the routine clinical practice, including allopurinol, febuxostat and topiroxostat [33]. Their action is aimed in decreasing UA production at the background of proper hygienic and dietary regimen – optimal fluid intake, decreasing the intake of UA-generating foods (meat, alcohol, fructose-rich food). Urine alkalization leads to increase in UA solubility and dissolves uric acid stone along with increasing the excretion of UA. Xantine oxidase inhibitors should not be combined with azathioprine because of the risk of cytopenia/agranulocytosis, and allopurinol should not be given with mercaptopurine, mycophenolatmofetil, cyclosporin, aluminum hydroxide, theophylline or Warfarin [34].

Uricosuric Medications

Uricosuric medications inhibit the reabsorption of UA via several transporting systems, including URAT1 (SLC22A12) and GLUT9 (SLC2A9). These medications include URAT1 blockers probenecid, benzbromarone, lesinurad and verinurad, URAT2 and OAT4 blocker arhalofenate (it also modulates PPAR-gamma pathway and leads to decrease in the liberation of IL1ß, stimulated by MSU crystals [33]. Uricosuric medications are not indicated in the presence of renal stones and in patients with CKD. Several other types of medications also decrease uric acid have UA-lowering effect, including pegloticase - recombinant, pegylated mammalian uricase that has been demonstrated to lower significantly serum urate, have beneficial effect on tophi size and improve the course of gout arthritis, reduce blood pressure without effect on renal function [33]. Pegloticase could be immunogenic and should not be administered in individuals with glucose-6-phosphate dehydrogenase because of the risk of hemolytic crisis.

Other Agents

Many medications have uricosuric properties, losartan (angiotensin II receptor blocker) and fenofibrate (antihypirlipidemic drug, the last 2 probably binding URAT1) that have not been designed for and are not indicated for the treatment of high UA levels have uricosuric effect [34]. Many plant extracts act on different steps of UA synthesis, excretion and action and have xantine oxidase inhibiting, uricosuric and anti-inflammatory effects (inhibition of tumor necrosis factor alpha (TNFa) and IL1b expression and pathway activation) leading to improvement in UA levels and gout symptoms and evolution [35].

A promising new class of medications that decreases UA levels but is aimed at treatment of diabetes, CKD and heart failure are sodium-glucose co-transporter 2 (SGLT2) inhibitors. These medications, including dapagliflozine [36], empagliflozine [37] and canagliflozin [38], inhibit the re-uptake of sodium and glucose via cotransporter in the proximal tubule and increase urinary excretion of uric acid (probably via inhibition of GLUT9) [39] and possibly inhibit xantine oxidase via reduction of reactive oxygen species, thus decreasing serum UA levels [36, 37, 38]. This class of medications has significant cardio-renal and metabolic benefits: they ameliorate glucose homeostasis, decrease intraglomerular pressure and have nephroprotective effect beyond glycemic control, and decreased sodium and water retention. Moreover, SGLT2 inhibitors have additional anti-inflammatory effect via inhibition of IL1β and reduce oxidative stress due to activation of SIRT1 signaling pathway, which additionally decreases xanthine oxidase activity [37].

Vitamin C (ascorbic acid) has uricosuric effects, mediated by inhibition of URAT1 transporter in the proximal tubule [33]. In vitro, salicyclic acid and its salts and indomethacin also inhibit the UA uptake by URAT1 [33, 39]. In low doses, salicylates inhibit UA renal tubular secretion, and in higher doses they inhibit both secretion and reabsorption. Therefore, in high doses, interference with reabsorption predominatesand the net effect is uricosuric, but high doses of salicylic acid pose the patient at risk for gastrointestinal bleeding.

Treatment of Comorbidities and Control of Risk Factors

As mentioned above, hyperuricemia is frequently associated with the metabolic syndrome and its components (visceral obesity, type 2 diabetes, arterial hypertension, dyslipidemia) and represents a risk factor for vascular complications and progression of CKD. Therefore, in patients with hyperuricemia and/or CKD all comorbidities should be treated adequately, along with control of the major risk factors for progression of CKD and for increased general and cardio-vascular morbidity and mortality, including:

- treatment of the components of the metabolic syndrome,
- treatment and prophylaxis of hyrercoagulation (if present),
- treatment of renal anemia and renal bone disease,
- treatment of the underlying kidney disease (glomerulonephritis, tubulointerstitial nephritis, etc.),
- timely and adequate treatment of intercurrent infections (urinary tract and other),
- minimization of the use of nephrotoxic substances, including non-steroid anti-inflammatory drugs (NSAIDs) and X-ray contrast media,
- adequate hydration of the patient and optimization of diuretic use.

In conclusion, hyperuricemia is a well-known risk factor for the development of acute and chronic renal diseases and for the progression of chronic kidney disease. A bidirectional relationship exists between hyperuricemia and renal diseases, as both hyperuricemia can harm the kidney, and renal diseases can lead to an increase in uric acid levels. The systemic and renal effects of hyperuricemia are mediated by a wide range of hemodynamic, oxidative stress and immune cascades, and the role of the immune response in the progression and perpetuation of both vascular and kidney complications is not completely understood. It has been speculated that in patients with acute and chronic nephropathies due to UA and with cardio-metabolic conditions, the liberation of danger-signals, such as ROS, extracellular ATP, UA, nucleic acids and matrix components, from the parenchymal structures can trigger NLRP3 activation with subsequent liberation of IL1β and IL18, further amplification of the inflammatory signal, engaging macrtophages/monocytes, neutrophils, fibroblasts and dendritic cells and development of local and systemic vascular and fibrotic complications due to uncontrolled synthesis and release of cytokines and other pro-inflammatory signals. These speculations require further verification and give suggestions for future research work aimed at finding novel treatment modalities and agent directed against inflammatory dysregulation, vascular and nephroprotection in hyperuricemia and kidney diseases.

References

[1] Manish K C, Leslie S W. *Uric Acid Nephrolithiasis*. [Updated 2023 May 30]. In: StatPearls [Internet]. Treasure Island (FL): StatPearls Publishing; 2023 Jan-. Available from: https://www.ncbi.nlm.nih.gov/books/NBK560726/Manish KC; Stephen W. Leslie.

[2] Russo E, Leoncini G, Esposito P, Garibotto G, Pontremoli R, Viazzi F. Fructose and Uric Acid: Major Mediators of Cardiovascular Disease Risk Starting at Pediatric Age. *Int. J. Mol. Sci.* 2020 Jun 24;21(12):4479. doi: 10.3390/ijms21124479.

[3] Ahmad M I, Masood S, Furlanetto D M and Nicolaou S (2021) Urate Crystals; Beyond Joints. *Front. Med.* 8:649505. doi: 10.3389/fmed.2021.649505.

[4] Gancheva, R., Kundurdjiev, A., Ivanova, M. Todor Kundurzhiev, Zlatimir Kolarov. Evaluation of cardiovascular risk in stages of gout by a complex multimodal ultrasonography. *Rheumatol. Int.* 37, 121–130 (2017). https://doi.org/10.1007/s00296-016-3556-6.

[5] Wiederkehr M R, Moe O W. Uric Acid Nephrolithiasis: A Systemic Metabolic Disorder. *Clin. Rev. Bone Miner. Metab.* 2011 Dec;9(3-4):207-217. doi: 10.1007/s12018-011-9106-6.

[6] El Ridi R, Tallima H. Physiological functions and pathogenic potential of uric acid: A review. *J. Adv. Res.* 2017 Sep;8(5):487-493. doi: 10.1016/j.jare.2017.03.003. Epub 2017 Mar 14.

[7] Bobulescu I A, Moe O W. Renal transport of uric acid: evolving concepts and uncertainties. *Adv. Chronic Kidney Dis.* 2012 Nov;19(6):358-71. doi: 10.1053/j.ackd.2012.07.009.

[8] Mei Y, Dong B, Geng Z, Xu L. Excess Uric Acid Induces Gouty Nephropathy Through Crystal Formation: A Review of Recent Insights. *Front. Endocrinol.* (Lausanne). 2022 Jul 14;13:911968. doi: 10.3389/fendo.2022.911968.

[9] Sugihara S., Hisatome I., Kuwabara M., Niwa K., Maharani N., Kato M. Depletion of uric acid due to SLC22A12 (URAT1) loss-of-function mutation causes endothelial dysfunction in hypouricemia. *Circ. J.* 2015;79(5):1125–1132.

[10] Iso T., Kurabayashi M. Extremely low levels of serum uric acid are associated with endothelial dysfunction in humans. *Circ. J.* 2015;79(5):978–980.

[11] Bainbridge S A, Roberts J M. Uric acid as a pathogenic factor in preeclampsia. *Placenta.* 2008 Mar;29 Suppl. A(Suppl A):S67-72. doi: 10.1016/j.placenta.2007.11.001. Epub 2008 Feb 21.

[12] Nery R. A., Kahlow B. S., Skare T. L., Tabushi F.I., do Amaral e Castro A. Uric acid and tissue repair. *Arq. Bras. Cir. Dig.* 2015;28(4):290–292].

[13] Kool M., Soullié T., van Nimwegen M., Willart M. A., Muskens F., Jung S. Alum adjuvant boosts adaptive immunity by inducing uric acid and activating inflammatory dendritic cells. *J. Exp. Med.* 2008;205(4):869–882.

[14] Kool M., Willart M.A., van Nimwegen M., Bergen I., Pouliot P., Virchow J.C. An unexpected role for uric acid as an inducer of T helper 2 cell immunity to inhaled antigens and inflammatory mediator of allergic asthma. *Immunity.* 2011;34(4):527–540.

[15] Hara K., Iijima K., Elias M. K., Seno S., Tojima I., Kobayashi T. Airway uric acid is a sensor of inhaled protease allergens and initiates type 2 immune responses in respiratory mucosa. *J. Immunol.* 2014;192(9):4032–4042.

[16] Gold M. J., Hiebert P. R., Park H. Y., Stefanowicz D., Le A., Starkey M. R. Mucosal production of uric acid by airway epithelial cells contributes to particulate matter-induced allergic sensitization. *Mucosal. Immunol.* 2016;9(3):809–820.

[17] Amaral K. B., Silva T. P., Malta K. K., Carmo L. A. S., Dias F. F., Almeida M. R. Natural *Schistosoma mansoni* infection in the wild reservoir *Nectomys squamipes* leads to excessive lipid droplet accumulation in hepatocytes in the absence of liver functional impairment. *Plos One.* 2016;11(11):e0166979.

[18] Tallima H, Dvořák J, Kareem S, Abou El Dahab M, Abdel Aziz N, Dalton JP, El Ridi R. Protective immune responses against Schistosoma mansoni infection by immunization with functionally active gut-derived cysteine peptidases alone and in combination with glyceraldehyde 3-phosphate dehydrogenase. *PLoS Negl. Trop. Dis.* 2017 Mar 27;11(3):e0005443. doi: 10.1371/journal.pntd.0005443.

[19] Rentzos M., Nikolaou C., Anagnostouli M., Rombos A., Tsakanikas K., Economou M. Serum uric acid and multiple sclerosis. *Clin. Neurol. Neurosurg.* 2006; 108(6):527–531.

[20] Wang L., Hu W., Wang J., Qian W., Xiao H. Low serum uric acid levels in patients with multiple sclerosis and neuromyelitis optica: an updated meta-analysis. *Mult. Scler. Relat. Disord.* 2016;9:17–22.

[21] Alvarez-Lario B., Macarrón-Vicente J. Is there anything good in uric acid? *QJM.* 2011;104(12):1015–1024.

[22] Fang P., Li X., Luo J. J., Wang H., Yang X. F. A double-edged sword: uric acid and neurological disorders. *Brain Disord. Ther.* 2013;2(2):109.

[23] Hernández Petzsche M R. 2021. *The Pathogenesis of Chronic Uric Acid Crystal Nephropathy. PhD diss.* Ludwig-Maximilians-Universität München.

[24] Johnson R J, Nakagawa T, Jalal D, Sánchez-Lozada L G, Kang DH, Ritz E. Uric acid and chronic kidney disease: which is chasing which? *Nephrol. Dial. Transplant.* 2013 Sep;28(9):2221-8. doi: 10.1093/ndt/gft029. Epub 2013 Mar 29.

[25] Mihai S, Codrici E, Popescu I D, Enciu A M, Albulescu L, Necula L G, Cristina Mambet, Gabriela Anton, Cristiana Tanase. Inflammation-Related Mechanisms in Chronic Kidney Disease Prediction, Progression, and Outcome. *J. Immunol. Res.* (2018) 2018:2180373. doi: 10.1155/ 2018/2180373.

[26] Fan, S., Zhang, P., Wang, A. Y. Wang X, Wang L, Li G, Hong. Hyperuricemia and its related histopathological features on renal biopsy. *BMC Nephrol.* 20, 95 (2019). https:// doi.org/10.1186/s12882-019-1275-4.

[27] Mahadita G W, Suwitra K. The Role of Hyperuricemia in the Pathogenesis and Progressivity of Chronic Kidney Disease. *Open Access Maced. J. Med. Sci.* [Internet]. 2021 Oct. 14 [cited 2023 Jun. 10];9(F):428-35. Available from: https://oamjms.eu/ index.php/mjms/article/view/7100.

[28] Choi W J, Hong Y A, Min J W, Koh E S, Kim H D, Ban T H, Kim Y S, Kim Y K, Shin S J, Kim S Y, Kim Y O, Yang C W, Chang Y K. The Serum Uric Acid Level Is Related to the More Severe Renal Histopathology of Female IgA Nephropathy Patients. *J. Clin. Med.* 2021 Apr 27;10(9):1885. doi: 10.3390/jcm10091885.

[29] Singh J A, Cleveland J D. Gout is associated with a higher risk of chronic renal disease in older adults: a retrospective cohort study of U.S. Medicare population. *BMC Nephrol.* 2019 Mar 15;20(1):93. doi: 10.1186/s12882-019-1274-5.

[30] Fang, B., Yu, Y., Dong, X. Lin Qi, Yan Wang, Fang Dai, Lan Wei, Yajie Kang. The relationship between serum uric acid levels and glomerular ischemic lesions in patients with Immunoglobin A nephropathy-a analytical cross-sectional study. *BMC Nephrol.* 23, 255 (2022). https://doi.org/ 10.1186/s12882-022-02880-x.

[31] Finn, W. F. (2016). Kidney Disease and Gout: The Role of the Innate Immune System. *The Open Urology & Nephrology Journal, 9*, 12-21.

[32] Goldberg A, Garcia-Arroyo F, Sasai F, Rodriguez-Iturbe B, Sanchez-Lozada LG, Lanaspa MA, Johnson RJ. Mini Review: Reappraisal of Uric Acid in Chronic Kidney Disease. *Am. J. Nephrol.* 2021;52(10-11):837-844. doi: 10.1159/ 000519491. Epub 2021 Oct 21.

[33] Cicero A F G, Fogacci F, Kuwabara M, Borghi C. Therapeutic Strategies for the Treatment of Chronic Hyperuricemia: An Evidence-Based Update. *Medicina.* 2021; 57(1):58. https://doi.org/10.3390/medicina57010058

[34] Jordan A, Gresser U. Side Effects and Interactions of the Xanthine Oxidase Inhibitor Febuxostat. *Pharmaceuticals (Basel).* 2018 May 25;11(2):51. doi: 10.3390/ ph11020051.

[35] Ling X, Bochu W. A review of phytotherapy of gout: perspective of new pharmacological treatments. *Pharmazie.* 2014 Apr;69(4):243-56.

[36] McDowell K, Welsh P, Docherty K F, Morrow D A, Jhund P S, de Boer R A, O'Meara E, Inzucchi SE, Køber L, Kosiborod MN, Martinez F A, Ponikowski P, Hammarstedt A, Langkilde A M, Sjöstrand M, Lindholm D, Solomon SD, Sattar N, Sabatine MS, McMurray JJV. Dapagliflozin reduces uric acid concentration, an independent predictor of adverse outcomes in DAPA-HF. *Eur. J. Heart Fail.* 2022 Jun;24(6):1066-1076. doi: 10.1002/ejhf.2433.

[37] Ferreira J P, Inzucchi S E, Mattheus M, Meinicke T, Steubl D, Wanner C, Zinman B. Empagliflozin and uric acid metabolism in diabetes: A post hoc analysis of the EMPA-REG OUTCOME trial. *Diabetes Obes. Metab.* 2022 Jan;24(1):135-141. doi: 10.1111/dom.14559. Epub 2021 Oct 4.

[38] Davies M J, Trujillo A, Vijapurkar U, Damaraju CV, Meininger G. Effect of canagliflozin on serum uric acid in patients with type 2 diabetes mellitus. *Diabetes Obes. Metab.* 2015 Apr;17(4):426-9. doi: 10.1111/dom.12439. Epub 2015 Feb 15.

[39] Chino Y, Samukawa Y, Sakai S, Nakai Y, Yamaguchi J, Nakanishi T, Tamai I. SGLT2 inhibitor lowers serum uric acid through alteration of uric acid transport

activity in renal tubule by increased glycosuria. *Biopharm. Drug Dispos.* 2014 Oct;35(7):391-404. doi: 10.1002/bdd.1909. Epub 2014 Aug 6.

Biographical Sketch

Name: ***Milena Krasimirova Nikolova***

Affiliation: University Hospital St. Ivan Rilski, Sofia, Bulgaria, EU
Education: Medical University-Sofia
Business Address: University Hospital St. Ivan Rilski, Clinic of Nephrology, 15 Iv. Evst Geshov blvd, 1612, Sofia, Bulgaria, EU

Research and Professional Experience

More than 20 years of experience in the field of Internal Medicine and Nephrology

Professional Appointments

Assistant and Chief Assistant Professor, Associate Professor at the Medical Univeristy – Sofia, Bulgaria

Publications from the Last 3 Years

1) Baleva M, Lesichkova S, Gesheva N, Mihailova S, Gerova V, Vladimirov B, Penchev P, Nikolova-Vlahova M, Naumova E. Common variable immune deficiency, central diabetes insipidus, and anemia. *Cent. Eur. J. Immunol.* 2020;45(3):351-354. doi: 10.5114/ ceji.2020.101267. Epub 2020 Nov 1. IF 2.085.
2) Nikolova-Vlahova M K, Kamburova M, Hristova J, Vasileiou D, Bogov B, Krastev R, Hadjiev E, Tsvetkova G, Vasileva C, Houbanov N. Biclonal myeloma presenting with renal failure. *Centr. Eur. J. Immunol.* 2020;45(1):122-124. IF 2.085.
3) Genov, D., Kundurdgiev, A., Ivanova, I., Nikolova, M., Pencheva, V., Hristova, M., Koleva, N., Kostadinova, A. and Vutova, Ts.. "Role of Serum Uromodulin in the Early Diagnosis of Chronic Kidney Disease" *Acta Medica Bulgarica,* vol.48, no.1, 2021, pp.13-16. https://doi.org/10.2478/amb-2021-0002.

4) Nikolova, M., Angelova, I., Kotseva, V., Kostadinova, A., Genov, D., Vutova, C., Koleva, N., Todorov, J., Chupetlovska, K., Penkov, M., Ananiev, J., Milenova, V. and Kundurdzhiev, A.. "Acute Kidney Injury and Acute Renal Failure in Coronaviral Infection" *Acta Medica Bulgarica*, vol.49, no.3, 2022, pp.38-42. https://doi.org/ 10.2478/amb-2022-0028.
5) Nikolova, M., Kotseva, V., Monov, D., Genov, D., Voikova, P., Ananiev, J., Tanova, R., Kundurdjiev, A., Gancheva, R. and Vlahov, Y. (2022) Rhabdomyolysis after the Intake of Illicit Drugs as a Cause of Acute Renal Failure. *Open Journal of Nephrology*, **12**, 482-488. doi: 10.4236/ojneph.2022.124047.
6) Mihaylova A, Lesichkova S, Baleva M, Nikolova-Vlahova M, Kundurzhiev T, Kolevski A, Naumova E. Durability of humoral and cell-mediated immune response after SARS-CoV-2 mRNA vaccine administration. *J. Med. Virol.* 2023 Jan;95(1):e28360. doi: 10.1002/jmv.28360.

Chapter 5

Surgical Treatment of Uric Acid Stones

Kaloyan M. Davidoff[1]
Milena K. Nikolova[2,*]
and Yordan D. Vlahov[3]

[1]Clinic of Urology, Sofiamed University Hospital, Faculty of Medicine, Sofia University St. Kliment Ohridski, Sofia, Bulgaria
[2]Clinic of Nephrology, University Hospital St. Ivan Rilski, Medical University-Sofia, Bulgaria
[3]Clinic of Endocrinology and Metabolic Diseases, Sofiamed University Hospital, Faculty of Medicine, Sofia University St. Kliment Ohridski, Sofia, Bulgaria

Abstract

Uric acid stones are common in patients with metabolic syndrome and it components, such as obesity, arterial hypertension and diabetes. This type of renal stones is becoming more common in the industrial world. Advanced age, certain climate characteristics, male sex and decreased urine volume with more acidic urinary pH are risk factors for their formation. In the majority of cases, uric acid stones can be dissolved by changing the urinary pH and the patient's hygienic and dietary regimen, lifestyle and accompanying medical treatment. Nevertheless, in approximately one third of the patients with uric acid stones conservative treatment fails and surgical interventions are indicated.

The development of urinary tract obstruction with superimposed infection of the kidney and/or forniceal rupture represents a medical emergency and requires urgent desobstruction. Urinary tract

* Corresponding Author: Dr. Milena Nikolova, MD, PhD, MBA, Assoc. Prof. Clinic of Nephrology, University Hospital St. Ivan Rilski Medical University-Sofia, Bulgaria, EU; e-mail: milena_i_dani@abv.bg.

In: Hyperuricemia
Editor: Warren Y. Salinas
ISBN: 979-8-89113-239-9

desobstruction may be achieved with endoscopic placement of double J ureteric stent or percutaneous nephrostomy. The authors discuss the main surgical techniques for the treatment of uric acid stones, including extracorporeal shock wave lithotripsy, ureteroscopic laser fragmentation and percutaneous nephrolithotomy, and the strategies for emergency desobstruction of the urinary tract.

Keywords: uric acid stones, urinary tract obstruction, forniceal rupture, surgical management

Introduction

Uric acid (UA) is the final metabolite of purines in humans as a product of xantine oxidase pathway. It originates from three main processes: degradation of cellular nucleic acids (from cell turnover), liver synthesis, and the intake of food rich in purines and/or fructose (the latter is metabolized to UA) [1,2]. Purines are metabolized to xantine which is further converted to uric acid via the xantine oxidase pathway. UA is excreted by the kidneys (in 60-70%) and by the intestines (in 30-40%) with subsequent intraintestinal metabolism by the gut microbiota. Renal excretion encompasses four major processes: glomerular filtration, tubular reabsorption, tubular secretion and postsecretory reabsorption. UA is water soluble, but it can crystallize in the form of monosodium urate (MSU) in the tissues and in the urinary tract under certain conditions when the solubility threshold is exceeded (oversaturation) and/or precipitating factors are present [3]. The risk of crystallization increases in dehydration, acidosis, decreased blood flow/stasis, hypothermia and local tissue damage. MSU crystals can deposit in joints, soft tissues (tophi), and kidneys, (Figure 1). MSU can crystallize in the form of urinary tract stones with subsequent sedimentation and crystallization of calcium oxalate, and in the tubular and interstitial spaces and induce local inflammatory reaction, leading to the development of granuloma-like tissue reaction and secondary nephrocalcinosis and perpetuation of low-grade inflammation that further increases both tissue damage and cardiovascular risk [3, 4, 5].

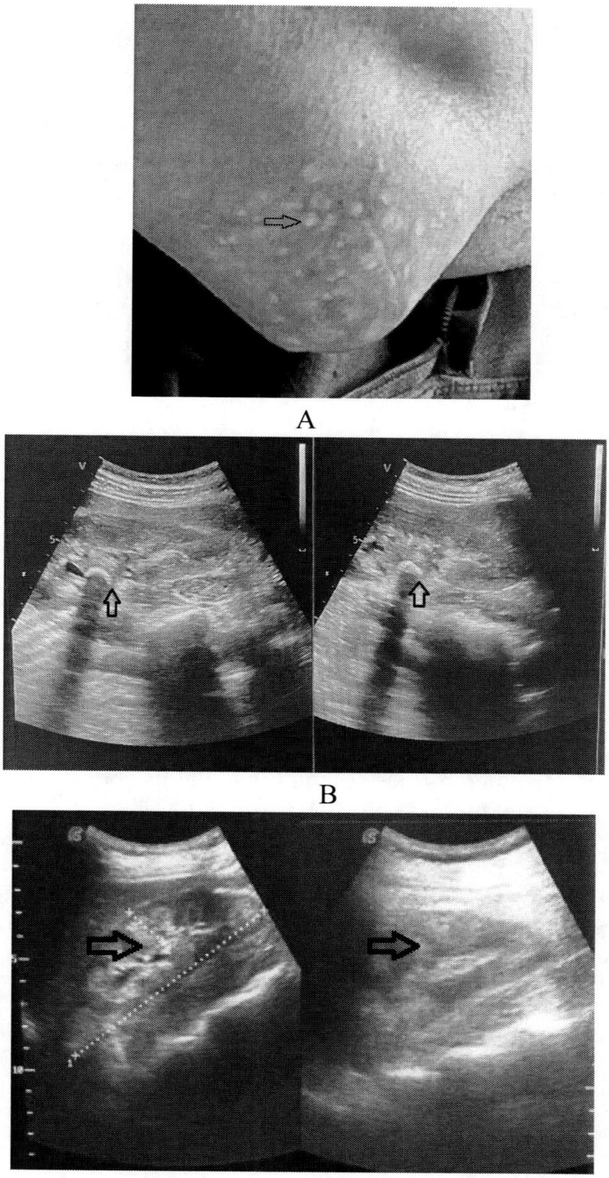

Figure 1. Deposition of UA in the soft tissues in the form of tophi on the elbow (arrow) (A), in the pyelocaliceal system in the form of stones (arrows) (B) and nephrocalcinosis secondary to renal parenchymal damage in UA-associated tubulointerstitial nephritis (arrows) (C).

Uric acid stones are particularly common in humans, affecting in 2-10% of the population, more frequently developing in men, in certain ethnic groups, and in areas with hot/tropical climate [1]. UA was first described approximately 250 years ago as the main component of bladder stones by C. Scheele, a Swedish pharmacist [5]. These stones account for up to 40% of urinary calculi in humans and develop more frequently in men, probably because of the protective role of estrogens and the less alcohol consumption in women. UA levels are increased in the majority of patients with metabolic syndrome and uric acid lithiasis is particularly common in this population [6].

Classification and Etiology

According to the underlying cause or condition, UA stones can be classified as:

- Congenital: inborn metabolic defects (enzyme defects of purine synthesis, changes in urine stabilizer levels, tubulopathies with decreased urinary pH levels, familial hyperuricosuria, i.e., mutations in URAT1 transporter, Wilson's disease and inborn/hereditary hemolytic anemias and other diseases with high cell turn-over).
- Idiopathic – associated with metabolic disorders, including hyperuricemia, metabolic syndrome and its components and changes in urine alkalization.
- Acquired: in patients with increased UA production or decreased urinary excretion or urinary pH: in relation to gout, chronic diarrhea, decreased urinary stabilizers, overproduction in increased cell degradation (psoriasis, cancer, chemotherapy, etc.), high food UA and/or fructose intake, intake of substances that block UA renal reabsorption (uricosuric agents).

Pathophysiology

Uric acid can crystallize along the urinary tract in cases of oversaturation of the urine (hyperuricosuria, usually when more than 800 mg/day are excreted in the absence of aciduria and hyperuricemia), decrease in urinary pH (high meat intake, inborn or acquired tubular defects with aciduria, urinary tract infections with acidic urine), low fluid intake/hypovolemia with decreased dieresis of highly concentrated/saturated urine, in the presence of nuclei of crystallization (for instance, mucus or leukocyte/bacterial aggregates in urinary tract infections), and in decreased urinary levels of urine stabilizers and crystallization inhibitors (citrate, glycosaminoglycans, etc.) [1, 6, 7]. UA can also serve as nidus for crystallization for calcium oxalate or destabilize the urine and cause precipitation of calcium oxalate, thus forming stones of mixed type [1].

Clinical Manifestations

UA stones can remain silent or manifest with renal colic. The colic is usually caused by migration of the stone from the renal calyces or pelvis down the ureters to the urinary bladder and through the urethra. The migration of stones can cause severe pain, vegetative symptoms (changes in pulse rate, blood pressure, vomiting, nausea) and/or obstruction of the urinary tract with the development of infection with pyonephrosis or forniceal rupture.

Pyonephrosis develops in the presence of complete block of urinary flow through the affected ureter and development of bacterial infection inside the obstructed renal pelvis. The clinical picture is dramatic, with high fever and severe pain in the affected flank area, intoxication and sepsis. The diagnosis is based on imaging studies. Pyonephrosis requires urgent desobstruction.

Forniceal rupture (FR) is a rupture of the pyelo-calyceal system developing in cases of increased intracavitary pressure due to obstruction. It usually develops in protracted renal colics, especially in small stones that block the ureteric flow, or in malignant obstruction due to pressure from outside the ureter or in ureteric cancer. FR can lead to leakage of urine around the kidney or in the retroperitoneal space with the formation of urinoma and/or inflammatory complications, such as paranephral abscessus, phlegmona of the retroperitoneal space and/or urosepsis. The diagnosis is based on the results of imaging studies (abdominal echography and contrast-enhanced computed tomography). Treatment can be conservative (implantation of DJ ureteric stent, extirpation of the stone, antibiotics and spasmo-analgesics) or surgical – correction of the defect and draining of the retroperitoneal fluid collection.

Diagnosis

UA stones are visible on ultrasound examination (Figure 2) but because they lack calcium, they cannot be visualized on plain X-ray or computed tomography (CT) of the abdomen without the use of contrast media. In patients with renal colic hydronephrosis may be visible on both ultrasound (Figure 2) and CT scans. Contrast-enhanced CT is required in all patients with urinary tract abnormalities (ectopic kidneys, congenital or acquired urological abnormalities), renal transplant allograft, complex stone anatomy, neurological disorders and altered body habitus, urinary diversion or prior urological surgeries. All patients should be evaluated for the presence of infection, including complete blood count, erythrocyte sedimentation rate and C-reactive protein, urinalysis and urinary microbiological investigation, and renal function.

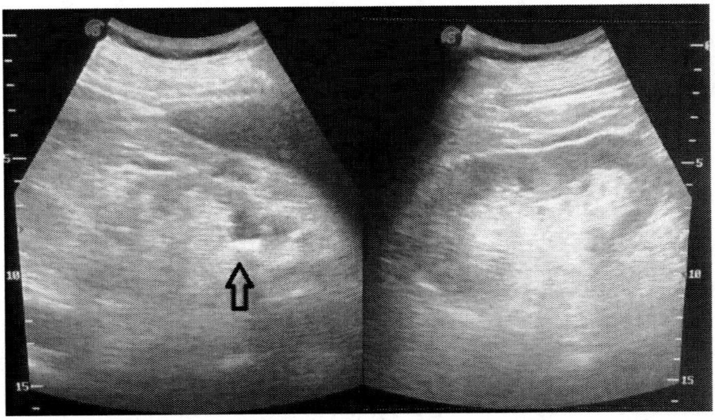

A

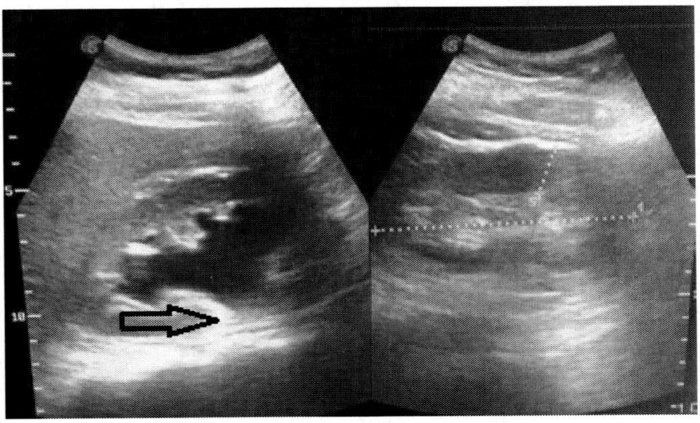

B

Figure 2. Abdominal ultrasound in uric acid stones. A) Renal stone without obstruction of the urinary flow (arrow). B) Right-sided hydronephrosis and hydroureter (arrow) due to urinary tract obstruction in migrating stone.

Differential Diagnosis

Renal stones should be differentiated from renal parenchymal calcifications and other hyperechogenic lesions, such as angiomyolipoma. Renal colic should be differentiated from all acute vascular and inflammatory processes in the abdomen, pelvis and retroperitoneal space, renal papillary necrosis, acute pyelonephritis, subcapsular renal hematoma, retroperitoneal fibroses and other masses in the retroperitoneal space, renal cancer, ovarian cyst, endometriosis, pleuritis, myocardial infarction, neuromuscular diseases, neurological conditions, spine pathology.

Therapeutic Approach

The therapeutic approach in UA stones depends on the presence of acute complications (renal colic, infection, forniceal rupture), the size of the calculus and the presence of comorbidities.

Treatment of Hyperuricemia and Strategies to Dissolve UA Stones

The dietary interventions aimed at decreasing the formation of UA stones and dissolving the existent stones include optimal fluid intake, decrease purine-rich and fructose-rich foods, urine alkalization – intake of lemon juice or alkalizing substances.

The medical management of hyperuricemia, hyperiuricosuria and UA stones consists in:

- Decrease of UA synthesis – xantine oxidase inhibitors - allopurinol, febuxostat and topiroxostat. It is important to note that uricosuric medications should not be administered in patients with nephrolithiasis because they can stimulate the formation of stones via increase in UA crystallization.
- Urine alkalization – sodium and potassium citrate, sodium bicarbonate, acetazolamide

Conservative Treatment of Renal Colic

The degree of hydronephrosis and the severity of clinical symptoms (pain, vomiting, vegetative symptoms) do not predict the likelihood of spontaneous passage of the stone. Overall, if hydronephrosis is mild to moderate and in the absence of intense pain, in small stones (< 8-9 mm) with low volume, and absence of significant thickening of the ureteral wall, signs of pyonephrosis or forniceal rupture, the stone is most probably passable. In these cases, conservative approach is indicated, including spasmo-analgesics, anti-inflammatory agents (both non-steroid anti-inflammatory drugs (NSAIDs) and low-dose corticosteroids), alpha-blockers (tamsulosin), optimization of fluid intake, symptomatic treatment, and antibacterial agents, if indicated.

In general, calculus size, location, and patient's symptoms could predict the likelihood of spontaneous stone passage of a renal stone [1, 7]. Approximately 90% of stones less than 5 mm eventually pass within four weeks, and in the majority of cases the stones larger than 8 mm require intervention to pass [7].

Surgical Treatment of Renal Colic and UA Stones

The indications for surgical treatment are:

- failure of conservative treatment,
- presence of severe hydronephrosis and complete obstruction of the affected ureter and kidney with severe pain and/or,
- presence of complications: pyonephrosis, forniceal rupture,
- infected stones.

There are no specific indications for surgical treatment of stones below 5 mm in size that do not cause obstruction or lead to forniceal rupture, but elective surgery should be undertaken in certain circumstances, such as frequent travelling (including pilots), planning pregnancy, avoiding symptomatic stones that are expected to require surgery.

Indications for emergency surgery: ureteric obstruction with manifested or suspected infection, bilateral obstruction/obstruction of single functioning kidney with acute kidney injury.

Indications for elective surgery (according to the 2016 American Urological Association/Endourological Society guidelines) [8, 9]: ureteral stones >10 mm in size (not expected to pass spontaneously); uncomplicated stones in the distal ureter below 10 mm in size that have not passed spontaneously for 4-5 weeks with or without expulsive therapy; symptomatic kidney stones with pain without other apparent cause; pregnancy, when the watchful waiting/observation has failed; persistent renal obstruction due to stone(s);

When considering elective surgery, it is worth mentioning the predictors for poor chance of spontaneous elimination of a kidney [1, 7]: ureteral stone length of 9 mm or more, stone volume > 0.2 cc, higher stone density (> 700 Hounsfield units – in calcium and magnesium-containing stones), ureteral wall thickness > 2 mm, extrarenal pelvis and/or stenosis of the pyelo-ureteral junction or other anatomical abnormalities of the urinary tract, anterior-posterior diameter of the renal pelvis > 18 mm.

The main modalities of surgical treatment of UA stones are [1, 8, 9]:

- Extracorporeal shock wave lithotripsy (ESWL): X-ray positive stones – calcium containing radio-opaque kidney stones less than 20 mm in size. As UA stones are radiolucent, for the ESWL they will need X-ray contrast – either intravenous, or retrograde urography to make them clearly visible.
- Ureteroscopic (URS) stone laser fragmentation and subsequent retrieval: for kidney and ureteral stones less than 20 m in size.
- Percutaneous nephrolithotomy (PNL): for larger kidney stones (greater than 20-25 mm in size).
- Laparoscopic and robot-assisted surgical techniques.
- Open surgery.
- Sometimes ureteric desobstruction with JJ (or double J, DJ) ureteral stents is needed.

The main goals of surgical treatment are [1, 8, 9]: relief of patient's symptoms, treatment of infection and restoration of renal function developing or worsening due to obstruction/infection. Following terms should be clarifies:

1) Treatment success – the patient becoming stone-free with stone removal and absence of residual fragments below 4 mm in size,
2) Complications pre-, intra- and postoperative.
3) Improvement of patient's quality of life.

There are no specific contraindications for surgical desobstruction caused by kidney stones and the general surgical guidelines apply. Obese patients, pregnancy and uncontrolled hemorrhagic diathesis are contraindications for shock wave lithotripsy [8, 9].

Beside the clinical-laboratory, imaging and microbiological investigations, following perioperative considerations should be made when undertaking surgical treatment of renal stones [8, 9]:

- Evaluation of the indications for interventional approach against watchful waiting and conservative treatment,
- Antibiotic prophylaxis: indicated in patients with suspected or proven urinary tract infection, in elective ureteroscopy (URS) or percutaneous nephrolithotomy (PNL) – as purely prophylactic, not routinely indicated in ESWL.
- Removal of secondary stones (asymptomatic stones, detected on imaging studies – ipsy- or contralateral): there is no consensus on this issue, but the removal of these stones can decrease morbidity and make the patient stone-free. According to G.M. Preminger [8], when removing an obstructing or symptomatic stone by URS or PNL, ipsilateral asymptomatic stones are to be removed during the same procedure, as this does not prolong the duration of the procedure and does not increase significantly the operation time (approximately 30 to 60 minutes) or morbidity attributable to the procedure. However, the author does not recommend routine removal of asymptomatic contralateral stones [8], because in URS this would lead to bilateral placement of JJ catheters and could increase morbidity.

Shock Wave Lithotripsy

SWL is the most commonly used procedure for the treatment of kidney stones worldwide, especially in kidney and proximal ureteral stones. As UA stones are radiolucent, requires additional contrast administration – intravenous or retrograde. SWL approach is associated with delayed fragment elimination and is contraindicated in obese individuals, pregnant and patients with hemorrhagic diathesis [8, 9]. SWL is not indicated if infected calculi are present or suspected. It can be performed as outpatient procedure, requires anesthesia and has low rate of complications – ureteral blockage develops in approximately 5% of the cases, and 2% may develop urinary tract infections, transient hematuria, septic and bleeding complications are rare [8].

Ureteroscopy

URS is a treatment of choice in the middle and distal ureteral stones, especially in terms of severe obstruction and or suspected forniceal rupture. It is also applicable in patients in whom SWL has been unsuccessful. It can be performed in obese individuals, during pregnancy, in patients with hemorrhagic diathesis and in the presence of hard obesity, hard of infected stones [8, 9]. URS can be performed in the outpatient settings, requires anesthesia and allows dilation of stenoses, use of stone baskets or grasping forceps to remove stones, and intracorporeal fragmentation of the stone with holmium and thulium laser [8, 9]. Multiple URS can be performed if needed. Sometimes JJ stents are placed after the procedure to prevent ureteric obstruction from postprocedural edema or passage of a stone fragment. Ureteral discomfort due to the stent (in up to 25% of the cases), infections (5%), ureteral wall injury (5%) and strictures (3%), sepsis or ureteral avulsion (< 1%) have been reported as complications of URS [8].

Percutaneous Nephrolithotomy

PNL is considered to be more effective than SWL or URS for most patients, with a higher rate of complications [8] and is therefore preserved as a method of choice in large (> 20 mm), staghorn or complex stones, or when the other two methods are unsuccessful. It is performed under general anesthesia, can be combined with intracorporeal laser litothripsy and requires a short hospital stay of 1-3 days. Mini- and micro-PNL techniques with smaller incisions and tissue trauma have been developed [8]. Moreover, a patient's position can be changed in order to facilitate stone removal. Nephrostomic tube can be placed to ensure adequate proper drainage of the kidney and access for subsequent PNL aimed at removal of residual stone fragments. If the patients are stone-free after the first PNL and no complications or subsequent PNL are planned, the procedure can be "tubeless" and no JJ stent is required ("stentless"), which further reduces post-PNL morbidity. As it is more invasive, PNL is associated with a higher complication rate than SWR and URS. The major complications of PNL are bleeding (8%), perforation of renal pelvis (3%), and hydrothorax (2%), more common with larger stones [8], infections.

Laparoscopic and Robot-Assisted Surgery

These approaches are much less invasive than open surgical techniques and represent reasonable alternative options in large or complex kidney stones. The post-procedure complications and morbidity are less than in open surgery patients, but mor prevalent than in SWL, URS, and PNL. Thus, laparoscopic and robot-assisted methods are indicated in cases when minimal-invasive techniques have either failed or are not applicable [8]. They are an alternative to ESWL, URS and PNL in large proximal stones.

Open Surgery

This method is indicated in large and/or complex and infected kidney stones that cannot be removed by minimally invasive techniques, or would require a large number of the latter, in patients in whom endoscopic or minimally invasive approaches have failed and/or have severe or complex urinary tract or kidney anomalies, in patients with morbid obesity [8].

Placement of Ureteral Stent (JJ Stent)

Ureteral stents are aimed at preventing ureteric obstruction and pain and ensuring proper urine drainage when passing a stone or stone fragment. Routine placement of stents after uncomplicated URS is not indicated [8, 9]. According to the 2016 American Urological Association guidelines, ureteral stent placement in URS for renal colic can be omitted *in the presence of all of the following criteria* [9]: no suspected ureteric injury during URS, no evidence of ureteral stricture or other anatomical impediments to stone fragment passage, normal contralateral kidney, no renal functional impairment, no secondary URS procedure planned. The routine placement of a ureteral stent before URS (prestententing) is not advisable because of the risk of complications and the discomfort to the patient [9]. Routine ureteral stenting should *not be performed* in patients undergoing SWL, because this approach has not shown to be superior to no placement [8, 9]. Following complications have been described after placement of JJ stent: stent discomfort (ameliorated with alpha-blockers, e.g., tamsulosin, and spasmolytic muscarine agents); ureteral obstruction due to accumulation of stone fragments (treated either by laser fragmentation via URS approach, or in the past – via placement of nephrostomic tube); urinary tract infections (treated with antibiotics); residual stone fragments (require second procedure).

Renal Colic During Pregnancy

Renal colic during pregnancy is a rare medical emergency, but still represents the most common non-obstetric indication for hospitalization in this population [10]. It develops in approximately 1:1500 pregnancies and could turn into a serious challenge for both urologists and gynecologists because of the adverse effects of ionizing radiation and of many medications on the embryo and fetus. Pregnancy is both pro-lithogenic and pro-colic state, because of hormonal changes and smooth muscle relaxation in combination with physiological dilation of ureters due to the increased size of the pregnant uterus. The differential diagnosis between physiological and stone-related hydronephrosis in pregnancy can be made using X-ray methods, but as UA stones are radiolucent, Doppler-ultrasound can aid to the differentiation, because in renal colic renal resistive index (RI) is increased in the obstructed and/or dysfunctional kidney and the DeltaRI shows increase [11].

The most common clinical presentation is flank pain with or without hematuria. Abdominal ultrasound reveals hydronephrosis and hydroureter on the affected side, but, as mentioned above, physiological dilation of renal pelvices and ureters can be seen in normal pregnancy, especially in late term. Therefore, Doppler ultrasound is a method of choice in the differentiation, as in renal obstruct/dysfunction it reveals asymmetrical increase in renal resistive index on the side of the colic. Low-dose X-ray and CT and magnetic resonance imaging are also methods of choice. In general, the initial management, in the absence of complications, must be conservative. The success rate of conservative approach in this population is 70-80% [10]. In the presence of complications of if the stone cannot pass, JJ ureteral stent placement or percutaneous nephrostomic catheter implantation are methods of choice for pelvic and ureteral desobstruction, and the definitive management can be postponed until after birth [10]. In the presence of complications that cannot be managed via these two methods, ureteroscopic approach is indicated, and if this method fails of is not applicable, classical surgical techniques (open surgery) with cautious choice of anesthetic should be undertaken [10]. Shock wave lithotripsy is not routinely used in pregnant women [10].

In conclusion, uric acid stones are a frequent clinical problem, requiring team approach with the joint efforts of urologist, nephrologist/internal medicine specialist, radiologist and sometimes anesthesiologist. If conservative treatment and watchful waiting approaches fail and in the presence of persistent obstruction, severe urinary tract infection, acute kidney injury or surgical complications (pyonephrosis, forniceal rupture, etc.), invasive treatment is indicated. The choice of invasive strategy depends on the size of the stones, the presence of urological anomaly, the presence of complications/pregnancy/obesity and the previous therapeutic approaches used. Surgical treatment frequently requires anesthesia and the more invasive the modality is, the more and the more serious the complications could develop. Still, surgical treatment remains the gold standard if the conservative approach fails, in the presence of complications and in kidney and/or ureteric obstruction during pregnancy.

References

[1] Manish K C, Leslie S W. *Uric Acid Nephrolithiasis.* [Updated 2023 May 30]. In: StatPearls [Internet]. Treasure Island (FL): StatPearls Publishing; 2023 Jan-. Available from: https://www.ncbi.nlm.nih.gov/books/NBK560726/Manish KC; Stephen W. Leslie. Accessed on May 30, 2023.

[2] Russo E, Leoncini G, Esposito P, Garibotto G, Pontremoli R, Viazzi F. Fructose and Uric Acid: Major Mediators of Cardiovascular Disease Risk Starting at Pediatric Age. *Int. J. Mol. Sci.* 2020 Jun 24;21(12):4479. doi: 10.3390/ijms21124479.

[3] Ahmad MI, Masood S, Furlanetto DM and Nicolaou S (2021) Urate Crystals; Beyond Joints. *Front. Med.* 8:649505. doi: 10.3389/fmed.2021.649505.

[4] Gancheva, R., Kundurdjiev, A., Ivanova, M. Todor Kundurzhiev, Zlatimir Kolarov. Evaluation of cardiovascular risk in stages of gout by a complex multimodal ultrasonography. *Rheumatol. Int.* 37, 121–130 (2017). https://doi.org/10.1007/s00296-016-3556-6.

[5] Wiederkehr M R, Moe O W. Uric Acid Nephrolithiasis: A Systemic Metabolic Disorder. *Clin. Rev. Bone Miner. Metab*. 2011 Dec;9(3-4):207-217.

[6] Scales C D, Smith A C, Hanley J M, Saigal C S., Urologic Diseases in America Project. Prevalence of kidney stones in the United States. *Eur. Urol.* 2012 Jul;62(1):160-5.

[7] Patti L, Leslie S W. Acute Renal Colic. [Updated 2023 May 30]. In: *StatPearls* [Internet]. Treasure Island (FL): StatPearls Publishing; 2023 Jan-. Available from: https://www.ncbi.nlm.nih.gov/books/NBK431091/. Accessed on May 30, 2023.

[8] Preminger G M. *Kidney stones in adults: Surgical management of kidney and ureteral stones.* Uptodate. https://www.uptodate.com/contents/kidney-stones-in-adults-surgical-management-of-kidney-and-ureteral-stones. Accessed on May 30, 2023.

[9] Assimos D, Krambeck A, Miller N L, Manoj Monga, M Hassan Murad, Caleb P Nelson, Kenneth T Pace, Vernon M Pais Jr, Margaret S Pearle, Glenn M Preminger, Hassan Razvi, Ojas Shah, Brian R Matlaga. Surgical Management of Stones: American Urological Association/Endourological Society Guideline, PART II. *J. Urol.* 2016; 196:1161.

[10] Blanco L T, Socarras M R, Montero R F, Diez E L, Calvo A O, Gregorio S A Y, Cansino J R, Galan J A, Rivas J G. Renal colic during pregnancy: Diagnostic and therapeutic aspects. Literature review. Cent European *J. Urol.* 2017;70(1):93-100. doi: 10.5173/ceju.2017.754. Epub 2016 Oct 28.

[11] Shokeir A A, Mahran M R, Abdulmaaboud M. Renal colic in pregnant women: role of renal resistive index. *Urology.* 2000 Mar;55(3):344-7. doi: 10.1016/s0090-4295(99)00475-6.

Index

A

B

C

D

E

F

G

H

N

O

P

R

S

U

V

W

Z

β